# Dictionary of
# Veterinary Terms

Vet-Speak Deciphered for the Non-Veterinarian

## Jennifer Coates, DVM

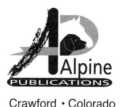

**Alpine**
PUBLICATIONS

Crawford · Colorado

*Dictionary of Veterinary Terms: Vet-speak deciphered for the non-veterinarian*

ISBN 10:  1-57779-090-1
ISBN 13:   978-1-57779-090-7

Library of Congress Cataloging-in-Publication Data

Coates, Jennifer, 1970-
Dictionary of veterinary terms : vet-speak deciphered for the non-veterinarian / Jennifer Coates.
p. cm.
ISBN 978-1-57779-090-7 (pb)
1. Veterinary medicine--Dictionaries. I. Title.

SF609.C63 2007
636.089'03--dc22
2007030847

This book is available at special quantity discounts for clubs and organizations, or for educational use. Write for details or email alpinecsr@aol.com.

Cover Design: Laura Newport

1 2 3 4 5 6 7 8 9 0

Printed in the United States of America.

Many thanks are owed to Debbie Richardson,
Richard Easterbrook and Judy Coates. Your love, support and
invaluable assistance are appreciated more than you know.
Finally, I would also like to thank Betty McKinney
and the staff of Alpine Publications
for making this idea a reality.

# Contents

About the Author     vi

Guide for Readers     vii

Alphabetical Listings     1 - 285

I.    **Commonly Prescribed Drugs:** Including their actions,     286
side effects and alternate names

II.    **Acronyms and Abbreviations**     307

III.    **Weights, Measures and Conversions**     312

IV.    **Normal Physiologic Parameters:** Including average life     313
expectancies, body temperatures and heart and respiration rates

V.    **Normal Reproductive Parameters:** Including age     314
at sexual maturity, time in heat, estrous cycle
duration and pregnancy length

Sources for More Information     315

# About the Author

Jennifer Coates, DVM, graduated with honors from the Virginia-Maryland Regional College of Veterinary Medicine. She worked as an associate veterinarian and chief of staff in Petersburg, Virginia and now practices in Jackson, Wyoming, where she is often praised for her ability to communicate with clients and staff.

Prior to graduating from veterinary school, Jennifer worked as a veterinary receptionist, assistant, and technician. It was then that she became aware of the frustrations caused by veterinary jargon. Pet owners were confused and upset by their lack of understanding. Receptionists were unable to answer client's questions. Technicians had trouble deciphering medical orders. Animal owners, veterinary support staff, and animal care workers needed a clear and concise resource to explain terminology in plain English. The skill and knowledge gained through years spent immersed in all aspects of veterinary care gave Jennifer an exceptional perspective from which to write the *Dictionary of Veterinary Terms*.

An animal owner for most of her life, Jennifer resides in Etna, Wyoming, with her husband, daughter, dogs, cats, and horses. When she is not at work in the clinic she enjoys hiking, horseback riding, skiing and traveling.

# A Guide for Readers

Over the last several decades, veterinary medicine has become overwhelmingly complex. On a daily basis, veterinarians now use technologies, diagnostic tests, surgical procedures and medicines that rival those offered in modern human medicine. As a result, veterinary care is vastly superior to what was available in the past.

But the new language of veterinary medicine is creating a barrier between veterinarians, pet owners and people who work with animals just when clear communication is more essential than ever. In *The Dictionary of Veterinary Terms* I will attempt to answer the frequently asked question, "What did the vet mean by that?"

The layout of this reference is outlined in the table of contents. Please note that the majority of information regarding abbreviations, drugs and physiological data can be found in the appendices.

The material contained in this book is intended to cover the veterinary profession only, including diseases common to North America and important foreign diseases. Other meanings for some of the terms are possible in different situations.

If a complex term cannot initially be located, looking up the root of the word or a single term in a compound name can be helpful. For example, "anal sac expression" can be understood through the individual definitions for "anal sac" and "express."

It should be remembered that every animal and every situation is unique. Questions regarding the health care of specific animals should be directed to a veterinarian.

We believe that animal owners and those who work in the veterinary field or with animals will find this book helpful.

*Jennifer Coates, DVM*

# A

**abaxial** adj. located away from the midline of the body or body part. *Compare* axial.

**abdomen** n. the part of the body between the chest and the pelvis that contains the stomach, intestines, liver, urinary bladder and other organs - **abdominal** adj.

**abdominal breathing** n. the abnormal use of abdominal wall muscles to assist in moving air to and from the lungs. Diseases affecting the respiratory system can cause abdominal breathing.

**abdominal effusion** n. abnormal fluid buildup around the organs in the abdominal cavity, which may be caused by liver and heart disease, infections, cancer and many other disorders. The belly of the affected animal often is visibly enlarged. Removing and analyzing a sample of the fluid can be helpful in diagnosis.

**abdominal wall** n. the muscles, bones and other tissues that combine to encircle the abdominal cavity and protect it from the outside environment.

**abdominocentesis** n. insertion of a hollow needle into the abdomen to withdraw fluid. Samples are usually removed to be analyzed and help with diagnosis.

**abduct** v. to move a structure (e.g., a leg) away from the midline of the animal. *Compare* adduct.

**abiotrophy** n. early and progressive loss of function of an organ or tissue. Usually refers to inherited diseases, especially of the nervous system.

**ablate** v. to completely remove, usually surgically - **ablation** n.

**abomasal torsion** n. an especially severe form of a displaced abomasum in which the organ rotates and flips thereby blocking its blood supply and the outflow of fluid. The condition is fatal unless surgically corrected. *Also called* abomasal volvulus.

**abomasopexy** n. a procedure in which the abomasum is affixed to the abdominal wall. This surgery is often performed after correction of a displaced abomasum to prevent recurrence.

**abomasum** n. one of the four chambers of the ruminant stomach - **abomasal** adj.

**aboral** adj. in a direction away from the mouth within the gastrointestinal tract.

**abortion** n. birth of a fetus before it can survive outside of the uterus. Abortions may occur for many reasons, including infections, poor nutrition and trauma.

**abortion storm** n. a cluster of abortions affecting a large number of individuals in a herd.

**abrasion** n. a wound in which only the surface of a tissue is lost.

**abscess** n. a localized pocket of pus within a tissue. Abscesses can be painful and lead to high fevers. They may spontaneously rupture releasing pus or require surgical drainage. Additional treatment often includes flushing of the pocket with an antiseptic and antibiotics. *Compare* cellulitis.

**absolute polycythemia** n. *See* polycythemia vera.

**acanthomatous epulis** n. a type of tumor affecting the gums of dogs that can grow aggressively into local tissues, including bone. Complete surgical removal is curative but often difficult. *Also called* canine peripheral ameloblastoma or canine acanthomatous ameloblastoma.

**acanthosis nigricans** n. a condition affecting dogs in which the skin of the armpits, groin and possibly other regions loses hair and becomes dark, thickened and/or flaky. Dachshunds are predisposed, but any breed of dog can be affected due to chronic irritation of the skin. Treatment is usually not necessary unless the condition is severe and uncomfortable.

**acariasis** n. infestation of the surface of the body with ticks or mites. See entries for specific diseases (e.g., demodicosis and sarcoptic mange) for details.

**acaricide** n. a substance that kills ticks or mites.

**accommodation** n. the process whereby the lens of the eye changes shape to focus an image on the retina.

**ACE inhibitors** n. *See* angiotensin converting enzyme inhibitor.

**acetabulum** n. the part of the pelvis that acts as the socket for the hip joint.

**acetaminophen toxicity** n. poisoning by ingestion of sufficient quantities of the drug acetaminophen to cause disease. Cats are especially sensitive, but any species is at risk if enough of the drug is absorbed. Affected animals may drool, exhibit facial swelling, vomit, breath rapidly and have brown or yellow-tinged mucous membranes and dark urine. Treatment varies with the time elapsed since ingestion but can include medications that induce vomiting or absorb the drug, supportive care and specific antidotes.

**acetonemia** n. *See* bovine ketosis.

**acetylcholine (ACh)** n. a substance present in the body that primarily acts to transmit signals from one nerve to another.

**acetylcholinesterase** n. an enzyme that breaks down acetylcholine. *Also called* cholinesterase.

**achalasia** n. a failure of certain muscles in the gastrointestinal tract to relax and allow food to pass. Vomiting or regurgitation may result.

**Achilles tendon** n. a group of tendons connecting muscles of the upper leg to the hock. *Also called* common calcaneal tendon. *See also* dropped hock.

**acholic feces** n. stool that is grey or beige due to a lack of normal bile in the feces. Acholic feces may indicate blockage of the duct that drains bile from the liver into the intestinal tract.

**acid** n. a substance with a pH less than seven. Some acids are essential to normal body function (e.g., gastric acid) but may also cause damage when they are overproduced - **acidic** adj. *Compare* base.

**acid-base balance** n. the normal condition in which the body's natural acids and bases are in equilibrium. Many diseases can cause an acid-base imbalance, which disrupts body functions and is potentially fatal if severe enough and left untreated. *See also* acidosis and alkalosis.

**acidosis** n. the condition in which the body's tissues and fluids have a pH that is lower than normal. Many diseases can cause acidosis. Severe acidosis can lead to abnormal muscle movements, heart arrhythmias, coma and death. *Compare* alkalosis.

**acorn poisoning** n. ingestion of sufficient quantities of green acorns or young oak leaves to damage the kidneys and gastrointestinal tract. Affected animals can exhibit dehydration, increased thirst and urination, loss of appetite, constipation and diarrhea. Treatment is difficult unless caught early, and many severely affected animals die. *Also called* oak bud poisoning.

**acquired** adj. describes a quality that arises because of influences of the outside environment on the body. *Compare* congenital.

**acquired bursa** n. *See* hygroma.

**acral lick dermatitis** n. thickening and inflammation of the skin, usually affecting a dog's lower front leg. Acral lick dermatitis is caused by excessive licking, either psychologic in origin or due to discomfort. Treatment is often difficult and may not be necessary if the lesion is only superficial and not infected. *Also called* lick granuloma.

**acromegaly** n. a condition most often seen in cats suffering from diabetes mellitus in which the pituitary gland over-secretes growth hormone. Affected individuals develop abnormally large bones, muscles and organs. Treatment is difficult. *Also called* gigantism and hypersomatotropism.

**ACTH stimulation test** n. a blood test that checks the function of the adrenal glands by measuring the body's response to a stimulatory injection. An ACTH stimulation test is most often used to diagnose Cushing's or Addison's disease. *Also called* ACTH response test.

**actinic dermatitis** n. inflammation and lesions on the skin that develop in response to sunlight exposure. *Also called* solar dermatitis.

**actinic keratoses** n. areas of thickened, hardened and sometimes red skin, which develop in response to sunlight exposure. Some of these lesions can progress to cancer. *Also called* solar keratosis.

**actinobacillosis** n. a disease caused by infection with a type of *Actinobacillus* bacteria. Symptoms vary depending on which bacteria and which species is involved. Cattle can develop a form of actinobacillosis that causes abscesses, thickening and hardening of the tongue. Treatment may include surgical removal of infected tissues and antibiotics. *Also called* wooden tongue.

**actinomycosis** n. a disease caused by infection with a type of *Actinomyces* bacteria. Symptoms vary depending on which bacteria and which animal is involved. Cattle can develop a form of actinomycosis that causes abscesses around the head. Treatment may include surgical removal of infected tissues and antibiotics. *Also called* lumpy jaw.

**activated clotting time (ACT)** n. a test that measures the clotting ability of blood. A prolonged ACT indicates abnormalities affecting particular coagulation factors.

**activated partial thromboplastin time (APTT)** n. *See* partial thromboplastin time.

**active immunity** n. resistance to disease that develops as a result of exposure to microorganisms or vaccines. *Compare* passive immunity.

**active labor** n. the stage of birth during which the female pushes to expel the fetus from the womb.

**acupuncture** n. a form of therapy during which small needles are inserted at specific points on the body in order to treat a wide range of disorders. Acupuncture has been used for thousands of years in eastern cultures and is gaining wider acceptance in western veterinary medicine.

**acute** adj. describes a condition in which symptoms develop quickly, usually over the course of a day or two. *Compare* chronic.

**acute abdomen** n. a syndrome with many underlying causes (e.g., infection and inadequate blood supply to abdominal organs), all of which result in the rapid onset of severe abdominal pain. In some cases of acute abdomen, an animal's condition can rapidly deteriorate and become life threatening.

**acute bovine pulmonary edema and emphysema** n. *See* bovine atypical interstitial pneumonia.

**acute bronchointerstitial pneumonia** n. a disease of foals that can cause a high fever, difficulty breathing, blue-tinged mucous membranes and may rapidly lead to death. The cause is unknown. Treatment may include antibiotics, medicines to reduce fever and inflammation and to dilate airways, oxygen therapy and supportive care.

**acute hepatic atrophy** n. *See* Theiler's disease.

**acute renal failure (ARF)** n. the sudden loss of the kidneys' ability to perform their normal functions, including excreting waste and conserving water. Affected animals often drink and urinate more than normal, stop eating and are lethargic. In later stages, individuals may stop urinating completely. Acute renal failure can develop because of infections, toxins (especially antifreeze) or other causes. Treatment differs depending on the cause, but intravenous fluid therapy is an essential component. *Compare* chronic renal failure.

**ad libitum** adj. without restrictions. Often used to describe a feeding system in which food is continually available.

**adactyly** n. the condition of being born without fingers or toes.

**Addisonian crisis** n. the development of severe vomiting, diarrhea, dehydration, weakness, collapse and possibly death in an undiagnosed Addisonian animal or when a previously well-regulated Addisonian experiences stress. *See also* Addison's disease.

**Addison's disease** n. a disease in which the adrenal glands do not secrete enough of the hormones necessary for normal fluid and electrolyte balance and response to stress.

Affected animals often exhibit vomiting, diarrhea, dehydration, weakness and collapse. Treatment includes normalizing the body's fluid and electrolyte levels and medications that replace the missing hormones. *Also called* hypoadrenocorticism and adrenocortical insufficiency.

**adduct** v. to move a structure (e.g., a leg) towards the midline of the animal. *Compare* abduct.

**adenitis** n. inflammation of a gland.

**adenocarcinoma** n. a type of cancer that either arises from a gland or consists of tissues that have characteristics of a gland. Most adenocarcinomas are malignant.

**adenoma** n. a type of cancer that either arises from a gland or consists of tissues that have characteristics of a gland. Most adenomas are benign.

**adhesion** n. an abnormal connection that can develop between two tissues after surgery or injury. Adhesions may develop in the abdomen preventing normal intestinal function or in a tendon sheath causing lameness.

**adipose tissue** n. body fat. Adipose tissue stores energy, maintains body temperature and protects other organs from injury.

**adjuvant** n. most often refers to a substance added to vaccines that increases the body's immune response. Some adjuvants have been implicated in the development of cancer at injection sites in cats.

**adrenal androgen panel** n. a blood test most commonly used to diagnose adrenal disease in ferrets.

**adrenal gland** n. one of the organs that lies near each kidney and produces many hormones essential to normal body function. An adrenal gland consists of two parts, the medulla that produces epinephrine and norepinephrine, and the cortex that secretes some sex hormones, glucocorticoids and mineralocorticoids.

**adrenalectomy** n. the surgical removal of an adrenal gland. An adrenalectomy is often used to treat tumors of the adrenal glands.

**adrenaline** n. *See* epinephrine.

**adrenergic** adj. having activity similar to that of epinephrine or causing the release of epinephrine.

**adrenocortical insufficiency** n. *See* Addison's disease.

**adrenocorticotrophic hormone (ACTH)** n. a hormone produced by the pituitary gland that stimulates the adrenal glands to secrete other hormones, most notably corticosterone. *Also called* corticotropin.

**adult onset** adj. describes a condition that develops in a mature animal. *Compare* juvenile onset.

**adulticide** n. a drug that kills mature heartworms. The most common adulticide now used is melarsomine.

**advance** v. to move something in the desired direction. For example, a skin flap may be advanced to cover a wound or a catheter advanced into a vein.

**advanced** adj. usually describes a disease that is in its later stages, often indicating a poorer prognosis.

**adventitious sounds** n. abnormal noises made by air moving in and out of the lungs that can be heard with a stethoscope. Adventitious sounds may be an increase in the intensity of the noises that are normally heard or sounds like wheezes or crackles that are never normal.

**adverse drug reaction** n. any unwanted response of a patient to a drug that has been administered. In many cases, stopping the drug is curative, but hospitalization or treatment with other medicines may be necessary.

**aerobic** adj. requiring oxygen.

**aerophagia** n. the swallowing of large amounts of air.

**aerosol** n. small droplets of liquid or small solid particles that can easily move through the air.

**afebrile** adj. having a normal body temperature.

**aflatoxin** n. the toxin produced by an *Aspergillus* fungus that can cause liver damage and death when ingested. The fungus may grow on grains or nuts stored under warm or wet conditions.

**afterbirth** n. the placenta and other substances that are expelled from the uterus after a fetus is born.

**agalactia** n. an inability to produce normal amounts of milk.

**agammaglobulinemia** n. a disorder in which the body does not produce antibodies, which leads to recurrent infections. *See also* combined immune deficiency.

**aganglionosis** n. a disease in which the body fails to develop a specific type of nerve cell. There is no treatment. *See also* ileocolonic agangliosis.

**agar** n. a gel used to grow microorganisms in the lab. Different substances can be added to agar to promote or inhibit the growth of particular species.

**agenesis** n. the complete absence of a structure or organ due to its failure to develop in the embryo.

**agglutination** n. the clumping together of normally separate items. For example, red blood cell agglutination can be seen with some diseases or when incompatible blood types are mixed.

**aggression** n. the tendency of an animal to attack or act like it will attack other animals or people. See specific types of aggression (e.g., fear, dominance or food) for details.

**aggressive** adj. 1. *See* aggression. 2. describes a disease (e.g., cancer) that tends to spread or worsen rapidly. 3. describes a treatment plan in which multiple therapeutic options are employed at the same time to increase the likelihood of a successful outcome. *Compare* conservative.

**agonal** adj. pertaining to death.

**agonal breathing** n. a reflex that can cause an animal to take deep breaths at the time of death.

**agonist** n. a substance that binds to a receptor and produces an effect in the body. *Compare* antagonist.

**air bronchogram** n. a finding on a chest radiograph indicating that some parts of the lung that are normally filled with air are instead filled with fluid.

**air embolism** n. the introduction of a bubble of air into the bloodstream. Small air emboli generally cause no harm, but if large enough, they can interrupt blood flow to various organs and potentially cause death.

**air sacs** n. balloon-like structures in multiple areas of a bird's body that allow continuous flow of air through the respiratory system.

**air sac mite** n. small insects that can infest the air sacs and other parts of the respiratory tract of some types of birds. If many mites are present the bird may have difficulty breathing and can die when stressed. Medications are available to kill the mites.

**air sacculitis** n. inflammation of the air sacs of birds often caused by infection with bacteria or fungi.

**airplane wing** n. rotation of the end of a bird's wing, often caused by a broken bone that healed abnormally. The end of the wing sticks out from the body at rest rather than lying flat.

**airway** n. *See* upper and lower airway.

**alanine aminotransferase (ALT)** n. a substance measured in blood, the levels of which can rise with liver disease or damage.

**albino** n. an individual lacking the pigments normally found in the skin, hair and eyes. True albino animals are rare and have pink eyes and skin.

**albumin** n. a small protein produced by the liver that plays an important role in wound healing and the ability of an animal's blood to hold fluid within the circulatory system. Low blood levels may indicate disease of the gastrointestinal tract, kidneys or liver. High urine levels are seen with kidney disfunction.

**albuminuria** n. the abnormal presence of albumin in the urine, often indicating kidney disfunction.

**aldosterone** n. a hormone produced by the adrenal glands that helps maintain fluid and electrolyte balance. Lack of aldosterone production is a key component of Addison's disease.

**Aleutian disease** n. a contagious viral disease of ferrets that can cause weight loss, weakness, pale mucous membranes, neurological abnormalities, high blood protein levels and death. Treatment is limited to supportive care.

**algal poisoning** n. a disease caused by ingestion of cyanobacteria that can form large blooms in warm, stagnant water. Toxins produced by the bacteria can cause muscle tremors, neurologic abnormalities, difficulty breathing and rapid death. Supportive treatment is often successful if the animal is quickly removed from the source of the poisoning.

**alimentary tract** n. *See* gastrointestinal tract.

**alkaline** adj. describes a substance with a pH greater than 7. *Also called* basic.

**alkali disease** n. *See* selenium toxicosis.

**alkaline phosphatase (ALP)** n. a substance measured in blood, the levels of which can rise with liver disease, bone disease or growth, drug therapy, Cushing's disease or age.

**alkaline phosphatase isoenzyme test** n. a laboratory test that may help identify the cause of a high blood alkaline phosphatase level.

**alkalosis** n. the condition in which the body's tissues and fluids have a pH that is higher than normal. Many diseases can cause alkalosis. *Compare* acidosis.

**allantois** n. a part of the placenta that forms a sac and is filled with a urine-like liquid produced by the fetus.

**allergen** n. a substance that in some individuals can cause an allergic reaction. Common allergens include pollens, molds, dust mites and some types of food.

**allergic inhalant dermatitis** n. *See* atopic dermatitis.

**allergy** n. an abnormal reaction of the body's immune system to substances that often do not incite a similar reaction in other individuals. Allergic symptoms in animals can include itching, hives, skin disorders, coughing and difficulty breathing - **allergic** adj. *See also* anaphylaxis.

**alloimmune hemolytic anemia** n. *See* neonatal isoerythrolysis.

**alopecia** n. abnormal thinning or lack of hair. *Also called* hypotrichosis.

**alopecia X** n. a syndrome causing hair loss and poor hair regrowth in plush-coated dog breeds (e.g., Pomeranian, Samoyed and Siberian Husky), the cause of which is not fully understood. Hair loss is progressive, usually starting on the dog's rear end. Some dogs may respond to neutering, hormone supplements or other therapies. Oftentimes hair regrowth is temporary. Many other terms are used to describe alopecia X, often referring to the assumed cause or effective treatment (e.g., growth hormone responsive alopecia).

**altered** adj. 1. neutered or spayed. 2. describing a mental state in which an animal does not respond normally to stimuli.

**alternative medicine** n. a group of therapies including acupuncture, homeopathy and herbal medicine that have not been traditionally utilized in veterinary medicine as it is practiced in western countries. *Also called* complementary medicine.

**altitude sickness** n. *See* high mountain disease.

**alveolar pattern** n. a finding on a chest radiograph indicating that some parts of the lung that are normally filled with air are instead filled with fluid.

**alveolus** n. 1. the bony socket that surrounds the roots of teeth. 2. one of many microscopic, air-filled sacs within the lung through which gasses are transferred to and from the bloodstream - **alveoli** pl.

**Amazon tracheitis** n. a contagious, viral disease of Amazon parrots and some other birds that causes discharge from the eyes and nose, difficulty breathing and coughing. Treatment includes supportive care and antibiotics for secondary bacterial infections.

**ambulatory** adj. able to walk.

**amebiasis** n. a disease caused by infection with *Entamoeba* protozoal parasites producing diarrhea that varies in severity. Treatment can be difficult but includes medications to kill the parasites and supportive care. *Also called* amebiosis and entamebiasis.

**amelia** n. the condition of being born without front limbs.

**American Kennel Club (AKC)** n. an organization devoted to the registration, advancement and promotion of purebred dogs with an emphasis on conformation.

**ameroid constrictor** n. a device that is used in the treatment of portosystemic shunts. It is surgically placed around the abnormal blood vessel and expands over the next month to gradually restrict blood flow.

**amino acid** n. a molecule that in combination with other amino acids forms proteins. Animals can synthesize many amino acids within their bodies. Some species cannot make certain types (called essential amino acids), and these are required in the diet.

**aminoglycoside** n. a class of antibiotics, including gentamicin and amikacin, the improper use of which can damage the kidneys and the ability to hear.

**ammonia** n. a waste product of digestion that is removed from the blood by the liver.

**ammonia tolerance test (ATT)** n. a test measuring the liver's ability to remove ammonia from the bloodstream that can be used to help diagnose a portosystemic shunt or other liver abnormalities.

**ammonia toxicosis** n. *See* non-protein nitrogen poisoning.

**ammoniated forage poisoning** n. *See* non-protein nitrogen poisoning.

**amniocentesis** n. the insertion of a hollow needle through the abdomen of a pregnant female to remove a sample of the fluid that surrounds the fetus. The fluid is often analyzed to help determine fetal health.

**amnion** n. a membrane that encircles the fetus while in the uterus.

**amniotic fluid** n. the fluid surrounding a developing fetus that is contained within the amnion.

**amorphous** adj. without a recognizable shape.

**amphibian** n. a class of animals that can live on land or in the water, including frogs, toads and salamanders - **amphibious** adj.

**amputation** n. the surgical removal of an appendage such as a limb, toe or tail - **amputate** v.

**amylase** n. a substance usually measured in blood, the levels of which can rise with pancreatitis, other forms of pancreatic disease or with kidney disease.

**amyloid** n. an abnormal protein that can be deposited within the body and disrupt organ function.

**amyloidosis** n. a disease caused by the deposition of amyloid within the kidneys or other parts of the body. If enough amyloid is present the function of the affected organ can be disrupted leading to illness and sometimes death. Treatment is difficult.

**anabolic steroids** n. hormones (e.g., testosterone) that tend to increase muscle mass. Anabolic steroids are sometimes used to increase strength in older animals.

**anaerobic** adj. not requiring oxygen or requiring an absence of oxygen. *Compare* aerobic.

**anal atresia** n. *See* atresia ani.

**anal gland** n. the tissues producing the foul smelling material that is stored in anal sacs.

**anal sac** n. a storage area on either side of the anus that holds foul smelling material released with defecation as a form of territorial marking in some species. If the sacs do not regularly empty, they can become distended, painful and may rupture.

**anal sacculectomy** n. the surgical removal of one or both anal sacs.

**analgesia** n. relief or absence of pain - **analgesic** adj.

**anamnestic response** n. the process by which the immune system responds to a stimulus that it has been exposed to in the past. The anamnestic response creates a superior and longer lasting immunity than was initiated by the first response.

**anaphylaxis** n. an extreme allergic reaction that can cause difficulty breathing, low blood pressure, collapse and death. Immediate treatment with epinephrine and diphenhydramine can be life saving. *Also called* anaphylactic shock.

**anaplasmosis** n. a disease caused by infection with *Anaplasma* bacteria often transmitted through tick bites. The disease in cattle can lead to pale or yellow mucous membranes, difficulty breathing, high heart rates and abortion. Treatment may include antibiotics and blood transfusions. *Also called* gall sickness. *See also* equine granulocytic anaplasmosis.

**anasarca** n. widespread accumulation of fluid within the tissues under the skin. *See also* edema.

**anastomosis** n. a connection between two tubes. For example, a surgical anastomosis can be performed to connect the cut ends of intestine after a section of bowel has been removed.

**anatomy** n. the physical structure of an animal.

**ancillary tests** n. additional tests or procedures that are often ordered after preliminary testing has failed to lead to a diagnosis.

**androgen** n. a type of hormone that produces typically male traits in an animal.

**anemia** n. a lower than normal number of red blood cells in circulation. Anemia can be caused by blood loss and destruction or lack of production of red blood cells. Animals that are anemic often have pale mucous membranes, rapid breathing, fast heart rates and are lethargic and weak - **anemic** adj.

**anemia of chronic disease** n. a symptom of many different diseases of long duration. Generally, the individual's red blood cell count is not low enough to cause any symptoms or require specific treatment.

**anencephaly** n. the condition of being born without a large portion of the brain.

**anesthesia** n. a lack of the ability to feel pain. Anesthesia often refers to the physiologic state induced by drugs in which an animal is without most of its senses and can undergo a painful procedure such as surgery without discomfort - **anesthetic** adj.

**anesthetic depth** n. the degree to which an animal is being affected by anesthesia. An animal that is "light" generally is at a lower risk of complications but may be able to feel pain as compared to an animal that is "deep."

**anesthetic risk** n. the degree to which an animal can be expected to develop complications from anesthesia. In most cases, healthy individuals have a lower anesthetic risk than do animals affected by concurrent disease or injury.

**anestrus** n. a period of time during which the female does not cycle in and out of heat. Anestrus can be normal in some species (e.g., mares in the winter) or can be an indication of disease. *Compare* estrus and diestrus.

**aneurysm** n. an abnormal outpouching of a blood vessel or part of the heart. Aneurysms can rupture and bleed, or they can be associated with clots that disrupt circulation of blood.

**angiocardiogram** n. a radiograph of the heart and its associated blood vessels that is taken after an animal is injected with a substance that highlights these structures.

**angioedema** n. the sudden development of areas of swelling under the skin that is often associated with an allergy. Treatment can include antihistamines, corticosteroids and epinephrine if the condition is potentially life-threatening. *Also called* angioneurotic edema.

**angioendothelioma** n. *See* angiosarcoma.

**angiogram** n. a radiograph of blood vessels that is taken after an animal is injected with a substance that highlights these structures.

**angioma** n. a benign tumor of blood or lymph vessels. *See also* hemangioma and lymphangioma. *Compare* angiosarcoma.

**angioplasty** n. the surgical reconstruction or replacement of blood or lymph vessels.

**angiosarcoma** n. an aggressive cancer of blood or lymph vessels. *See also* hemangiosarcoma and lymphangiosarcoma. *Also called* angioendothelioma. *Compare* angioma.

**angiotensin** n. a chemical within the body that raises blood pressure and reduces blood flow to the kidneys thereby decreasing the amount of fluid lost in the urine.

**angiotensin converting enzyme (ACE) inhibitor** n. a class of drugs that dilates blood vessels and is used to lower blood pressure, treat heart failure and promote kidney function. Enalapril is a commonly used ACE inhibitor.

**angular limb deformity** n. a disorder of fetal development or growth in a young animal that causes the individual to have an abnormally bent leg or legs. Defects affecting the bones or soft tissues around joints are the most common causes of angular limb deformities. Treatment can include splints or casts, exercise restriction and surgery.

**anhidrosis** n. a lack of the ability to sweat, which is most often seen in horses and can limit their ability to exercise.

**Animal and Plant Health Inspection Service (APHIS)** n. the U.S. federal government agency responsible for protecting and promoting agricultural health, administering the Animal Welfare Act and carrying out wildlife damage management activities.

**anion** n. a negatively charged atom or group of atoms. Common anions in the body include chloride and bicarbonate *Compare* cation.

**anion gap** n. a calculation of the difference between the amounts of cations and anions in the blood. An abnormal anion gap indicates a disturbance in the acid-base balance of the animal.

**aniridia** n. the condition of being born without an iris, either in whole or in part.

**anisocoria** n. unequal pupil size. Anisocoria can be seen with some types of neurologic disease or with disorders of the eye.

**ankyloblepharon** n. the sticking together of the upper and lower eyelids. This condition is normal in puppies and kittens up to about 10 days of age.

**ankylosis** n. a partial or complete fusion of a joint, which limits its range of motion. Ankylosis can be caused by severe osteoarthritis.

**anodontia** n. the condition of being born without some or all of the normal number of teeth.

**anogenital distance** n. the space between the anus and the penis or vulva that can be observed to help determine the sex of some newborn animals. For example, a male kitten has a larger anogenital distance than does a female kitten.

**anointing** n. *See* anting.

**anomaly** n. an abnormal finding or condition.

**anophthalmos** n. the condition of being born without an eye or eyes. Sometimes an abnormal and nonfunctional structure that in some ways resembles an eye may be present.

**anorchid** adj. describes a male animal that was born without two testicles. Individuals may be missing one or both testicles. *Compare* cryptorchid.

**anorectal** adj. pertaining to the anus, rectum and surrounding tissues.

**anorexia** n. an abnormal lack of appetite for food. Anorexia is a symptom of many diseases or may be brought about if the offered food is unpleasant or the animal is somehow discouraged from eating.

**anoxia** n. *See* hypoxia.

12

**antacid** n. a class of drugs that reduce the level of acid within the stomach. Some antacids (e.g., aluminum hydroxide) can also be used to reduce the amount of phosphorous in the body.

**antagonist** n. a substance that counters the effect of another substance - **antagonize** v. *Compare* agonist.

**antebrachium** n. the region of the front limb between the elbow and the wrist that is comparable to the forearm in humans.

**antemortem** adj. pertaining to the time before death.

**antenatal** adj. *See* prenatal.

**anterior** adj. in front of or pertaining to the front end. *Compare* posterior.

**anterior chamber** n. the part of the eye that is located in front of the iris and behind the cornea and filled with aqueous humor.

**anterior enteritis** n. a disease affecting horses in which the initial part of the small intestine becomes inflamed for unknown reasons. Affected animals have abdominal pain, may develop laminitis and can die even with appropriate therapy. Treatment can include procedures or surgery to relieve distension of the stomach and small intestine, fluid therapy, pain relief and medications that stimulate motility of the gastrointestinal tract. *Also called* proximal enteritis-jejunitis and duodenitis-jejunitis.

**anterior presentation** n. a description of the birth of a fetus in which the head and front limbs emerge from the uterus first. This is the normal position for delivery in many species, including horses and cattle. *Compare* breech presentation.

**anterior uveitis** n. inflammation often associated with infection of the anterior chamber and iris of the eye. Affected eyes are often red, cloudy and painful. Treatment depends on the underlying cause but may include antibiotics, anti-inflammatories and drugs to dilate the pupil. *Also called* iridocyclitis.

**anthelmintic drug** n. a type of medicine that kills or otherwise aids in the removal of worms from the body.

**anthrax** n. a disease caused by infection with *Bacillus anthracis* bacteria. Affected animals may die suddenly before any clinical signs develop or can exhibit high fevers, bloody diarrhea and swellings throughout the body. Treatment with antibiotics can be successful, and preventative vaccines are available. The disease is transmissible to humans and must be reported to appropriate regulatory agencies. Anthrax bacteria form spores that can survive for many years in the environment.

**anthropomorphism** n. the tendency to attribute human characteristics to animals.

**antiarrhythmic drug** n. a medicine that can improve abnormal heart rhythms.

**antibacterial** adj. having properties that kill or inhibit the growth of bacteria.

**antibiotic** n. a type of drug that kills some types of microorganisms, especially bacteria, or prevents them from reproducing.

**antibody** n. a type of protein that is manufactured by cells called lymphocytes and is essential to the function of the immune system. Different antibodies are developed against specific stimulants called antigens. Sometimes antibodies are inappropriately produced and stimulate an immune response against parts of the animal's own body. *Also called* immunoglobulin or gamma globulin.

**anticholinergic** adj. reducing the activity of the parasympathetic nervous system. Some anticholinergic drugs are used to increase heart rates or treat vomiting and diarrhea. *Also called* parasympatholytic and vagolytic.

**anticoagulant** n. a substance that decreases the ability of blood to clot. Some anticoagulants are poisons while others are used in the laboratory or as medicines to prevent blood clots when they are undesirable.

**anticoagulant rodenticide toxicity** n. ingestion of some types of poisons (e.g., brodifacoum and warfarin) that are used to kill mice and rats and hinder the ability of blood to clot. Affected animals often bleed or bruise easily and may die. Treatment can include vitamin K supplementation and sometimes blood transfusions.

**anticonvulsant** n. a type of drug that reduces the frequency and/or severity of seizures.

**antidepressant** n. a type of drug that may be used to treat a variety of behavioral problems in animals.

**antidiuretic hormone (ADH)** n. a hormone manufactured by the pituitary gland that causes the kidneys to limit water loss from the body through the urine. *Also called* vasopressin.

**antidiuretic hormone (ADH) response test** n. a test of the kidneys' ability to concentrate urine after administration of antidiuretic hormone. Test results help to differentiate between two types of diabetes insipidus, one arising from the kidney and the other from the pituitary gland.

**antidote** n. a substance that can be given to an animal to reverse the effects of a poison.

**antiemetic drug** n. a type of medicine that reduces vomiting.

**antifreeze toxicity** n. *See* ethylene glycol toxicosis.

**antifungal** adj. having properties that kill or inhibit the growth of fungi.

**antigen** n. a substance that invokes a response from the immune system. Antigens may be parts of microorganisms, proteins or the animal's own cells - **antigenic** adj.

**antihistamine** n. a medicine that eases the symptoms of allergies. Some antihistamines can also be used to treat motion sickness or as a sedative.

**anti-inflammatory drug** n. a type of medicine that reduces pain, swelling, heat and redness. Anti-inflammatories are often used after surgery or injury and to ease the discomfort of infections and arthritis.

**antimicrobial** adj. having properties that kill some types of microorganisms or prevent them from reproducing.

**anting** n. a behavior seen in hedgehogs during which they produce large quantities of saliva in order to taste a new object to which they're been exposed. *Also called* anointing.

**antinuclear antibodies (ANA)** n. antibodies directed against part of an animal's own cells that can be seen in some autoimmune diseases.

**antinuclear antibody (ANA) test** n. a laboratory test used to help diagnose systemic lupus erythematosus. Because other disorders can cause an abnormal ANA test, results must be interpreted in conjunction with other clinical findings.

**antioxidant** n. a substance that reduces the damage to the body caused by free radicals.

**antipyretic** adj. having properties that can reduce a fever.

**antiseptic** adj. having properties that kill or reduce the growth of microorganisms on the surface of objects or the body.

**antiserum** n. serum obtained from an animal that contains antibodies against a specific antigen, which then may be given to another animal to prevent or treat a disease.

**antispasmodic** adj. having properties that reduce painful, involuntary muscle contractions. *Also called* spasmolytic.

**antitoxin** n. an antibody directed against a toxic substance (e.g., tetanus or botulinum toxin) that can be used in the treatment of a particular disease.

**antitussive** adj. having qualities that reduce coughing.

**antivenin** n. an antitoxin used to treat the bite or sting of a poisonous animal.

**anuric** adj. not producing urine.

**anus** n. the sphincter located at the back end of the digestive tract - **anal** adj.

**anxiety** n. a feeling of nervousness, uneasiness or apprehension.

**anxiolytic** adj. having properties that relieve anxiety.

**aorta** n. the large blood vessel exiting the heart that carries blood into other arteries.

**aortic stenosis** n. a narrowing around the valve between the left ventricle of the heart and the aorta that prevents normal flow of blood away from the heart. Affected animals may tire easily, faint, develop congestive heart failure or die suddenly. Medicines can ease the effects of the narrowing.

**aortic thromboembolism** n. *See* saddle thrombus.

**aortic valve** n. the structure between the left ventricle of the heart and the aorta that prevents backward flow of blood into the heart.

**apathy** n. a loss of interest in things that once would have attracted an animal's attention.

**aphakia** n. the lack of a lens in the eye - **aphakic** adj.

**apex** n. the pointed end of a structure - **apical** adj.

**aplasia** n. abnormal development leading to the complete absence of a tissue or the formation of a rudimentary, nonfunctional structure in its place - **aplastic** adj.

**aplasia cutis** n. *See* epitheliogenesis imperfecta.

**aplastic anemia** n. a disease of the bone marrow characterized by a lack of production of red blood cells and sometimes white blood cells and platelets. If the disease is a result of infection, drug administration or other reversible causes, recovery is possible with appropriate therapy. Repeated blood transfusions or bone marrow transplantation is necessary in cases where the bone marrow fails to respond to treatment.

**apnea** n. a lack of breathing - **apneic** adj.

**apocrine gland** n. specific types of tissues that can be found associated with the hair follicles, anal sacs or ears and can produce oily and waxy substances, sweat and fluids used for territorial marking and sexual attraction.

**aponeurosis** n. a wide sheet of fibrous material connecting a muscle to another structure.

**appose** v. to bring structures into contact with one another (e.g., the edges of a wound) - **apposition** n., **apposable** adj.

**aqueocentesis** n. the insertion of a hollow needle into the eye to remove aqueous humor, either to be analyzed or to reduce pressure within the eye.

**aqueous flare** n. an abnormal cloudiness to the aqueous humor, which is often seen with infections involving the interior of the eye.

**aqueous humor** n. the liquid located in the anterior chamber that maintains eye pressure and nourishes parts of the eye.

**Arabian fading syndrome** n. the progressive and patchy loss of pigment in the skin and hair sometimes seen in Arabian horses as they mature. There is no effective treatment, but the disorder does not adversely affect most animals. *Also called* vitiligo, pinky syndrome and lavender foal.

**arachnoid cyst** n. an abnormal fluid-filled structure arising from one of the layers of the membrane covering the brain and spinal cord. As it grows it presses on and hinders normal function of nearby nervous tissue. Surgical removal can be curative, but regrowth is possible.

**arbovirus** n. a virus that reproduces within and is transmitted by ticks, mosquitos or other insects.

**arcade** n. commonly refers to the rows of teeth located around the upper and lower jaws.

**arrhythmia** n. an abnormal heart rhythm. See specific arrhythmias (e.g., tachycardia and respiratory sinus arrhythmia) for details. *Also called* dysrhythmia.

**arsenic poisoning** n. disease caused by ingestion of arsenic found in some types of pesticides, wood preservatives, feed additives or from other sources. Affected individuals can experience diarrhea, abdominal pain, weakness, collapse and may die. Treatment includes supportive care and administration of medicines that bind to and help remove arsenic from the body.

**arteriovenous fistula** n. an abnormal connection between an artery and a vein that disrupts normal circulation of blood. Effects vary depending on the location. For example, an arteriovenous fistula in the leg may cause local swelling while in the liver it can lead to the buildup of fluid in the abdomen and toxic substances in the blood.

**arteritis** n. inflammation of an artery. *See also* equine viral arteritis.

**artery** n. a vessel carrying blood away from the heart - **arterial** adj. *Compare* vein.

**arthritis** n. inflammation of a joint. Arthritis is painful and can affect any joint in the body. It may develop due to infection, autoimmune disease, trauma or joint instability. See specific types of arthritis (e.g., septic arthritis, osteoarthritis and rheumatoid arthritis) for details.

**arthrocentesis** n. the insertion of a hollow needle into a joint, usually to remove a sample of joint fluid for analysis.

**arthrodesis** n. the surgical fusion of a joint to prevent movement and pain.

**arthrogryposis** n. a condition in which a joint or joints are flexed and unable to be straightened. Some cases or arthrogryposis are caused by birth defects that may be related to viral infections, exposure to toxins or genetic disorders.

**arthropathy** n. any disease affecting a joint.

**arthroplasty** n. the surgical reconstruction or replacement of a joint.

**arthroscope** n. a tubular instrument including a light source and viewing device that can be placed into a joint to allow the veterinarian to see inside of the structure, take samples and repair some types of abnormalities.

**articular** adj. pertaining to a joint or joint surface.

**articular fracture** n. a bone break that extends to the surface of the bone involved in a joint. Articular fractures often lead to arthritis.

**artifact** n. a diagnostic procedure or test result that does not relate to the individual being examined but is a consequence of the test itself.

**artificial insemination (AI)** n. the placement of semen into the female's reproductive tract via an instrument rather than through natural mating.

**artificial respiration** n. a procedure used to move air into and out of the lungs when breathing has stopped. Artificial respiration can be performed using devices like a respirator or via mouth to mouth and mouth to nose techniques.

**artificial tears** n. a lubricant used when tear production is not sufficient to protect the health and comfort of the eye.

**artificial vagina** n. an apparatus used to collect semen from a male animal that simulates natural breeding and leads to ejaculation.

**arytenoid chondritis** n. inflammation of structures on either side of the larynx, which can cause loud breathing and reduced ability to exercise.

**ascarid** n. a type of parasitic worm that usually infests the small intestine. *See also* roundworm.

**ascites** n. abnormal fluid buildup around the organs in the abdominal cavity. Ascites may be caused by many disorders, including liver and heart disease and low blood protein levels. The belly of the affected animal often is visibly enlarged.

**ascorbic acid** n. *See* vitamin C.

**aseptic** adj. not involving infection or contamination with microorganisms - **asepsis** n. *Also called* sterile.

**aseptic meningitis** n. *See* steroid-responsive meningitis.

**aseptic necrosis of the femoral head** n. *See* Legg-Calvé-Perthes disease.

**aseptic technique** n. performance of a procedure in such a manner as to reduce the possibility of infection or contamination. Aseptic surgical technique includes cleaning the skin with antimicrobial solutions, wearing sterile gloves and gowns, using sterile instruments and performing the procedure in a very clean environment.

**ash** n. often refers to a component of cat foods that was once thought to play a role in the development of urinary stones. Current research indicates that ash is not an important factor in this disorder.

**aspartate aminotransferase (AST)** n. a substance measured in blood, the levels of which can rise with damage to the liver, muscle tissue or destruction of red blood cells. *Also called* serum glutamic-oxaloacetic transaminase (SGOT).

**aspergillosis** n. a disease caused by infection with an *Aspergillus* fungus. Most infections involve the respiratory tract including the guttural pouches of horses, nasal passages of dogs and lungs of birds, but other species and organs may be affected (e.g., the placenta of cattle causing abortion). Treatment can include physical removal of the fungus and administration of antifungal drugs.

**aspermatogenesis** n. a lack of sperm production.

**aspermia** n. a lack of sperm production or inability to ejaculate semen.

**asphyxia** n. inability to inhale and/or absorb sufficient quantities of oxygen to sustain life.

**aspiration** n. 1. the removal of material through suction, often with a needle - **aspirate** v. 2. the act of inhaling.

**aspiration pneumonia** n. inflammation and often infection of the lungs that develops due to inhalation of foreign material (e.g., food or orally administered liquids). Treatment may involve antibiotics, anti-inflammatories, oxygen therapy and procedures and drugs to loosen material in the chest. *Also called* inhalation pneumonia.

**assay** n. a laboratory test, specifically one that analyzes the amount, components or activity of a substance.

**Association of American Feed Control Officials (AAFCO)** n. an organization that works to develop and implement regulations, standards, and enforcement policies for the manufacture, distribution and sale of animal feeds.

**asthma** n. a disease most commonly seen in cats that is characterized by recurring episodes of constricted airways. Affected animals have to work harder to breath, especially to exhale, and may wheeze or cough. Possible triggers for an asthma attack are numerous, but allergies are often responsible.

**astrocytoma** n. a tumor most commonly affecting the brain of dogs. Astrocytomas arise from cells that are often associated with blood vessels. Treatment is difficult.

**asymmetric** adj. describes the situation in which opposite sides of a structure appear dissimilar when they should be alike.

**asymptomatic** adj. not displaying clinical signs despite having a medical condition.

**asystole** n. lack of a heart beat. *See also* cardiopulmonary arrest.

**ataxia** n. unsteady and irregular walking movements that are caused by neurologic abnormalities - **ataxic** adj.

**atelectasis** n. the loss of air from lung tissue that is caused by pressure on the area or an airway becoming blocked. Difficulty breathing results, the degree of which is determined by the amount of lung that is involved. *Also called* collapsed lung.

**atlantoaxial subluxation** n. a disease that is most often seen in dogs and is caused by a malformed vertebra in the upper neck. Abnormal movement of the spinal column results, causing pain and damage to the spinal cord. Affected animals may be weak, stagger or become paralyzed. Surgery to stabilize the neck can be successful. *Also called* atlantoaxial instability.

**atlas** n. the first vertebrae of the spinal column located in the upper neck.

**atonic** adj. without normal muscle tone, which can cause weakness. For example, an atonic bladder cannot contract and expel urine normally - **atony** n.

**atopic dermatitis** n. inflammation of the skin that is caused by a genetic tendency to have allergic reactions, often to pollen, molds and dust mites. Affected animals are itchy and have an increased tendency to develop skin and ear infections. Symptoms may be seasonal at first but often progress and are observable year round. Treatment can include medicated baths, antihistamines, steroids or other medications that reduce itching and inflammation and a series of injections of the inciting allergen to desensitize the animal to its affects. *Also called* allergic inhalant dermatitis.

**atopy** n. a genetic tendency towards allergic reactions that often cause itchy skin - **atopic** adj. *See also* atopic dermatitis.

**atresia** n. the failure of a fetus to develop an opening that should normally be present.

**atresia ani** n. the failure of a fetus to develop the normal opening between the rectum and the anus. Affected newborns cannot defecate and often strain and exhibit abdominal pain. Surgery to create an opening from the rectum to the anus can be successful. *Also called* anal atresia.

**atresia coli** n. a lack of normal development of the colon resulting in a gastrointestinal tract that is sealed before feces can enter the rectum. Affected newborns cannot defecate and often strain and exhibit abdominal pain. Corrective surgeries can be attempted but are often unsuccessful.

**atria** n. *See* atrium.

**atrial fibrillation** n. very fast and uncoordinated contractions of the atria that decrease the ability of the heart to move blood around the body. Atrial fibrillation most often is a symptom of diseases that cause enlargement of the atria. Treatment can include medications to slow the heart rate.

**atrial flutter** n. abnormally rapid contractions of the atria, which may cause weakness and exercise intolerance. Treatment can include medications or procedures to slow the heart rate.

**atrial septal defect (ASD)** n. an abnormal hole in the portion of the heart that separates the right and left atria. Affected individuals develop heart enlargement, a murmur and heart failure if the hole is large enough. Surgical repair is difficult but can be attempted. Treatment for heart failure can improve the quality of life.

**atrial standstill** n. lack of contraction of the heart's atria resulting in a very slow heart rate. Causes include high blood potassium levels and infections or scarring of the heart muscle.

**atrioventricular block (AV block)** n. an irregular heart rhythm that results from a lack of normal conduction of impulses through a specific portion of the heart. AV blocks come in three types (i.e., first, second and third degree) ranging from the least to the most serious forms of the disease. Affected animals may faint. Treatment can include medications that increase the heart rate or implantation of a pacemaker. *Also called* heart block.

**atrioventricular valves** n. the valves in the heart that control blood flow from the atria into the ventricles. The mitral valve is located on the left side of the heart and the tricuspid valve on the right.

**atrium** n. a chamber, most notably one in the heart that receives blood from the body (i.e., right atrium) or the lungs (i.e., left atrium) - **atria** pl., **atrial** adj.

**atrophic rhinitis** n. a disease of pigs caused by environmental contaminants and infections. Affected individuals may exhibit sneezing, tear-staining and changes to the shape of the upper jaw. Vaccination, antibiotics and controlling dust and ammonia can limit the effects of this disease.

**atrophy** v. to waste away and diminish in size - **atrophic** adj.

**atropine response test** n. a test that aids in the diagnosis of narcolepsy or certain types of arrhythmias. Atropine is administered to an animal, and changes in its behavior or heart rhythm are noted.

**attenuate** v. to weaken - **attenuation** n.

**attenuated vaccine** n. *See* modified live vaccine.

**attitude** n. an animal's general demeanor (e.g., bright, alert and responsive) or body position.

**atypical** adj. occurring in a different way than what is normally observed.

**auditory** adj. relating to the sense of hearing.

**Aujeszky's disease** n. *See* pseudorabies.

**aura** n. the period directly before a seizure during which an individual may begin to act abnormally.

**aural** adj. pertaining to the ear.

**aural hematoma** n. a swelling within the flap of the ear caused by a ruptured blood vessel. Aural hematomas often occur in dogs that shake their head or scratch their ears excessively because of ear infections. Surgery to remove the blood clot and join together the layers of the ear flap is usually necessary, as is treatment of the underlying ear infection. *Also called* auricular hematoma.

**aural plaque** n. raised, light-colored lesions involving the inner surface of a horse's ear caused by a virus that is probably transmitted by black flies. The lesions usually go unnoticed by the horse but can be unsightly. Treatment is difficult, and fly control is the best prevention. *Also called* papillary acanthoma and ear papillomas.

**auricle** n. 1. the external flap of the ear - **auricular** adj. *Also called* pinna. 2. one of the ear-shaped extensions that are connected to the atria of the heart.

**auriculopalpebral nerve block** n. an injection of local anesthetic around a nerve running between the ear and eye to prevent movement of the eyelids. This allows for easier and more thorough examination and treatment of the eye and its associated structures.

**auscultation** n. the act of listening to the sounds produced by the body, often with a stethoscope – **auscultate, auscult** v.

**autoagglutination** n. usually describes the abnormal clumping together of red blood cells that can result from the production of antibodies directed against them. *See also* Coombs test.

**autoantibodies** n. abnormal antibodies produced by an animal that are directed against some of its own cells.

**autoclave** n. a device used to sterilize surgical instruments and other items.

**autogenous** adj. originating from an animal's own body.

**autoimmune disease** n. a condition in which the immune system attacks cells within an animal's own body.

**autoimmune hemolytic anemia (AIHA)** n. *See* immune mediated hemolytic anemia.

**autoimmune thrombocytopenia** n. *See* immune mediated thrombocytopenia.

**autonomic nervous system (ANS)** n. the part of the nervous system that cannot be consciously controlled and regulates the actions of glands, heart muscle and smooth muscle.

**autonomy** n. the ability of reptiles to break off a part of their own body, usually the tail, in order to escape an attack.

**autotransfusion** n. the removal of blood from an animal's own body and its subsequent infusion back into the circulatory system. For example, an animal that is bleeding into its abdomen may have that blood removed, filtered and then replaced into a vein.

**AV block** n. *See* atrioventricular block.

**avascular** adj. without a blood supply.

**aversive conditioning** n. a method of training animals in which a startling and disagreeable response is the quick result of an unwanted behavior.

**avian** adj. pertaining to birds.

**avian influenza** n. a contagious virus infecting poultry and other species of birds. Symptoms can include discharge from the eyes and nose, discolored skin, difficulty breathing, neurologic disorders and death. Outbreaks must be reported to appropriate regulatory agencies. Some strains can infect people.

**aviary** n. an enclosure used to house birds.

**AVID® chip** n. a microchip made by a particular company that can be injected under the skin and scanned to help identify the animal.

**avitaminosis** n. a disorder that results from a lack of a specific vitamin or vitamins in the diet.

**avulse** v. to pull a structure or part of a structure off its attachments - **avulsion** n.

**avulsion fracture** n. a break in a bone that is caused when a ligament or tendon pulls a piece of bone off the rest of the structure.

**awn** n. a long and sharp bristle on the surface of some grass seeds that can penetrate the skin and move surprising distances within the body, causing chronic infections. They can also be found under the eyelids, leading to wounds and infections on the surface of the eye.

**axial** adj. located toward the midline of the body or body part. *Compare* abaxial.

**axilla** n. the armpit.

**axis** n. 1. the second vertebra of the spinal column located in the upper neck. 2. a line through the center of a structure.

**Azo® stick** n. a laboratory test that helps determine whether an animal's kidneys are functioning normally. An Azo® stick can also be used to test whether abnormal fluid in the abdomen is urine.

**azotemia** n. higher than normal blood levels of creatinine and/or blood urea nitrogen. Azotemia can indicate dehydration, kidney disease, a rupture in the urinary tract or other problems - **azotemic** adj. *Also called* uremia.

**azoturia** n. *See* exertional rhabdomyolysis.

## B

**B cell** n. a type of lymphocyte (i.e., white blood cell) that is primarily responsible for making antibodies. *Compare* T cell.

**babesiosis** n. a disease that is spread by ticks carrying the protozoal parasite *Babesia*. Infected animals can have a fever, pale or yellow mucous membranes, discolored urine, rapid breathing, weakness and may die. Treatment can include supportive care, blood transfusions and medications to kill the parasite or to reduce the body's immune response. *Also called* piroplasmosis.

**bacillary hemoglobinuria** n. a disease most often affecting cattle caused by infection with the bacteria *Clostridium haemolyticum*. Affected animals may have a fever, pale or yellow mucous membranes, dark red, foamy urine, difficulty breathing, abdominal pain, diarrhea and can die suddenly. Treatment may include antibiotics, fluid therapy and blood transfusions. Vaccines are available. *Also called* red water disease.

**back at the knee** n. a conformation flaw usually described in horses in which the middle of the front leg appears to bow backward when viewed from the side. *Also called* calf knee. *Compare* over at the knee.

**bacteremia** n. the presence of bacteria within the blood. Affected individuals can develop a fever, extreme lethargy, low blood pressure and may die without prompt and aggressive treatment. *Also called* blood poisoning or septicemia.

**bactericidal** adj. having the ability to kill bacteria. *Compare* bacteriostatic.

**bacterin** n. a vaccine that contains killed bacteria.

**bacteriology** n. the science and study of bacteria and the diseases that they cause.

**bacteriostatic** adj. having a tendency to slow the reproduction of bacteria. *Compare* bacteriocidal.

**bacterium** n. a particular type of single-celled microorganism that is ubiquitous in the environment but can cause disease under the right conditions - **bacterial** adj., **bacteria** pl.

**bacteriuria** n. the abnormal presence of bacteria in the urine.

**Baermann float** n. a laboratory technique used to identify parasitic larvae, usually in a sample feces.

**balanitis** n. inflammation of the penis.

**balanoposthitis** n. inflammation of the penis and the surrounding sheath.

**ball and socket joint** n. a type of connection between two bones that allows for rotational movement and consists of a round structure tightly fitting into a cup.

**balling gun** n. an instrument used to give pills to livestock.

**balloon catheter dilatation** n. a procedure used to dilate an abnormally narrowed structure during which a flexible tube is maneuvered into position and the balloon-like tip is inflated to stretch the affected area.

**ballottement** n. a technique of pushing or tapping on the abdomen of an animal in order to feel if a structure (e.g., a fetus) or a fluid wave bounces back and strikes the hands through the abdominal wall.

**band** n. 1. an immature neutrophil in the blood, which indicates the presence of infection within the body. 2. a device placed around the leg of a bird to aid in identification. *See also* elastrator.

**bandage** n. layers of material applied to a body part that can be used to control bleeding, protect a wound or provide support to an injured area.

**bandage scissors** n. scissors that have a blunt structure on the end of one of the blades allowing it to slide between the skin and a bandage without injuring the animal.

**barbering** n. a behavioral problem in which an animal will chew on and damage its own fur or that of another individual to which it has access.

**barber's pole worm** n. *See* hemonchosis.

**barbiturate** n. a type of drug that can be used as a short-acting general anesthetic or to treat seizures.

**barium** n. a substance that can be introduced into the gastrointestinal tract to highlight the structures when a radiograph is taken. Barium permits identification of physical abnormalities (e.g., a tumor) or physiological disorders (e.g., delayed emptying of the stomach) that can be invisible on traditional radiographs.

**barker** n. an animal that makes an abnormal, very loud noise while breathing, which resembles the sound of a dog's bark. *See also* neonatal maladjustment syndrome.

**barn itch** n. *See* sarcoptic mange.

**barren** adj. not able to become pregnant or not currently pregnant.

**barrow** n. a castrated male pig.

**bars of the foot** n. the raised parts on the underside of a horse's foot that extend from the heels towards the toe on either side of the frog.

**bars of the mouth** n. the parts of a horse's lower jaw that have no teeth and are located between the canine teeth and molars on both sides of the mouth. The bit typically rests on the bars of the horse's mouth.

**basal cell tumor** n. a skin tumor most often seen in dogs and cats. One type is a benign epithelioma, and surgery is usually curative. Complete removal of the more aggressive type, called a basal cell carcinoma, can be difficult. Neither form tends to spread to other organs.

**basal metabolic rate** n. the energy required to fuel an animal's body when it is at rest.

**base** n. 1. a substance with a pH greater than seven - **basic** adj. *Compare* acid. 2. the wide, supportive or bottom part of a structure - **basilar** adj.

**base narrow** adj. a description of an animal's conformation in which its feet are placed too close together. *Compare* base wide.

**base wide** adj. a description of an animal's conformation in which its feet are placed too far apart. *Compare* base narrow.

**basement membrane** n. the deepest layer of some tissues, such as the cornea or the skin.

**bask** v. to rest in the sun or under an artificial light source. Basking is especially important for reptiles because they use external heat sources to regulate their body temperature - **basking** n.

**basopenia** n. a lower than normal number of basophils in the blood.

**basophil** n. 1. a cell or structure that is easily stained with certain types of dye. 2. a specific type of white blood cell that plays an important role in allergic reactions and other immune functions.

**basophilia** n. a higher than normal number of basophils in the blood.

**bastard strangles** n. infection of horses with the bacteria *Streptococcus equi equi*. Bastard strangles specifically refers to a form of the disease in which lymph nodes other than those around the head and neck are affected. *See also* strangles.

**behavioral modification** n. a protocol that is used to alter an animal's undesirable behaviors. Training, changes in the animal's environment and medications can all play a role in behavioral modification.

**Bence Jones proteinuria** n. the abnormal presence of a specific type of protein in the urine, which is usually associated with myelomas.

**bench knee** n. a conformation flaw usually described in the front leg of a horse in which the cannon bone is placed too far to the outside of the knee. *Also called* offset cannon.

**benign** adj. describes a disease (e.g., cancer) that does not have the tendency to spread or worsen appreciably. *Compare* malignant.

**benign prostatic hyperplasia (BPH)** n. enlargement of the prostate commonly seen in male dogs that have not been neutered. Affected individuals may have difficulty defecating and blood in their urine. Castration is usually curative. Medicines can help control the disease if the animal is to be used for breeding. *Also called* benign prostatic hypertrophy.

**bent leg** n. a disease of young goats caused by a dietary imbalance of calcium and phosphorous. The front legs of affected individuals often bend to the inside or outside of the body. Animals may be in pain and reluctant to move. Correcting the diet will usually improve the situation but may not be curative. *Also called* epiphysitis.

**beta-blocker** n. a class of drugs most often used to slow the heart rate and lower blood pressure.

**bezoar** n. *See* phytobezoar and trichobezoar.

**bicarbonate** n. a natural chemical that helps maintain an animal's acid-base balance. If a disease has caused a low blood bicarbonate level, the compound may be given to normalize the individual's condition.

**biceps** n. a muscle having two heads, usually referring to a muscle in the front limb that helps flex the elbow joint - **bicipital** adj.

**bicipital bursitis** n. inflammation of a fluid-filled sac that lies between a tendon and bone in the upper front leg. The condition is usually caused by trauma, and the individual will often avoid extending the affected leg. Treatment can include prolonged rest and medications to decrease inflammation.

**bicipital tenosynovitis** n. a condition most often seen in large-breed dogs that is caused by inflammation of the tendon connecting the biceps muscle to the shoulder. Treatment can include rest, medicines to decrease inflammation or surgery.

**bicuspid valve** n. *See* mitral valve.

**bifurcation** n. the part of a structure where a separation into two branches occurs.

**big head** n. *See* miller's disease.

**bilateral** adj. pertaining to both sides of the body or structure. *Compare* unilateral.

**bile** n. the liquid produced by the liver that is emptied into the intestinal tract to aid in digestion - **bilious, biliary** adj. *Also called* gall.

**bile acid test** n. a laboratory test used to assess liver function. The amount of bile acid in the bloodstream is usually measured before and after a meal.

**bile duct** n. the tube that connects the gall bladder (or in the horse, the liver) to the intestinal tract and carries bile.

**biliary system** n. the parts of the liver, the gall bladder and ducts that all serve to produce, store or transport bile.

**bilious vomiting syndrome** n. a disorder seen in dogs that causes vomiting of bile or bile-stained mucous when the stomach is empty. After more serious diseases have been ruled out, treatment may include feeding smaller, more frequent meals or medications to help control the vomiting.

**bilirubin** n. a breakdown product of hemoglobin produced by red blood cell destruction and removed from the blood by the liver.

**bilirubinuria** n. the presence of bilirubin in the urine. Healthy, male dogs may have small amounts of bilirubin in their urine. Otherwise, bilirubinuria usually indicates liver disease or increased destruction of red blood cells.

**bioavailability** n. the degree to which a drug that is given to an animal will be absorbed and able to exert its desired effect.

**biochemical profile** n. a group of laboratory tests that measure the level of many different substances in the blood, often including those produced by the kidneys, liver and pancreas as well as proteins, electrolytes and other elements and compounds. The results of a biochemical profile can aid in diagnosis. *Also called* chemistry panel.

**biological** adj. 1. pertaining to biology. 2. n. a type of medication that is made from a living organism or its products. For example, many vaccines contain portions of microorganisms and are considered biologicals.

**biological response modifier** n. a type of medication given to an animal to alter the activity of the immune system.

**biopsy** v. to surgically remove a section of tissue that will be analyzed in order to aid in diagnosis.

**biosecurity** n. measures taken to prevent the spread of infectious organisms.

**biotin** n. a type of vitamin B, a deficiency of which can cause skin problems and poor quality hair, nails and hooves.

**birth canal** n. the passage, including the uterus and vagina, through which a fetus must travel during birth.

**bitch** n. a female dog.

**bite evaluation** n. an examination of the mouth to determine if the teeth align normally.

**Black disease** n. a disease primarily affecting sheep caused by infection with the bacteria *Clostridium novyi* associated with liver flukes. Individuals usually die suddenly. Vaccines are effective. *Also called* infectious necrotic hepatitis.

**black fly** n. a type of small flying insect that can be intensely irritating to grazing animals and may transmit some diseases, including onchocerciasis.

**black walnut poisoning** n. a condition most frequently seen in horses housed on bedding containing even a small amount of black walnut shavings. Affected individuals can develop laminitis, swelling of the lower legs, colic and rapid breathing. Treatment includes removing the contaminated shavings, anti-inflammatories, medications that improve blood flow to the damaged tissues and therapeutic hoof trimming and shoeing if laminitis is severe.

**black water** n. *See* exertional rhabdomyolysis.

**blackleg** n. a disease of cattle and sheep caused by infection with the bacteria *Clostridium chauvoei*. Affected individuals develop soft swellings, often with palpable air bubbles, in heavily muscled areas. The animals are lethargic, febrile, in pain, and their condition can quickly deteriorate to include death within a matter of hours. Preventative vaccination is effective, while treatment of ill animals with antibiotics often is not.

**bladder** n. a balloon-like structure that can fill with fluid, usually referring to the organ that holds urine.

**bladder prolapse** n. the movement of the urinary bladder through a tear in the vaginal wall to become located in or protrude from the vagina. Bladder prolapse is most often seen in cows after a difficult birthing process. The bladder can be replaced through the tear, which is then surgically repaired.

**bladder stone** n. an accumulation of minerals and other substances within the urinary bladder that form a hard object. Bladder stones often are associated with bloody urine, straining or inability to urinate and infections. Some types can be dissolved with special diets or medications while others must be removed surgically. *Also called* urolith and cystic calculus. *See also* struvite, calcium oxalate, urate and cystine uroliths.

**bladder tumor antigen test** n. a laboratory test performed on urine that is helpful in the diagnosis of the most common type of canine bladder tumor.

**blast cell** n. usually refers to a precursor cell located in the bone marrow or lymph nodes that can divide and mature to produce the different types of blood cells. Abnormal numbers of blast cells can be seen with some types of cancer.

**blastomycosis** n. a disease caused by infection with a *Blastomyces* fungus. Effects vary depending on where the infection develops but difficulty breathing, skin lesions, enlarged lymph nodes and eye disease are possible. Treatment with an antifungal medication is often successful, but relapses can occur.

**bleb** n. usually describes a small pocket of fluid injected under the skin.

**bleeder** n. 1. a horse that bleeds into its respiratory tract during periods of extreme exertion. *See also* exercise-induced pulmonary hemorrhage. 2. a blood vessel that bleeds profusely when cut.

**blenderized** adj. describes food that has been processed in a blender to give it a thinner consistency, usually so it can be more easily passed through a feeding tube.

**blepharitis** n. inflammation of the eyelids.

**blepharoedema** n. swelling of the eyelids.

**blepharoplasty** n. the surgical reconstruction of an eyelid.

**blepharorrhaphy** n. the suturing of an eyelid.

**blepharospasm** n. squinting of the eyelids, usually indicating pain within the eye or the surrounding structures.

**blepharotomy** n. a surgical incision into an eyelid.

**blind** adj. lacking the sense of sight. Blindness can occur because of disorders of the eye or of the nerves and parts of the brain that receive input from the eye - **blindness** n.

**blind quarter** n. one section of an udder that is not producing milk while the other parts are lactating.

**blind spot** n. a portion of an animal's field of vision where objects are invisible. Some animals, such as horses, are unable to see objects at a certain distance directly in front or in back of them because of the wide placement of their eyes. Another blind spot is associated with the area on the retina through which the optic nerve leaves the eye.

**blind staggers** n. behavior characterized by continual, unsteady walking (often in circles), blindness, the tendency to become stuck in corners and other neurologic abnormalities. Blind staggers can be caused by selenium toxicosis in cattle, leukoencephalomalacia in horses or other conditions affecting specific parts of the brain.

**blink reflex** n. the normal, involuntary response of an animal to close its eyelids when an object quickly moves toward an eye. The loss of a blink reflex can indicate blindness or abnormalities affecting the nerves or part of the brain that control the eyelids.

**blister** n. a pocket of serum that forms under the surface of a tissue.

**blister beetle poisoning** n. *See* cantharidin poisoning.

**blister disease** n. *See* scale rot.

**blistering** n. the process of applying an irritating substance to the skin to encourage healing of deeper tissues such as tendons or ligaments. Blistering traditionally has been used to treat injuries affecting horses' legs but is of questionable value and may not be humane in many cases.

**bloat** n. the accumulation of gas within the gastrointestinal tract, usually the stomach or rumen, to the point of distention and pain. Passage of a stomach tube or surgery to remove the gas is necessary to provide relief. *See also* frothy and free gas bloat (cattle) and gastric dilatation and volvulus (dog).

**block vertebra** n. an abnormal fusion of two spinal vertebrae that is present at birth. Some individuals have no problems associated with a block vertebra while others may require surgery to relieve instability of the spine or pressure on the spinal cord.

**blocked cat** n. obstruction of the urethra with a plug of mucus, protein, cells and/or crystals most often seen in neutered male cats. Affected individuals strain but are unable to urinate and may exhibit abdominal pain, become depressed and die without rapid treatment. Therapy can include placement of a urinary catheter, fluid therapy, supportive care and sometimes a perineal urethrostomy surgery.

**blood** n. the liquid containing cells, chemicals and dissolved gasses that is pumped by the heart and carried by vessels throughout the body. Blood carries nourishment to and waste products from tissues.

**blood feather** n. *See* pin feather.

**blood gas analysis** n. a laboratory test that analyzes the levels of oxygen and carbon dioxide in and the pH of an animal's blood. Blood gas analysis can be performed to evaluate an individual's acid-base balance or the function of its respiratory system.

**blood glucose** n. the level of glucose (a type of sugar) in the blood. Blood glucose measurements are often taken to monitor the condition of diabetic animals or if low blood sugar is suspected in young or extremely ill individuals. *Also called* blood sugar.

**blood group** n. *See* blood type.

**blood poisoning** n. the presence of bacteria and/or toxins released by damaged or dead bacteria within the circulatory system. Affected individuals can develop a fever, extreme lethargy, low blood pressure and may die without prompt and aggressive treatment. *Also called* septicemia or endotoxemia.

**blood pressure** n. a measurement of the force exerted by blood within arteries and veins. High blood pressure can be seen with certain diseases (e.g., kidney failure). Low blood pressure may result from blood loss, heart failure, anaphylaxis, severe infection or extreme dehydration. Prolonged high or low blood pressure can damage many organs within the body.

**blood smear** n. a spot of blood spread across a glass slide that is stained and examined with a microscope to evaluate the numbers and condition of the cells.

**blood spavin** n. swelling of a horse's hock that is caused by bleeding into the joint.

**blood sugar** n. *See* blood glucose.

**blood type** n. a classification system that identifies the kinds of red blood cells produced by different individuals. Transfusions of the blood of one type to an individual with blood of another type can cause a potentially fatal transfusion reaction. *Also called* blood group.

**blood urea nitrogen (BUN)** n. a substance measured in blood, the levels of which can be altered by a variety of disorders. Elevations can be seen with kidney disease, dehydration and some types of infection and reductions with liver disease.

**blood vessel** n. a tube that carries blood to and from the heart and throughout the body.

**blood worm** n. *See* large strongyle.

**blood-brain barrier** n. the partial separation that exists between the brain and its blood supply, which allows some substances access to brain tissues while others are excluded. The blood-brain barrier can lessen the ability of some drugs to treat the brain.

**blow fly** n. a type of fly that lays its eggs in wounds, on skin soiled with urine or feces or on carcasses. The larvae feed on the tissue of their host ani-

mal and can cause irritation, illness and death. Treatment includes clipping and cleansing the affected areas, medications to kill the larvae and supportive care.

**blue Doberman syndrome** n. *See* color dilute alopecia.

**blue eye** n. a clouding of the cornea seen in some dogs infected with canine adenovirus (CAV-1) or given an outmoded type of CAV-1 vaccine. *See also* infectious canine hepatitis.

**bluetongue** n. a viral disease seen primarily in sheep that is transmitted by the bites of *Culicoides* insects. Affected individuals may exhibit a fever, swelling, lesions of and discharge from the nose and mouth, a blue discoloration to the tongue, lameness, abnormal wool growth and death. Vaccination and insect control can help prevent the disease. Treatment is difficult.

**blue-green algae** n. *See* cyanobacteria.

**blunt dissection** n. a surgical technique during which tissues are separated but not cut.

**blunt force trauma** n. an injury that is caused by an animal being struck by an object that does not pierce the skin. Blunt force trauma can lead to bruising, bleeding, fractures and damage to internal organs and tissues.

**boar** n. an unaltered male pig that is of breeding age.

**board certified** adj. describes a veterinarian who has successfully completed additional training, tests and license requirements and is considered an expert in a specialized aspect of veterinary medicine (e.g., dermatology, ophthalmology, internal medicine or surgery).

**body condition score (BCS)** n. a numerical rating system that assesses the weight of an animal in association with its body type. A scale of one to five or one to ten is often used, with the middle number indicating an ideal weight. Lower numbers correspond to varying degrees of leanness or emaciation and higher numbers designate an overweight or obese condition.

**body surface area** n. a measurement of the size of an animal that can be used instead of body weight in the calculation of drug dosages.

**bog spavin** n. a soft swelling of a horse's hock that is caused by an increased amount of fluid within the joint often associated with inflammation. Affected individuals are rarely lame. If the bog spavin is a result of a transient event (e.g., trauma) it will usually resolve over a period of weeks to months. If poor conformation is to blame, the condition can recur.

**boil** n. *See* furuncle.

**bolus** n. a cohesive mass of medication, food or another substance that is given to an animal all at one time or passes through the intestinal tract as a unit.

**bone** n. the rigid, mineralized tissue that forms the individual parts of the skeleton.

**bone marrow** n. the tissue encased within many bones that produces red and white blood cells and platelets.

**bone marrow aspiration** n. a procedure during which a sample of marrow is removed from within a bone via a needle or similar instrument. The tissue is then analyzed to determine it's health.

**bone scan** n. *See* scintigraphy.

**bone spavin** n. a hard swelling of a horse's hock that is associated with osteoarthritis. Individuals often have lameness in the affected leg that improves with exercise but worsens with rest. Pain relievers and anti-inflammatories can be helpful. The joint may fuse on its own or surgery can hasten the process at which point the animal's pain is lessened.

**bone spur** n. *See* exostosis.

**booster** n. a subsequent injection of a vaccine that raises the level of immunity provided by previous vaccinations.

**borborygmi** n. the noises made by the gastrointestinal system. Decreases, increases and changes in these sounds can be heard with specific diseases.

**border disease** n. a contagious, viral disease primarily affecting sheep that may cause abortions, low birth weights, excessively hairy fleeces, bony abnormalities and tremors in newborn lambs. Only the offspring of animals newly exposed to the virus during early pregnancy are at risk. No effective treatment or vaccine exists. *Also called* hairy shaker disease.

**Bordetella** n. a type of bacteria that causes a contagious respiratory disease in many species. Effects may range from a mild, self-limiting cough to pneumonia and death. Therapy can include antibiotics and cough suppressants. Vaccination helps prevent the disease in some species. *See also* kennel cough.

**borreliosis** n. *See* Lyme disease.

**botryomycosis** n. chronic infection of the skin, usually with *Staphylococcus aureus* bacteria that form nodules of inflammation and infection and can spread to deeper tissues.

**bots** n. the larvae of various types of flies. *See also* nasal bots, hypodermosis, cuterebriasis and gasterophilosis.

**bottle jaw** n. fluid accumulation under the jaw, most often describing a condition of ruminants that have a low blood protein level because of heavy infestation with intestinal parasites.

**botulism** n. a disease caused by a toxin produced by *Clostridium botulinum* bacteria. The toxin is usually absorbed when animals eat decaying material or the maggots feeding on it. Affected individuals exhibit progressive weakness and paralysis. Treatment can include antitoxin administration and supportive care. Some animals may recover without treatment if not too severely affected. *Also called* forage poisoning and limberneck. *See also* toxicoinfectious botulism.

**bounding pulse** n. the feel or sight of blood coursing through an artery that is more evident than normal. A bounding pulse can be an indication of some types of heart disease, high blood pressure or other problems, or it may be normal if the animal is very excited or has just exercised.

**bovine** adj. pertaining to cattle.

**bovine atypical interstitial pneumonia** n. a disease of cattle often seen soon after they have been given access to lush pasture. Individuals have difficulty breathing and high respiratory rates and if severely affected, may die when stressed. Milder cases generally resolve in a few days. *Also called* acute bovine pulmonary edema and emphysema and fog fever.

**bovine bonkers** n. *See* non-protein nitrogen poisoning.

**bovine ketosis** n. a disease most commonly seen in overweight dairy cows when they are producing a lot of milk. Affected cattle exhibit loss of appetite, depression and sometimes abnormal behavior. Treatment may include glucose infusions and corticosteroid injections. Prevention is aided by maintaining cattle at their optimum weight and encouraging feed intake during early and peak lactation. *Also called* ketonemia and acetonemia.

**bovine leukemia virus (BLV)** n. the virus that can cause bovine leukosis.

**bovine leukosis** n. a disease of cattle that is often caused by the bovine leukemia virus. Many infected individuals do not become sick, but some animals develop cancer of their lymphocytes leading to enlarged lymph nodes and/or tumors in almost any organ. No effective treatment exists. *Also called* bovine lymphosarcoma and bovine malignant lymphoma.

**bovine respiratory disease complex (BRD)** n. describes a disease of cattle that is a result of a combination of stress, environmental irritants (e.g., dust and ammonia) and infection with a variety of viruses and bacteria. Affected individuals can develop a fever, cough, nasal and ocular discharge and difficulty breathing. Therapy includes antibiotic administration and relieving the stress and environmental irritants. *Also called* shipping fever.

**bovine spongiform encephalopathy (BSE)** n. a disease of adult cattle usually caused by ingestion of a type of abnormal protein called a prion contained in contaminated feed. Affected animals can develop unusual behaviors, difficulty walking and eventually die. There is no treatment, and suspected cases must be reported to appropriate regulatory agencies. Ingestion of BSE contaminated tissues is associated with a neurologic disease in humans. *Also called* mad cow disease.

**bovine ulcerative mammillitis** n. a contagious, viral disease of cattle. Affected animals develop painful ulcers and scabs on their teats and udders that can take weeks to heal. No effective treatment exists.

**bovine viral diarrhea (BVD)** n. a contagious, viral disease of cattle that can cause fever, diarrhea, nasal and ocular discharge, difficulty breathing, ulcers, abortion, birth defects and death. Treatment is limited to supportive care. Effective vaccines exist. *See also* mucosal disease.

**bowed legs** n. describes limbs that curve toward the outside of the body in the middle of the leg.

**bowed tendon** n. inflammation of a tendon in the lower, back part of a horse's leg often caused by rupture of some of the tendon fibers. Bowed tendons may develop because of overextension of the leg due to fatigue or poor footing. Treatment usually involves rest, cold compresses or baths, bandaging, anti-inflammatories and a gradual return to exercise. Many other procedures may also be tried. *Also called* tendinitis.

**bowel** n. the part of the intestinal tract between the stomach and the anus incorporating both the small and large intestines.

**brachial plexus** n. a network of nerves that runs to and from the spinal cord and front limb through the armpit.

**brachial plexus avulsion** n. an injury that pulls nerves running through the armpit from their attachments to the spinal cord. Affected individuals lose the ability to use their front limb normally and may have Horner's syndrome. Recovery from a less severe form of brachial plexus injury is possible, but the damage caused by a true avulsion is permanent, and amputation may be required.

**brachycephalic** adj. describes a facial structure that consists of an extremely short snout, wide head and prominent eyes (e.g., a Bulldog). *Compare* dolicocephalic.

**brachycephalic airway syndrome** n. a combination of anatomic abnormalities (e.g., narrowed nasal openings and windpipe, long soft palate and excess tissue in the back of the throat) seen in brachycephalic animals, which can lead to difficult and noisy breathing. Surgery to repair some of these problems is possible and often greatly improves the affected individual's quality of life.

**brachygnathism** n. a shorter than normal lower jaw. Mild cases may be insignificant to the animal, but severe abnormalities can lead to oral injuries and pain. A variety of dental procedures can be used to shorten teeth or change their orientation so that they no longer cause damage. *Also called* parrot mouth and overshot jaw. *Compare* prognathism.

**brachytherapy** n. a type of cancer therapy involving delivery of radiation directly into a tumor through implantation of a device or other methods that will treat the disease for a prolonged period of time.

**bracken fern poisoning** n. ingestion of sufficient quantities of the bracken fern plant to cause disease. Horses develop difficulty walking, loss of appetite, trembling, neurologic abnormalities and will sometimes die. Treatment with thiamine supplements can be successful if the disease is caught early. Affected cattle have blood that fails to clot normally, can bleed throughout their body and often die. Treatment is difficult. *See also* bright blindness (sheep) and enzootic hematuria.

**bradyarrhythmia** n. an irregular and slow heart rhythm. *Compare* tachyarrhythmia.

**bradycardia** n. an abnormally slow heart rate. *Compare* tachycardia.

**bradycardia-tachycardia syndrome** n. *See* sick sinus syndrome.

**bradypnea** n. an abnormally slow rate of breathing. *Compare* tachypnea.

**brain** n. the organ that is encased within the skull and is responsible for regulating an animal's nervous system.

**brain herniation** n. the abnormal movement of a portion of brain tissue through an opening at the base of the skull, which is often caused by increased intracranial pressure. Treatment is difficult.

**brain stem** n. the portion of the brain that connects with the spinal cord. Parts of the brain stem help control some of the most basic aspects of body function, including breathing and heart rates.

**brainstem auditory evoked response test (BAER)** n. a procedure that measures the brain's responsiveness to noise, which can be used to evaluate the function of the brainstem or as a hearing test.

**bran disease** n. *See* miller's disease.

**brand** n. a permanent, identifying mark put on the skin of an animal, usually through application of a very hot or very cold instrument.

**breast blister** n. a fluid or pus-filled sac that can develop over the prominent breastbone of birds in response to repeated trauma to this area.

**breech presentation** n. a description of the birth of a fetus in which the hind legs or rump emerge from the uterus first. This is an abnormal position for delivery in some species, including horses and cattle, and may require that the fetus be turned or a cesarian section performed to complete the birthing process. *Also called* posterior presentation. *Compare* anterior presentation.

**breed** n. a group of individuals that are genetically and physically more similar to each other than they are to other members of the same species.

**breed standard** n. a description of the characteristics of an ideal individual of a certain breed.

**breeding soundness exam** n. a series of evaluations and laboratory tests performed to determine the likelihood of an individual successfully reproducing.

**bright blindness** n. a progressive blindness seen in sheep that eat bracken fern. Affected individuals have eyes that are more reflective than normal when a light is shone on them. No treatment exists.

**brisket disease** n. *See* high mountain disease.

**brittle diabetic** n. an animal with diabetes mellitus whose blood sugar levels do not stabilize with insulin treatment as well as expected. Diabetic animals that have concurrent diseases can be difficult to regulate.

**brodifacoum** n. *See* anticoagulant rodenticide poisoning.

**broken wind** n. *See* recurrent airway obstruction.

**bromethalin toxicity** n. ingestion of sufficient quantities of the mouse and rat poison bromethalin to cause excitement, tremors, seizures, depression and sometimes death. Lower, repeated doses may cause vomiting, difficulty walking and tremors. Treatment is difficult if several hours have elapsed since the animal ate a large amount of the poison.

**bromide level** n. a laboratory test used to determine if an animal taking potassium bromide for the treatment of seizures is receiving the correct amount of the drug.

**bronchi** n. *See* bronchus.

**bronchial pattern** n. a finding on a chest radiograph seen when the walls of airways within the lungs thicken, often because of inflammation.

**bronchiectasis** n. an irreversible dilation of airways within the lung often associated with chronic lung disease.

**bronchitis** n. inflammation of the large passageways for air leading from the trachea into the lungs or carrying air throughout the lungs. Bronchitis may be caused by infections, allergies or inhaled irritants and usually causes an animal to cough. Treatment may include cough suppressants, antibiotics and medicines to thin mucous and dilate airways.

**bronchoalveolar lavage (BAL)** n. a procedure that uses a bronchoscope to take samples of mucus, other fluids and cells from within the small airways of the lungs. The material is then analyzed to help determine the cause of a respiratory disorder.

**bronchoconstriction** n. a narrowing of the airways within the lung, often due to an allergic response.

**bronchodilator** n. a type of drug that widens a constricted airway within the lung and eases breathing.

**bronchopneumonia** n. inflammation of lung tissue and airways often associated with viral and/or bacterial infections, though other causes and organisms can be involved. Affected individuals may cough, be lethargic and have difficulty breathing and nasal discharge. Treatment can include antibiotics, medicines to reduce fever and inflammation and to dilate airways and thin mucus, oxygen therapy, procedures to loosen mucus within the airways and supportive care.

**bronchoscopy** n. the use of a tubular instrument including a light source and viewing device placed into the trachea and bronchi, which allows the veterinarian to see abnormalities, remove foreign objects and take samples of tissue or fluid for analysis.

**bronchovesicular sounds** n. the noises made by air passing through the airways and lungs that can be heard with a stethoscope. Decreases, increases and changes in these sounds can be heard with specific diseases.

**bronchus** n. any of a number of large passageways for air leading from the trachea into the lungs or carrying air throughout the lungs - **bronchi** pl., **bronchial** adj.

**brooder pneumonia** n. a disease of young chickens, turkeys and some other birds caused by infection of the respiratory system with *Aspergillus* fungi. Affected birds have difficulty breathing, lethargy, weight loss and may develop neurologic abnormalities. Antifungal medications can be effective. *Also called* aspergillosis.

**broodiness** n. the tendency of birds to want to sit on their eggs until they hatch. Broodiness can be a problem for egg producers because birds that are sitting on their eggs are not producing new ones.

**broodmare** n. a female horse that is used primarily to produce foals.

**brown stomach worm** n. *See* ostertagiasis.

**brucellosis** n. a disease caused by infection with *Brucella* bacteria. Most affected individuals display reproductive problems such as abortion and retained placentas in females and infections of the testicles and associated glands in males. The bacteria can cause problems in other parts of the body as well (e.g., fistulous withers in horses or infections of the spine in dogs). Antibiotics can help control the disease, but infection may persist despite treatment. In cattle, preventative vaccination is very effective, eradication programs exist and infected animals must be reported to appropriate regulatory agencies. Human infections are possible.

**bruise** n. *See* contusion.

**bruised sole** n. an injury to the bottom of a horse's hoof caused by stepping on a sharp, hard object like a stone. The affected area is usually red and painful. Treatment involves rest, pain relief and monitoring for the development of an abscess.

**bruxism** n. grinding of the teeth that can be displayed by some animals (e.g., cattle) that are in pain or are neurologically abnormal.

**buccal** adj. pertaining to or oriented towards the cheeks. *Compare* lingual.

**buccal mucosal bleeding time (BMBT)** n. a procedure used to test for the presence of an adequate number of functioning platelets in an animal's blood. A small incision is made in the mucous membrane of the lip and the time needed for a blood clot to form is measured.

**buck** n. 1. an unaltered male of several species, including goats, rabbits and deer. 2. a hopping and kicking motion of the rear legs, which is displayed by some animals (e.g., horses) when they are irritated or excited.

**buck knee** n. *See* over at the knee.

**bucked shin** n. a problem usually seen in young racehorses caused by intense exercise before the animal's bones can handle the stress. Small fractures, inflammation and pain develop at the front of the long bones of the lower leg. Treatment involves medication and therapies to relieve pain and inflammation and rest.

**budgerigar fledgling disease** n. a contagious, viral disease usually affecting young budgerigars (i.e., parakeets) and sometimes parrots that may cause lethargy, a distended crop, bruising, neurologic problems, abnormal feathers and death. Treatment includes supportive care and vitamin K supplements. A vaccine is available. *Also called Polyomavirus.*

**buffy coat** n. the layer containing white blood cells that lies between the red blood cells and serum when blood is centrifuged in a tube. Analyzing the buffy coat reveals the types and numbers of white blood cells in circulation.

**bull** n. an unaltered, male bovine animal of breeding age.

**bulla** n. a cavity filled with fluid or air - **bullae** pl., **bullous** adj. *See also* tympanic bulla.

**bulla osteotomy** n. surgery that opens a tympanic bulla to allow removal of diseased or damaged tissues and other treatments. *See also* total ear canal ablation.

**bullous emphysema** n. a disease characterized by the presence of air-filled cavities within the lung. The pockets can rupture and surround the lungs with air, making lung expansion and breathing difficult.

**bullous pemphigoid** n. a disease caused by an abnormal autoimmune reaction against some parts of an animal's skin. Affected individuals develop different types of skin lesions, most characteristically chronic reddened skin with pockets of fluid. Treatment with medicines to suppress the immune system can be effective.

**bumblefoot** n. infection of the feet of birds, guinea pigs, rabbits or other animals that are often housed on rough and dirty surfaces (e.g., wire mesh). Affected individuals have raised lesions on their feet and/or legs, which are often painful. Treatment includes antibiotics, cleaning wounds, surgical removal of diseased tissues and improving the animal's environment. *Also called* pododermatitis and sore hocks.

**buphthalmos** n. an abnormal enlargement of the eye, often seen as a result of glaucoma. *Also called* macrophthalmia.

**burn** n. an injury caused by heat, chemicals or radiation that damage tissue.

**bursa** n. a fluid-filled sac that protects tissues from rubbing against each other. A bursa is often located around joints in areas where tendons and ligaments pass over other structures. *See also* hygroma.

**bursitis** n. inflammation of a bursa, which is often caused by a traumatic injury. Affected animals are in pain and reluctant to move the affected joint. Treatment involves rest and anti-inflammatories. Infection can also cause bursitis, in which case drainage of the fluid and antibiotic therapy is also needed.

**butterfly vertebra** n. abnormal fetal development of a vertebra causing a cleft to form down the middle of the bone. Most individuals have no problems associated with a butterfly vertebra, though some may require surgery to relieve instability of the spine or pressure on the spinal cord.

**buttress foot** n. a bulging of the front surface of a horse's foot caused by injury to a bony process at the top of the bone encased by the hoof. Therapy depends on the type of underlying injury and may include rest, medicines to reduce pain and inflammation or surgery. Arthritis is a common consequence. *Also called* pyramidal disease and extensor process disease.

# C

**C-section** n. See Cesarian section.

**Cache Valley virus** n. a virus transmitted by mosquitoes that can cause birth defects and abortions. No vaccine or treatment exists.

**cachexia** n. extreme loss of body mass involving both muscle and fat.

**cage rest** n. strict restriction of activity by housing an animal almost exclusively in a cage just large enough to be comfortable but small enough to prevent unwanted movement. Cage rest is often used to prevent damage to a healing injury or to prevent exertion that may stress the heart and lungs.

**calcification** n. the deposition of calcium within a tissue. Calcification in abnormal areas can disrupt organ function and is seen in some cases of poisoning, hormonal imbalance and kidney disease.

**calcinosis cutis** n. abnormal deposition of calcium within the skin, which is sometimes associated with Cushing's disease.

**calcitonin** n. a hormone made by the thyroid gland that regulates the amount of calcium in the blood and bones.

**calcium** n. a mineral the correct levels of which are essential to maintaining normal bones, neurologic and muscular activity and many other body functions.

**calcium channel blocker** n. a type of drug used to slow the heart rate, improve heart function and to treat high blood pressure. Diltiazem is a commonly used calcium channel blocker.

**calcium oxalate urolith** n. a type of stone that can form within and disrupt the function of the urinary tract. Calcium oxalate uroliths may develop because of abnormal urinary pH or the presence of higher than normal levels of calcium in the urine. The stones must be physically removed through surgery or urohydropulsion. Dietary modifications can help prevent their return.

**calcium:phosphorous ratio** n. the relative levels of calcium and phosphorous in the diet. Adequate amounts and a balanced ratio of these minerals are essential to maintaining normal bones, neurologic and muscular activity and many other body functions.

**calciuria** n. an abnormally large amount of calcium in the urine, which can predispose an animal to the formation of some types of bladder stones.

**calculus** n. an abnormal, mineralized substance or stone found in the body. *See also* tartar and urolith - **calculi** pl.

**calf diphtheria** n. *See* necrotic laryngitis.

**calf knee** n. *See* back at the knee.

**calicivirus** n. a type of virus that can infect a variety of species causing different clinical signs. See the specific species or disease (e.g., feline and rabbit calicivirus and vesicular exanthema) for details.

**caliper** n. an instrument that can be used to measure the length, width, thickness or diameter of an object.

**callus** n. 1. an area of thick, hardened skin that often develops in response to repeated irritation. 2. bony tissue that forms around a broken bone to help stabilize and heal the fracture.

**caloric test** n. a test to determine if an animal's brainstem and vestibular system are functioning. The caloric test involves placing hot or cold liquid into the ear canal. Specific types of eye movement indicate a normal response.

**calorie** n. a unit of measurement used to quantify the energy content of food or energy expended by an animal.

**calvarium** n. the dome-shaped top of the skull.

**calving** n. the process through which a cow gives birth to a calf.

**calving paralysis** n. injury to nerves running into a cow's hind leg, which can occur during a difficult birth. Affected individuals are often unable to rise and are splay-legged. *Also called* obturator, ischiatic and sciatic nerve paralysis.

**camped out** adj. describes a body position in which the front legs are placed further forward and the rear legs are placed further back than is normal. This stance may be desirable when showing some breeds or may indicate musculoskeletal pain.

**campylobacteriosis** n. disease caused by infection with *Campylobacter* bacteria. Infection of the gastrointestinal tract causes diarrhea in many species. Some animals may carry and shed the bacteria in their feces without becoming ill themselves and are a source of infection for other animals or people. Treatment with antibiotics can be successful. Infection of the genital tract can cause sheep to abort and cows to lose their pregnancies early in gestation. Vaccinations and antibiotics can help eliminate the disease from cattle and sheep herds. *Also called* vibriosis.

**cancellous bone** n. the spongy and honeycomb-like bone tissue that surrounds and contains marrow within most bones. *Also called* trabecular bone. *Compare* cortical bone.

**cancer** n. disease caused by abnormal and uncontrolled growth of cells. Cancer may be caused by environmental factors (e.g., chemicals, cigarette smoke or sun exposure), viruses or an animal's own genes, but in many cases the specific reason cannot be pinpointed. Cancers can develop in almost any tissue and lead to a wide variety of symptoms. Therapy may include surgery, chemotherapy or radiation therapy with varying degrees of success depending on the type and progression of the disease - **cancerous** adj. *Also called* neoplasia.

**candidiasis** n. a disease caused by the fungus *Candida* that most often infects the digestive tract (e.g., a bird's crop) but can also involve other organ systems. Animals that are immunosuppressed or have been recently treated with antibiotics are at an increased risk for candidiasis. Affected individuals often are lethargic, lose their appetite and weight and may develop diarrhea. White plaques may be visible on infected tissues. Treatment can include antiseptics, antifungal medications and supportive care. *Also called* thrush and moniliasis.

**candling** n. the process of holding an egg in front of a light source to determine if there is an embryo within.

**canine** adj. pertaining to dogs.

**canine acanthomatous ameloblastoma** n. *See* acanthomatous epulis.

**canine adenovirus (CAV)** n. a type of virus causing infectious canine hepatitis (CAV-1) or kennel cough (CAV-2).

**canine coronavirus** n. a contagious virus causing mild diarrhea in infected puppies. Vaccines are available but rarely necessary.

**canine distemper** n. a contagious, viral disease of dogs, ferrets and some wildlife species. Affected individuals can develop a fever, discharge from the eyes and nose, loss of appetite, vomiting, diarrhea, coughing, difficulty breathing, neurological signs and thickening of the footpads and nose. Older dogs may develop neurologic abnormalities without any other clinical signs. Therapy can include supportive care and antibiotics for secondary bacterial infections, but successful treatment of dogs with neurologic signs and ferrets is difficult. Appropriate preventative vaccination is very successful. *Also called* hardpad disease.

**canine dysautonomia** n. a disease with an unknown cause that disrupts the autonomic nervous system. Affected individuals can have pupils that do not respond to light, third eyelid elevation, drooping upper eyelids, dry mucous membranes, weight loss and difficulty urinating. Treatment is difficult.

**Canine Eye Registry Foundation (CERF)** n. an organization dedicated to the elimination of heritable eye disease in purebred dogs through registration and research.

**canine fibrous histiocytoma** n. a raised mass affecting the eye and sometimes other tissues of dogs. It arises from inflammation of connective tissue and may be treated with corticosteroids. A severely affected eye that does not respond to medical management may need to be surgically removed. *Also called* collie granuloma, nodular fasciitis and proliferative keratoconjunctivitis.

**canine herpesvirus (CHV)** n. a contagious virus causing sudden death in young puppies that have not received immunity from their mothers. Bitches infected while pregnant can abort. No treatment or vaccine exists. Complete isolation of young, susceptible litters can prevent the disease.

**canine parvovirus (CPV)** n. a contagious virus of dogs that can cause vomiting, diarrhea often containing blood, secondary bacterial infections (e.g., pneumonia) and death. The disease is most often seen in young, inadequately vaccinated puppies. Treatment may include fluid therapy, antibiotics, antinausea medications and plasma transfusions. Vaccination on an appropriate schedule will usually prevent the disease.

**canine peripheral ameloblastoma** n. *See* acanthomatous epulis.

**canine tooth** n. one of the large, pointed teeth that is located between the incisors and premolars in most species.

**canker** n. 1. a lesion in which the surface of a tissue is damaged and lost. *Also called* ulcer. 2. chronic overproduction and subsequent loss of tissue on the bottom of a horse's foot. Treatment involves removal off all affected tissue and repeated cleansing and bandaging. 3. a specific infection of the upper digestive tract in birds. *See also* trichomoniasis.

**cannon bone** n. the long bone of the lower front and back legs of horses and ruminants located between the fetlock and the carpus or stifle.

**cannula** n. a hollow tube that can be inserted into a body opening (e.g., tear duct, nasal cavity or teat) and used to administer medications or for other treatments.

**canter** n. a specific way of moving described in horses in which three distinct beats or footfalls are evident. A canter resembles a slow gallop.

**cantharidin poisoning** n. a disease of horses caused by eating hay, usually alfalfa, contaminated with blister beetle insects. Affected individuals exhibit varying degrees of abdominal pain, depression, loss of appetite, frequent drinking, discolored urine and mucous membranes, sweating, fever and may die if enough toxin has been ingested. Treatment can include fluid therapy, mineral oil and activated charcoal administration, pain relief and supportive care. *Also called* blister beetle poisoning.

**canthoplasty** n. the surgical reconstruction of an eye's canthus.

**canthus** n. the junction of the upper and lower eyelids located at both corners of the eye.

**cap tooth** n. in the horse, an abnormally retained baby tooth that sits on top of the erupting adult tooth. The cap tooth should be removed to allow for normal chewing and tooth wear.

**capillariasis** n. a disease caused by infestation with a *Capillaria* worm. Various types of *Capillaria* can infest the digestive system, lungs and urinary tract of different animal species. Dewormers can be effective.

**capillary** n. one of the extremely small blood vessels that connect arteries and veins. The transfer of gasses, nutrients and other substances occurs through the thin walls of capillaries.

**capillary refill time (CRT)** n. a procedure that involves pressing a finger against an animal's mucous membrane (e.g., gum) and noting the amount of time necessary for the blanched tissue to return to a pink color. An elongated capillary refill time can indicate dehydration, shock or other problems.

**capnography** n. measurement of the amount of carbon dioxide in an animal's exhaled breath. Capnography may be performed on an anesthetized animal to monitor respiratory function.

**capped** adj. describes the abnormal presence of a fluid-filled sac over an animal's joint (e.g., elbow, hock or knee) that develops to protect the area from repeated trauma. It may be drained if unsightly or bothersome but will often recur unless the source of irritation is removed. *Also called* acquired or false bursa and hygroma.

**caprine** adj. pertaining to goats.

**caprine arthritis-encephalitis (CAE)** n. a contagious, viral disease of goats that causes swollen joints, lameness and sometimes neurologic abnormalities. No specific treatment exists, but supportive care and pain relief can improve the animal's quality of life.

**capsule** n. 1. a sheet of tissue that encircles another structure within the body. 2. a dissolvable casing that can be filled with medicine and given by mouth.

**capture myopathy** n. a disorder seen when an animal is severely stressed, struggles or is extremely active during capture. Affected animals are stiff, in pain, may be unable to rise and can die. Gentle handling and limiting stress to the animal is essential to avoiding capture myopathy. Treating severely affected animals can be difficult.

**carapace** n. the external, protective and supportive structure that encircles the top of some animals (e.g., turtles).

**carbamate toxicity** n. poisoning by exposure to carbamate chemicals, which are commonly used as insecticides. Affected animals may exhibit drooling, ocular discharge, urination, diarrhea, muscle tremors, weakness, depression, difficulty breathing and can die. Treatment includes washing the animal if the exposure was topical, treatments to limit absorption from the gastrointestinal tract if the poison was ingested, medications to block or reverse the effects of the poison and supportive care.

**carbohydrate** n. substances such as sugars and starches that are an important source of energy in an animal's diet.

**carbohydrate overload** n. *See* grain overload.

**carbon dioxide (CO$_2$)** n. a gas that is a byproduct of an animal's metabolism and is removed from the blood by the lungs and exhaled.

**carbon monoxide (CO)** n. a gas that when inhaled can reduce the oxygen carrying capacity of an animal's blood and lead to death. Treatment includes oxygen therapy and supportive care.

**carboxyhemoglobin** n. hemoglobin that has been bound to carbon monoxide rather than oxygen in an animal's blood.

**carbuncle** n. an area of multiple, connected abscesses under the skin. Treatment can include drainage, surgical removal of affected tissues and antibiotics.

**carcinogenic** adj. having the tendency to cause cancer - **carcinogen** n.

**carcinoma** n. a type of cancer arising from tissues that tend to line body surfaces or cavities (e.g. skin and the inner lining of the bladder). Carcinomas tend to spread readily to surrounding tissues or throughout the body.

**carcinomatosis** n. a cancer that has spread throughout the body or a body cavity.

**cardiac** adj. pertaining to the heart or the part of the stomach near the esophagus.

**cardiac arrest** n. lack of a heart beat. *See also* cardiopulmonary arrest.

**cardiac catheterization** n. placement of a long, flexible catheter into an artery or vein and threaded into the heart for purposes of taking samples or measurements.

**cardiac compressions** n. the application of rhythmic pressure to the outside of the heart either through the body wall or directly to the heart during surgery. Cardiac compressions can push blood from the heart to the rest of the body when the heart is not pumping on its own. *Also called* cardiac massage.

**cardiac glycosides** n. a class of medications that stimulate strong contractions of the heart muscle and slow the heart rate. Digoxin is a commonly used cardiac glycoside.

**cardiac silhouette** n. the outline of the heart that is visible on a radiograph of the chest. Specific changes in the cardiac silhouette can be seen with different diseases.

**cardiac tamponade** n. the presence of a liquid (e.g., blood) between the heart and its surrounding membrane that puts pressure on the heart preventing its normal function.

**cardinal signs** n. *See* vital signs.

**cardiocentesis** n. insertion of a hollow needle into the space between the heart and its surrounding membrane. Cardiocentesis is often performed to remove an abnormal buildup of fluid that is compromising the ability of the heart to pump blood around the body.

**cardiogenic shock** n. insufficient delivery of oxygen to tissues that is caused by the heart's inability to adequately pump blood throughout the body. Cardiogenic shock can result in organ failure and death. Treatment may include fluid and oxygen therapy, corticosteroids and medications to increase blood pressure and improve heart function.

**cardiomegaly** n. enlargement of the heart.

**cardiomyopathy** n. a disorder with many underlying causes in which the heart muscle loses its ability to contract normally. *See also* dilated cardiomyopathy, hypertrophic cardiomyopathy and restrictive cardiomyopathy.

**cardiopulmonary arrest** n. the lack of a natural, spontaneous heart beat and respiration. Cardiopulmonary arrest may be reversed with the rapid application of CPR, medicines to stimulate the heart and lungs and treatment of any underlying conditions.

**cardiopulmonary resuscitation (CPR)** n. a method of initially treating an animal that is not breathing on its own and does not have a heart beat. The sequence of CPR is to **A)** establish an **airway**, **B) breathe** for the patient and **C)** initiate **cardiac** compressions.

**cardiovascular** adj. pertaining to the heart and the vessels that move blood around the body.

**cardioversion** n. the application of a synchronized electrical shock to the heart in an attempt to treat an arrhythmia and reestablish a normal heart rhythm.

**caries** n. an area of tooth decay that creates a painful hole through the hard, protective covering of a tooth.

**carina** n. 1. the area where the trachea divides into two bronchi. 2. the

bony ridge that runs down the midline of a bird's chest. *Also called* keel.

**carnassial tooth** n. a large chewing and shearing tooth in the upper jaw of dogs and cats.

**carnitine** n. a substance found in some types of food (e.g., meat), the lack of which can cause heart disease in some dogs and may have other physiologic effects.

**carnivore** n. an animal that primarily eats other animals.

**carpal sling** n. a type of bandage that keeps the carpus flexed so that an animal cannot bear weight on the limb.

**carpitis** n. inflammation of the joint capsule and other structures of the carpus, which is most often seen in horses undergoing repeated exercise on a firm surface (e.g., race training). Therapy can include rest and treatments that remove excess fluid from the joint and reduce inflammation. *Also called* popped knee.

**carpus** n. the joint in the front limb between the elbow and the fetlock or foot. - **carpal** adj., **carpi** pl. *Also called* knee in large animals and wrist in small animals.

**carrier** n. an animal that is infected with a contagious, disease-causing organism but does not show any clinical signs of illness. Carriers are a source of infection for other individuals.

**cartilage** n. the tough, somewhat rigid tissue that is found throughout the body, chiefly as a part of joints or as supportive tissue. Cartilage is also the model through which normal bones develop in the fetus and young animal - **cartilaginous** adj.

**caseous lymphadenitis (CL)** n. a disease of sheep, goats and sometimes other species caused by infection with the bacteria *Corynebacterium pseudotuberculosis*. Animals are often infected through wounds that become contaminated with bacteria present in the environment. Affected individuals usually develop abscesses in the skin or lymph nodes, but bacteria can also spread to other organs. Treatment is difficult. Preventative vaccines are available.

**Caslick's procedure** n. the suturing together of the majority of the length of a mare's vulva to prevent air and foreign material from entering her reproductive tract. A Caslick's procedure may be performed to help a mare become and remain pregnant, but the operation must be reversed before she can give birth.

**cast** n. 1. a rigid form that encircles an injured area (e.g., a broken bone) to prevent motion and speed healing. 2. an abnormal tubular object seen in urine under the microscope that is often associated with kidney disease. 3. adj. describes an animal that has become trapped while lying down in a position that prevents it from standing.

**castrate** v. to surgically remove or otherwise disable the testicles. The term can also refer to the removal of the ovaries - **castration** n. *Also called* neuter.

**cat bag** n. a fabric bag into which a cat can be placed and secured to allow examination or minor procedures (e.g., nail trimming and blood collection)

while protecting the people handling a fractious animal.

**cat scratch disease** n. infection of humans by *Bartonella* bacteria often acquired through the bite or scratch of a cat. Affected individuals often develop redness and pustules at the site of the infection and swollen lymph nodes. Medical attention should be sought.

**cataplexy** n. the abnormal, rapid onset of temporary paralysis that is most often the result of a genetic disorder. Medications may decrease the severity of the attacks.

**cataract** n. loss of transparency of an eye's lens, which can develop due to disease (e.g., diabetes mellitus), injury or as an inherited disorder. If cataracts involve the entire lens of both eyes, blindness results. Surgical removal of the cataract can restore vision.

**catarrh** n. inflammation of and discharge from a mucous membrane (e.g., the inside of the nose) - **catarrhal** adj.

**catecholamine** n. one of a group of compounds (e.g., epinephrine and dopamine) that increase heart rate, blood pressure and blood sugar levels. Catecholamines are often secreted in response to fear, excitement or sudden stress.

**cathartic** adj. causing the release of feces from the body, sometimes in the form of diarrhea.

**catheter** n. a tube that can be inserted into part of the body (e.g., a blood vessel). Intravenous catheters can be used to administer fluids, give medication and sometimes take blood samples. Urinary catheters can allow urine to be drained or sampled from the bladder.

**cation** n. a positively charged atom or group of atoms. Common cations in the body include sodium and potassium. *Compare* anion.

**cattle grub** n. *See* warble.

**cauda equina** n. the collection of nerves that leave the back end of the spinal cord and continue through the vertebral canal and into the hind end of the animal.

**cauda equina neuritis** n. a disease of horses in which the nerves that leave the back end of the spinal cord become inflamed for an unknown reason. Other nerves may also be affected. Individuals can develop hind end weakness, difficulty walking, paralysis of the tail, incontinence and abnormal sensations. No effective treatment has been identified. *Also called* polyneuritis equi.

**cauda equina syndrome** n. a disease seen most frequently in dogs in which the nerves that leave the back end of the spinal cord are compressed by a narrowed vertebral canal. Affected individuals often are weak and painful in the hind end, have lameness in one or both hind legs and can be incontinent. Mild cases can respond to rest and medications to control pain and inflammation while more advanced cases may require surgery.

**caudal** adj. pertaining to or directed towards the hind end of an animal. *Compare* cranial.

**cautery** n. a surgical implement that uses heat, cold or chemicals to destroy tissue. Cautery can be used to remove small skin masses or to stop bleeding from small blood vessels - **cauterize** v.

**caval syndrome** n. a disease caused by the presence of heartworms in the vena cava and nearby blood vessels and heart chambers of a severely infested dog. Affected individuals may develop pale and yellow mucous membranes, discolored urine, weakness and difficulty breathing. Treatment is difficult. *See also* heartworm disease. *Also called* vena cava syndrome.

**cecal impaction** n. a type of equine colic in which intestinal materials become stuck within the cecum and surrounding large intestine causing intermittent abdominal pain. In severe or untreated cases, the cecum can rupture, releasing feces into the abdomen. Treatment may include aggressive fluid therapy, pain relief, administration of substances to soften the feces or surgery to remove the impaction.

**cecotrope** n. a specific type of stool that is produced within a rabbit's cecum and eaten by the rabbit to maintain normal digestion. *Also called* night feces.

**cecum** n. a pouch, often referring specifically to a structure located off the large intestine. The cecum may be small and of little significance in some species (e.g., dog) while in others (e.g., horse and rabbit) it is crucial for normal digestion - **cecal** adj.

**celiotomy** n. *See* laparotomy.

**cell** n. the smallest individual living unit able to survive on its own or combine with other cells to form increasingly complex tissues.

**cell mediated immunity** n. resistance to disease that is conferred through the body's T cells. *Compare* humoral immunity.

**cellulitis** n. inflammation that infiltrates a tissue and is often associated with infection. *Compare* abscess.

**Celsius (°C)** n. the system for measuring temperatures in which the freezing point of water is 0° and the boiling point of water is 100°. For a conversion equation to the Fahrenheit scale, see the appendices.

**centesis** n. the insertion of a hollow needle into a structure, usually to withdraw fluid. *Also called* tap.

**central** adj. pertaining to the middle or inner aspect of the body or other structure. *Compare* peripheral.

**central line** n. a long catheter that is inserted into one of the larger veins in the body (e.g., the jugular vein). Central lines can remain in place for a longer period of time and be used for more purposes than can shorter catheters placed into peripheral veins.

**central nervous system (CNS)** n. the brain and spinal cord. *Compare* peripheral nervous system.

**central venous pressure (CVP)** n. a measurement of an animal's blood pressure within the right atrium of the heart. This is a very accurate way to measure blood pressure but is more invasive than other methods.

**centrifuge** n. a device that spins fluids so that heavier objects within the

sample are separated to the bottom of a tube allowing for a more detailed analysis.

**cephalosporin** n. a class of antibiotics used to treat a variety of infections. Cephalexin is a commonly used cephalosporin.

**cerclage wire** n. a metal wire used in the surgical repair of bone fractures to hold pieces of bone closer to one another.

**cere** n. the fleshy connection between a bird's beak and face.

**cerebellar abiotrophy** n. a disorder in which young animals are normal at birth, but as they get older they develop progressively more trouble walking, tremors and other neurologic abnormalities due to destruction of nerves within the cerebellum. No treatment exists.

**cerebellar hypoplasia** n. failure of the fetal cerebellum to develop normally. A viral infection contracted during the pregnancy is often to blame. Affected newborns have difficulty walking, tremors and other neurologic abnormalities but do not tend to get worse as they age. No treatment exists.

**cerebellum** n. the part of an animal's brain that is located towards the back of the head and has a variety of functions, including control over some aspects of voluntary movement - **cerebellar** adj.

**cerebrocortical necrosis** n. a disorder seen in ruminants that is often associated with thiamine deficiency or high levels of sulfur in the diet. Affected individuals can develop blindness, twitching, difficulty walking, bizarre behavior, seizures, other neurologic abnormalities and may die. Treatment includes thiamine supplements and supportive and symptomatic care. *Also called* polioencephalomalacia.

**cerebrospinal fluid (CSF)** n. a liquid transported through and around the brain and spinal cord that is often sampled to help determine the health of the nervous system.

**cerebrovascular accident (CVA)** n. impairment of blood flow through the blood vessels of the brain leading to destruction of brain tissue. Some return of normal function can be seen with time and rehabilitation. *Also called* stroke.

**cerebrum** n. the part of an animal's brain that is located towards the front of the head and is responsible for controlling many of the so called "higher" functions such as reasoning, personality, sight, hearing, smell, touch and some aspects of movement - **cerebral** adj.

**cerumen** n. the waxy material produced by glands in the ear - **ceruminous** adj.

**cervical** adj. pertaining to the neck or to the uterine cervix.

**cervical line lesion** n. *See* feline odontoclastic resorptive lesion.

**cervical lymphadenitis** n. a disease of guinea pigs usually caused by bacteria (e.g., *streptococcus zooepidemicus*) that enter the body through wounds in the mouth. Affected individuals develop swellings around the neck. The infection may also involve other parts of the body. Treatment can include surgical drainage or removal of abscesses and antibiotics. *Also called* lumps or streptococcal lymphadenitis.

**cervical spondylomyelopathy** n. *See* cervical vertebral malformation-malarticulation syndrome.

**cervical stenotic myelopathy** n. a disorder seen most often in young, rapidly growing horses in which the spinal cord in the neck is compressed causing pain and difficulty walking. In early, mild cases, restricting exercise and caloric intake may be sufficient treatment while other individuals require surgery. *Also called* wobbler syndrome.

**cervical vertebral malformation-malarticulation syndrome** n. a disorder seen most often in young, large breed dogs in which the spinal cord in the neck is compressed by abnormalities in the vertebrae and/or intervertebral discs causing pain, difficulty walking and persistent flexion of the neck. Most cases require surgery to correct. *Also called* wobbler syndrome and cervical spondylomyelopathy.

**cervix** n. the narrowed area that divides the uterus from the vagina.

**Cesarian section** n. a surgical incision into the abdomen and uterus to remove a fetus. *Also called* C-section.

**chalazion** n. *See* meibomian gland adenoma.

**cheek pouch** n. large sacs on either side of a hamster's mouth that can be filled with food.

**cheek teeth** n. the premolar and molar teeth.

**cheilitis** n. inflammation of the lips.

**cheiloplasty** n. the surgical reconstruction of a lip.

**chelation therapy** n. the medical use of substances that bind metals (e.g., lead) and aid in their removal from the body.

**chemical restraint** n. the use of sedatives and anesthetics to restrict an animal's movements to allow for its safe handling.

**chemistry panel** n. *See* biochemical profile.

**chemodectoma** n. a tumor of the small organs that respond to changes in carbon dioxide and oxygen content of blood and help regulate breathing and circulation. The tumors are difficult to treat because they are usually attached to the heart or major blood vessels.

**chemosis** n. swelling of the eye's conjunctiva.

**chemotherapy** n. the use of medications to treat illness, often referring specifically to medical treatment aimed at killing or limiting the growth and spread of cancerous cells within the body.

**cherry eye** n. visible protrusion of the gland usually hidden at the base of the third eyelid. A genetic weakness of the structures that hold the gland in place is usually to blame. Surgery is required to replace or sometimes remove the gland. *Also called* third eyelid gland prolapse.

**chest tap** n. *See* thoracocentesis.

**chest tube** n. a hollow tube that is placed through the body wall and into the chest cavity, usually to remove an abnormal accumulation of fluid or air that is restricting the animal's ability to breath. Chest tubes may be sutured and remain in place for an extended period of time. *Also called* thoracostomy tube.

**chestnut** n. 1. the horny tissue located on the inside of a horse's front and rear legs. 2. a horse with a red coat color.

**cheyletiellosis** n. a contagious disease caused by a *Cheyletiella* mite. Affected individuals often have flaky skin and are itchy. Repeated treatment with medications to kill the mites is effective. *Also called* walking dandruff.

**Chiari type malformation** n. a birth defect in which the opening in the skull between the brain and the spinal cord is larger than normal causing compression of portions of the brain. Affected individuals often have difficulty walking, pain and other neurologic abnormalities. Treatment can include corticosteroids and surgery.

**chicken mite** n. *See* red mite.

**chigger** n. a very small insect found in many environments that can bite most mammals and birds causing skin lesions and intense itching. Medications to relieve itching can be helpful. *Also called* harvest mite and red bug.

**chin acne** n. solid or pus-filled bumps on the chin, which are most frequently seen in cats and some breeds of dogs. The condition can be allergy-related and may be treated with antibiotics and/or corticosteroids.

**chip fracture** n. small pieces of bone that are broken off of a larger bone. Chip fractures often affect the joints of horses. Individuals can be lame in the affected leg, in which case they usually require surgery to remove the chip. Rest and medications to control pain and inflammation can also be helpful.

**chiropracty** n. the treatment of disorders through manipulation of the spine. Chiropracty is based on the belief that many diseases are caused by abnormal pressure on nerves due to misalignment of vertebrae.

**chlamydiosis** n. a disease caused by infection with *Chlamydia* (also called *Chlamydophila)* bacteria. Eye infections are common, but *chlamydia* bacteria can also cause other problems, including abortions, pneumonia and arthritis. In many cases, supportive care and antibiotic treatment can be successful. Birds and aborting ruminants can infect humans. *See also* feline chlamydiosis, psittacosis (birds), enzootic abortion (sheep and goats) and transmissible serositis (ruminants and pigs). *Also called* chlamydophilosis.

**chlamydophilosis** n. a disease caused by infection with *Chlamydophila* bacteria (previously called *Chlamydia). See also* chlamydiosis.

**chloride** n. an important electrolyte, the correct levels of which are essential for maintaining normal body function.

**choana** n. one of the paired openings in the back of the mouth that connect the nasal and oral cavities - **choanae** pl., **choanal** adj.

**choanal atresia** n. the failure of normal development of one or both of the openings at the back of the mouth that connect the nasal and oral cavities. Affected newborns have difficulty breathing. Surgery can reconstruct these openings.

**chocolate toxicosis** n. ingestion of sufficient quantities of chocolate to cause illness. Affected individuals can develop vomiting, diarrhea, increased thirst and urination, hyperactivity, difficulty walking, tremors, seizures, irregular heart rhythms and may die. Treatment may include procedures to reduce absorption of the chocolate, medications to treat seizures and irregular heart rhythms, fluid therapy and supportive care.

**choke** n. 1. a condition most frequently seen in horses and ruminants in which a wad of food or other material becomes stuck in the esophagus. Affected animals often appear uncomfortable, have nasal discharge, cough, drool excessively, repeatedly swallow and have abdominal distension (ruminants). Treatment can include procedures to release gas from the rumen, sedation, medications to relax the esophagus, fluid therapy, passage of a tube into the esophagus, antibiotics, medications to help heal any resulting ulcers and modifications to diet. Possible complications include pneumonia and potentially irreversible damage to the esophagus. 2. v. to be unable to breath due to an obstruction of the airways.

**cholangiohepatitis** n. inflammation of the biliary system and liver. Cholangiohepatitis may develop secondary to infections, intestinal or pancreatic disease, immune disorders, parasites and stones within the biliary system. Affected individuals can demonstrate fever, loss of appetite and weight, abdominal pain, vomiting, jaundice and bizarre behavior. Treatment includes antibiotics, supportive care and addressing any underlying conditions.

**cholangitis** n. inflammation of the biliary system. *See also* cholangiohepatitis.

**cholecalciferol toxicity** n. disease caused by ingestion of a mouse and rat poison containing cholecalciferol. Affected individuals develop very high blood calcium levels, which can damage organs (e.g., the kidneys) and lead to loss of energy and appetite, increased thirst and urination, vomiting, constipation and bleeding. Treatment may include procedures to reduce absorption of the poison, fluid therapy and medications that reduce the accumulation of calcium within the body.

**cholecystectomy** n. the surgical removal of the gall bladder.

**cholecystitis** n. inflammation of the gall bladder.

**cholecystogram** n. a radiograph of the gall bladder and bile ducts taken after an animal is injected with a substance that highlights these structures.

**cholelithiasis** n. the presence of stones within the gall bladder, which can block the duct that drains bile. Affected individuals may develop weight loss, abdominal pain and jaundice. Treatment can include surgery to remove the stones, procedures to break the stones into very small pieces, fluid therapy, antibiotics and medications to treat pain and inflammation.

**cholestasis** n. the lack of normal movement of bile from the liver and gall bladder into the intestinal tract.

**cholesterol** n. a substance in the body the levels of which are often measured in blood to aid in the diagnosis of liver, thryoid and other diseases. The worries over high cholesterol levels and heart disease that are prevalent in human medicine are less meaningful in veterinary medicine.

**cholinergic** adj. increasing the activity of the parasympathetic nervous system. Some cholinergic drugs are used to treat bladder and gastrointestinal tract disfunction, glaucoma and other disorders. *Also called* parasympathomimetic.

**cholinesterase** n. *See* acetylcholinesterase.

**chondrodysplasia** n. abnormal growth and development of cartilage - **chondrodysplastic** adj.

**chondrodystrophic breeds** n. breeds of dogs including the Basset Hound and Dachshund that have abnormal cartilage development leading to short, bowed legs and often back problems.

**chondroma** n. a benign tumor arising from cartilage cells. Surgery to remove the tumor is usually curative.

**chondroprotective agent** n. a medicine that can help cartilage heal or protect itself from injury and improve the quality of joint fluid. Glucosamine is a commonly used chondroprotective agent.

**chondrosarcoma** n. a malignant tumor arising from cartilage cells.

Treatment can include surgery, but complete removal is often difficult.

**chordae tendineae** n. attachments between the atrioventricular valves and the heart wall that can rupture, leading to the sudden development of congestive heart failure and often death.

**chorea** n. muscle twitches that can be seen in dogs with canine distemper or other neurologic diseases.

**choriomeningitis** n. inflammation of the membranes that cover the brain and the organ that secretes cerebrospinal fluid.

**chorioptic mange** n. a disease affecting ruminants and horses caused by *Chorioptes* mites that produce skin lesions on the legs and sometimes other regions of the body. The disease is frequently worse in the winter and should be reported to appropriate regulatory agencies when diagnosed in ruminants. Various medications to kill the mites are effective. *Also called* leg mange.

**chorioretinitis** n. inflammation of the retina and surrounding tissues of the eye. Chorioretinitis can indicate disease (e.g., infection) that involves not just the eye but other parts of the body as well.

**chromodacryorrhea** n. the presence of greater than normal amounts of dark colored tears around the eyes. Chromodacryorrhea can indicate blockage of the ducts that normally drain tears away from the eyes or diseases affecting the glands that produce tears.

**chromosome** n. one of the paired structures located within the nucleus of cells that carry genetic information.

**chronic** adj. describes a long-lasting condition. *Compare* acute.

**chronic active hepatitis** n. any inflammatory disease of the liver that is present and continues to affect the organ for an extended period of time (months to years). Chronic active hepatitis is a term that covers several different types of liver disease. *Also called* chronic canine inflammatory hepatic disease.

**chronic bronchitis** n. a disease frequently associated with allergies, which causes a persistent cough that may be worse when pressure is applied to the trachea or with exercise. Treatment can include addressing any underlying allergies and medications to decrease inflammation, dilate airways and thin mucus.

**chronic obstructive pulmonary disease (COPD)** n. *See* recurrent airway obstruction.

**chronic renal failure (CRF)** n. the gradual loss of the kidneys' ability to perform their normal functions, including excreting waste and conserving water. Affected animals often drink and urinate more than normal, stop eating, vomit, lose weight and are lethargic. The underlying cause of the loss of kidney function is often not clear. Treatment can include fluid therapy, special diets and medications to lower blood pressure, decrease gastric acid secretion, raise red blood cell counts and help normalize levels of potassium and phosphorous in the blood. Some cats may be eligible for kidney transplantation. *Compare* acute renal failure.

**chronic superficial keratitis (CSK)** n. inflammation of the surface of the eye caused by dYsfunction of the immune system. Topical treatment with medications that suppress inflammation will usually control the disease. *See also* pannus.

**chronic valvular fibrosis** n. *See* endocardiosis.

**chronic wasting disease (CWD)** n. a contagious disease of deer and elk that is thought to be caused by a prion and leads to progressive neurologic dysfunction in adult animals. Affected individuals can develop weight loss, bizarre behavior, increased thirst and urination, difficulty walking, tremors and will die. No treatment exists.

**chute** n. a piece of equipment used to restrain large animals for examination and minor procedures (e.g., injections).

**chyle** n. a milky fluid formed in the intestines. Chyle transports fats and other materials from the gastrointestinal tract to the rest of the body - **chylous** adj.

**chylothorax** n. the abnormal presence of chyle surrounding the lungs within the chest cavity. Affected animals can have difficulty breathing. Treatment can include diet changes and drainage of the chyle.

**chyme** n. the partially digested mix of food, fluid and digestive secretions that leaves the stomach and enters the small intestines.

**cicatrix** n. a scar.

**cilia** n. 1. an eyelash. 2. a hair-like projection.

**circadian rhythm** n. the natural tendency for many biological process-es (e.g., the sleep/wake cycle) to occur on a 24 hour schedule.

**circling** n. the abnormal tendency to turn continually in one direction while walking, which may be an indication of a disorder affecting certain parts of the brain and/or inner ear.

**circling disease** n. *See* listeriosis.

**circulatory system** n. the heart, blood vessels and lymph channels that move fluids around the body.

**circumanal gland tumor** n. *See* perianal gland tumors.

**circumduction** n. 1. an abnormal, circular swinging of the leg while walking. 2. a circular motion of the eye.

**circumscribed** adj. limited to a particular area.

**cirrhosis** n. the replacement of normal liver tissue with scar tissue, eventually leading to disruption of liver function. Many diseases can cause cirrhosis. Affected individuals may develop loss of appetite, vomiting, jaundice, bizarre behavior, a distended abdomen and can die. Once the scar tissue is formed it cannot be removed. Therapy includes treatment of the underlying condition, medications to limit future scarring of the liver, special diets and supportive and symptomatic care.

**clamp** n. a surgical instrument used to grasp or apply pressure to tissues or other materials.

**claw** n. 1. the hard, curved structure that grows at the end of many species' toes. 2. one of the paired hooves that form the foot of cattle, sheep, goats and pigs.

**clear-eyed blindness** n. *See* elaeophorosis.

**cleft** adj. describes an abnormal split in a structure that should be fused. Often used to describe a congenital defect of the top of the mouth (palate) and/or lip.

**clinical sign** n. an abnormality caused by a disease that is observable in the sick animal. For example, the clinical signs of a dog infected with parvovirus usually include vomiting and diarrhea. *Also called* symptom.

**clitoris** n. an organ consisting of erectile tissue located within the vulva.

**cloaca** n. the end of the urinary, reproductive and gastrointestinal tracts that combine to form a common opening in birds, reptiles and amphibians. *Also called* vent.

**cloacal prolapse** n. eversion of the bird's cloaca, which can be caused by straining associated with intestinal parasites, begging for food or fecal retention. Treatment includes surgery to replace the cloaca and hold it in the normal position and addressing any underlying disorders.

**clonic-tonic seizure** n. a type of seizure during which periods of rigidity alternate with jerking movements.

**cloning** n. the production of an exact, genetic copy of cells, tissues or entire organisms using genetic material taken from an existing animal.

**closed fracture** n. an injury that includes a broken bone but no wounds through the overlying skin. *Also called* simple fracture. *Compare* open fracture.

**closed herd** n. a number of animals that are managed together without additions from outside of the group. Maintaining a closed herd reduces the likelihood of introducing infectious diseases. *Compare* open herd.

**clostridiosis** n. a disease caused by *Clostridia* bacteria and/or their toxins. *Clostridia* can infect wounds, the gastrointestinal tract and other sites, or the toxins alone may be ingested. *See also* bacillary hemoglobinuria, big head, black leg, botulism, enterotoxemia, Black disease, malignant edema and tetanus.

**clot** n. an accumulation of some of the components of liquid blood that form a solid mass and can stop bleeding. Clots may develop in inappropriate situations and block normal blood flow through a vessel.

**clotting factor** n. *See* coagulation factor.

**clotting times** n. a group of tests that evaluate the various processes that must occur for blood to clot normally. Some types of poisons or diseases that cause bleeding can be diagnosed by checking an animal's clotting times. *Also called* coagulation panel.

**club foot** n. an abnormally shaped hoof usually seen in horses with flexural limb deformities or chronic lameness. The affected hoof has an elongated heel, concave toe and a boxy appearance.

**cluster seizures** n. the occurrence of multiple seizures in rapid succession. Cluster seizures are potentially more dangerous for the animal than is an isolated seizure of short duration. *See also* seizure.

**coagulation** n. the process by which blood clots form - **coagulate** v.

**coagulation factor** n. one of a group of proteins that are required for normal blood clotting. Some types of poisons or diseases can disrupt the production of various coagulation factors and lead to bleeding. *Also called* clotting factor.

**coagulation panel** n. *See* clotting times.

**coagulopathy** n. any disorder that disrupts an animal's ability to form normal blood clots, potentially causing excessive bleeding and bruising.

**coaptation** n. the bringing and holding together of the ends of a broken bone so that they are aligned and can heal appropriately. Splints, casts and surgical devices can provide coaptation.

**cobalamin/folate test** n. the measurement of the blood levels of these two substances that are associated with vitamin B. Abnormal levels of cobalamin and/or folate can indicate intestinal or pancreatic disease.

**cocci** n. a type of bacteria that appears round under the microscope. Determining that bacteria are cocci can help diagnose and appropriately treat an infection. *Compare* rod.

**coccidioidomycosis** n. disease caused by infection with the fungus *Coccidioides immitis*. Affected individuals may develop a fever, loss of appetite and weight, a cough, difficulty breathing, skin lesions or other abnormalities depending on where the infection localizes. Treatment with antifungal medications can be suc-

cessful, especially if continued for a long period of time (e.g., 6-12 months). *Also called* valley fever.

**coccidiosis** n. disease caused by infection of the gastrointestinal tract with the one-celled parasite *Coccidia*. Affected individuals are often young and can develop diarrhea, vomiting, weight loss, dehydration and may die in severe cases. Treatment includes medications to kill or suppress the growth of the parasite and supportive care.

**coccidiostat** n. a medication that prevents *Coccidia* parasites from reproducing and allows the affected animal's immune system to eliminate the infection.

**coffin bone** n. the largest bone encased within a horse's hoof.

**Coggins test** n. a laboratory test performed on blood that checks for antibodies against the virus that causes equine infectious anemia.

**cognitive dysfunction** n. a change in the brain of some older dogs that can cause affected individuals to lose their housetraining, wander and interact differently with family members. Medicines may help improve the dog's behavior.

**coital exanthema** n. a contagious, viral disease of horses that is usually spread by sexual contact. Individuals develop lesions affecting the penis or vulva and surrounding skin. Other areas may also be involved. Treatment can include sexual rest and antibiotics to treat or prevent secondary bacterial infections. *Also called* genital horsepox and equine venereal balanitis.

**coitus** n. sexual intercourse. *Also called* copulation.

**cold agglutinin disease** n. a disease in which the immune system produces abnormal antibodies against an individual's red blood cells causing them to clump together. The reaction occurs in regions of low body temperature such as the ears, tail, toes and scrotum causing the skin in these areas to darken and die. The disease may be controlled with drugs that suppress the immune system but is often fatal. *Also called* cold hemagglutinin disease.

**colibacillosis** n. a disease caused by infection with the bacteria *Escherichia coli*. Affected individuals can develop diarrhea, fever, difficulty breathing, swollen and painful joints and many other clinical signs depending on where the infection localizes. If bacteria enter the bloodstream and overwhelm the immune system, septic shock and death can occur. Treatment often includes antibiotics, anti-inflammatories, fluid therapy and supportive care.

**colic** n. abdominal pain, usually referring to pain emanating from the gastrointestinal tract and less frequently the kidneys. Affected individuals often are restless, repeatedly lie down, paw, look at their sides and roll. Colic has a variety of causes. Mild cases often resolve with treatment that can include pain relievers, fluid therapy and passage of a stomach tube to relieve gas or fluid buildup and allow administration of medications. Severe cases that result from twisted or trapped loops of bowel, impacted food stuffs or other causes require surgery and can be fatal.

**coliform** adj. pertaining to certain types of bacteria that emanate from the gastrointestinal tract.

**colisepticemia** n. invasion of the bloodstream with the bacteria *Escherichia coli*. Affected individuals can develop depression, abnormal body temperature, collapse, diarrhea, difficulty breathing, swollen and painful joints or may die suddenly. Treatment includes aggressive use of intravenous fluids and antibiotics and supportive care.

**colitis** n. inflammation of the colon that may be initiated by bacteria, parasites, antibiotic use, autoimmune disease, ingestion of material that irritates the colon and other causes. Affected individuals often develop frequent episodes of straining to defecate and diarrhea, which may contain blood. Treatment can include dewormers, antibiotics, anti-inflammatory medications, fluid therapy and supportive care.

**colitis X** n. a disease of horses with an unknown cause. Affected individuals have often recently undergone a stressful episode (e.g., shipping) and develop profuse, watery diarrhea, dehydration, shock and usually die even with aggressive treatment.

**collagenous nevi** n. *See* focal adnexal dysplasia.

**collapse** n. a state of extreme physiological depression often associated with an individual falling to the ground and being unable to rise for a period of time. Lack of adequate oxygen supply to the brain and other parts of the body is often the cause.

**collapsed lung** n. *See* atelectasis.

**collapsing trachea** n. a disorder most often seen in older, small breed dogs, which causes a "honking" cough. The muscular section of the windpipe becomes weak and sags, narrowing the area through which air can flow. Treatment can include bronchodilators, cough suppressants, anti-inflammatories and antibiotics for secondary bacterial infections.

**collie eye anomaly** n. a genetic disorder of some breeds of dogs (e.g., Collies and Australian Shepherds) in which the eye does not develop normally. Severe cases may produce blindness. There is no treatment.

**collie granuloma** n. *See* canine fibrous histiocytoma.

**collie nose** n. *See* nasal solar dermatitis.

**collimate** v. to narrow a beam of radiation to produce a high quality radiograph and/or reduce the levels of radiation exposure - **collimation** n.

**colloid osmotic pressure (COP)** n. *See* oncotic pressure.

**colloidal fluid** n. a type of intravenous fluid that can be given to animals that require an increased ability to hold fluid within the circulatory system rather than having it diffuse into the tissues of the body. Plasma and hetastarch are commonly used colloidal fluids. *Compare* crystalloid fluid.

**coloboma** n. a defect in a part of the eye (e.g., iris or lens) that is caused by abnormal development and often appears as a hole surrounded by normal tissue.

**colon** n. the part of the gastrointestinal tract between the small intestine and rectum that absorbs water, holds feces and performs other digestive functions - **colonic** adj. *Also called* large intestine.

**colonoscope** n. a tubular instrument consisting of a light source and viewing device that is placed into the colon through the anus allowing the veterinarian to see the inside of this part of the gastrointestinal tract and take tissue samples.

**color dilute alopecia** n. a genetic disorder causing an abnormally light, often grey-blue coat color and sometimes recurrent skin infections, flaky skin and hair loss. Treatment for secondary skin infections and symptomatic therapy can be helpful, but the underlying genetic condition remains. *Also called* color mutant alopecia.

**colorectal** adj. pertaining to the colon and rectum.

**colostomy** n. the surgical creation of an opening from the colon directly to the outside of the body. A colostomy may be performed to allow evacuation of feces while bypassing a diseased or injured colon, rectum or anus.

**colostrum** n. the first milk produced by a female after giving birth, which transfers antibodies and immunity to the newborn. Prompt suckling of colostrum is extremely important in some species (e.g., horses).

**colt** n. a male horse under four years of age.

**coma** n. prolonged loss of consciousness from which an animal cannot be roused. Comas can develop due to brain injury, severe disease or poisons.

**comb** n. the fleshy structure on the top of the head of some birds (e.g., chickens and turkeys).

**combination therapy** n. the simultaneous use of multiple drugs or other therapies to treat a single disease.

**combined immunodeficiency disease (CID)** n. a genetic disease most commonly seen in Arabian foals in which many aspects of the immune system fail to develop normally. Affected newborns initially appear normal, but as the immunity that they received from their mother wanes, they develop multiple infections and die. There is no treatment.

**comedo** n. a dilated skin pore that is plugged with a dark, waxy substance - **comedones** pl.

**commensal** adj. describes organisms that live in a beneficial, close association with each other.

**comminuted fracture** n. a bone that has broken into multiple small pieces.

**commissure** n. a corner that is formed by the junction of two similar structures (e.g., the upper and lower eyelids or lips).

**common calcaneal tendon** n. *See* Achilles tendon.

**communicable** adj. *See* contagious.

**compact bone** n. the hard, outer layer of bones. *Also called* cortical bone. *Compare* cancellous bone.

**companion animal** n. dogs, cats, horses, birds, hamsters, rabbits and other species that people keep primarily for pleasure rather than to produce a marketable commodity.

**compartment syndrome** n. a disorder caused by swelling of muscles often due to injury or intense physical activity. The surrounding connective tissue becomes tight, disrupts blood supply and causes pain and muscle damage. Treatment can include surgery to relieve pressure on the affected muscles.

**compensated** adj. describes a situation in which the body has adjusted to a problem to the point where its clinical effects are minimal.

**complementary medicine** n. *See* alternative medicine.

**complete blood count (CBC)** n. a laboratory test measuring the numbers of red and white blood cells and platelets in a blood sample. Changes in an animal's CBC can help diagnose infections, anemia, some types of cancer, bone marrow disease, immune disorders and many other problems.

**complication** n. a problem that develops in addition to a patient's primary illness or injury making treatment more difficult.

**compound fracture** n. an injury that includes a broken bone and wounds through the overlying skin, thereby increasing the likelihood of infection at the fracture site. *Also called* open fracture. *Compare* closed fracture.

**compress** n. a bundle of material that may be soaked in warm or cold water or medication and applied to an injury to stop bleeding, speed healing or limit swelling.

**computed tomography (CT) scan** n. a method of imaging the body that takes radiographs through multiple sections of a structure and uses a computer to compile the information into detailed pictures.

**concave** adj. describes a structure that is inwardly depressed to form a dish-like surface. *Compare* convex.

**concentrate** n. 1. a mixture of vitamins, minerals, carbohydrates or other nutrients that are combined and added to the diet of an animal that normally eats hay or grass. Concentrates are often fed to increase growth, maintain body weight or supplement a diet that would otherwise be nutritionally deficient. 2. v. to increase the amount of a substance present in a mixture, often by removing fluid.

**conception** n. the fusion of a sperm and egg to form an embryo - **conceive** v. *Also called* fertilization.

**conceptus** n. the embryo or fetus and all of its surrounding membranes.

**concussion** n. a traumatic injury to the brain that can lead to a temporary loss of consciousness.

**conditioning** n. 1. repeated physical exercise used to prepare an athletic animal for competition. 2. behavioral modification or learning that results from repeated episodes of training.

**condyle** n. the rounded, protruding end of a bone involved in a joint - **condylar** adj.

**conformation** n. the physical appearance of an animal, particularly the presence or absence of flaws involving its musculoskeletal system.

**congenital** adj. describing a quality that is present at birth. *Compare* acquired.

**congestion** n. an abnormal buildup of fluid (e.g., blood) within an organ or tissue.

**congestive heart failure (CHF)** n. a possible result of many different types of heart disease. Congestive heart failure occurs when the heart is no longer able to pump blood efficiently, leading to fluid buildup in the lungs, abdomen or elsewhere throughout the body. Affected animals often cough, have difficulty breathing, are weak and tire easily. Treatment can include medications that improve heart function and remove excess fluid.

**conjunctiva** n. the mucous membrane lining the inner surface of the eyelids and parts of the eyeball.

**conjunctival flap** n. a surgery that cuts, moves and sutures a section of conjunctiva over a wound on the surface of the eye. The transposed conjunctiva strengthens the damaged area and promotes healing.

**conjunctival sac** n. the space between the eyelids and the eyeball that is lined with conjunctiva.

**conjunctivitis** n. inflammation of the conjunctiva that may or may not be associated with infection.

**connective tissue** n. the strong tissue found throughout the body that primarily serves to join and support other tissues. Tendons and ligaments are examples of connective tissue.

**conscious proprioception (CP)** n. the ability to sense where parts of the body are placed or have been moved. Loss of conscious proprioception is an indication of neurologic disease or damage.

**conservative** adj. describes a treatment or diagnostic plan in which only a few of the available options are employed. Conservative therapy is often chosen in milder cases of disease or when cost is a concern. *Compare* aggressive.

**consolidated** adj. describes a tissue that has become more dense than normal, specifically lung tissue in which air has been replaced by a fluid (e.g., pus).

**constant rate infusion** n. a method of administering medications resulting in a steady level of the drug being maintained in the body. Often the medicine is added to fluids that continually flow into the bloodstream through an intravenous catheter.

**constipation** n. abnormal retention of feces within the intestinal tract. Affected individuals may strain to defecate, act uncomfortable and lose their appetite. Treatment can include stool softeners, enemas, fluid therapy, medication to enhance muscular contractions of the colon and sometimes the physical removal of feces.

**constrict** v. to narrow or compress - **constriction** n.

**constricted toe syndrome** n. a condition seen in some young birds in which a band of tissue is present over joints in the toes blocking blood circulation. The cause is not known. Treatment may include removing or cutting the tissue band or toe amputation.

**contact allergies** n. an abnormal reaction of the body's immune system to substances that come in contact with body surfaces. Affected animals often develop red, itchy skin and rashes. Treatment can include removing the offending substance from the animal's environment, bathing and medications to reduce itching and inflammation.

**contact irritant dermatitis** n. inflammation of the skin arising from direct contact between the skin and an irritating substance. Removal of the substance from the animal's environment is curative.

**contagious** adj. able to be directly transmitted from one individual to another. *Also called* communicable and transmissible.

**contagious agalactia** n. a contagious disease of sheep and goats caused by infection with *Mycoplasma agalactiae* or other similar bacteria. Affected animals may exhibit fever, abnormal milk production, swollen and painful mammary glands and joints, conjunctivitis or other eye lesions, pneumonia and death. Antibiotics and vaccines can be effective, but often an infected herd is slaughtered to prevent spread of the disease.

**contagious ecthyma** n. *See* orf.

**contagious equine metritis (CEM)** n. a sexually transmitted disease of horses caused by the bacteria *Taylorella equigenitalis*. Newly infected mares develop profuse vaginal discharge and usually fail to become pregnant. Infected stallions and chronically infected mares do not show any clinical signs. Treatment can include topical application of antiseptic solutions.

**contagious pustular dermatitis** n. *See* orf.

**contaminated** adj. describes the unwanted presence of microorganisms or other substances on a surface or within a wound - **contamination** n.

**contour feather** n. the outermost feathers on a bird's body.

**contracted foal syndrome** n. a birth defect seen in horses causing foals to be born with abnormally twisted legs, spines and necks and sometimes with other abnormalities. Mares may have difficulty giving birth. No treatment is possible.

**contracted heel** n. an abnormal shape to a horse's hoof often precipitated by improper trimming or shoeing. Affected individuals have hooves with less frog than normal, an abnormally narrow heel, dry feet and are often lame. Treatment includes moisturizing the foot and corrective trimming and/or shoeing. *Also called* **contracted foot**.

**contracted tendons** n. *See* flexural limb deformity.

**contractility** n. the ability of a tissue or organ to temporarily constrict or shorten as a part of its normal function.

**contracture** n. an abnormal, often permanent tightening or constriction of a tissue that adversely affects its function or the function of surrounding structures.

**contraindicated** adj. describes a therapy or procedure that should not be performed under the circumstances because of the strong likelihood of an unwanted outcome.

**contralateral** adj. on the opposite side. *Compare* ipsilateral.

**contrast** n. the difference in the visual appearance between two structures on a radiograph. A high level of contrast is usually desirable to aid in diagnosis.

**contrast agent** n. a substance that can be injected into the patient to increase the contrast between an organ or tissue of interest and the surrounding tissues.

**contrast radiography** n. the taking of radiographs after injection of a contrast agent into the patient to highlight organs or tissue of interest. *Also called* contrast study.

**controlled drug** n. a medicine the prescribing and dispensing of which is regulated by the government, usually because of its potential to be abused.

**contusion** n. a dark discoloration of a tissue caused by leakage of blood from ruptured vessels, often secondary to a traumatic injury. *Also called* bruise and ecchymosis.

**convalescence** n. the period of time during which an animal is recovering from an illness, injury or surgery.

**convex** adj. describes a structure that is bowed outward to form a rounded surface. *Compare* concave.

**convulsion** n. an involuntary change in muscular activity throughout a large portion of the body. *See also* seizure.

**Coomb's test** n. a laboratory test that can be used to help diagnose immune mediated hemolytic anemia and other disorders.

**coonhound paralysis** n. *See* idiopathic polyradiculoneuritis.

**copper deficiency** n. disease caused by a lack of adequate amounts of copper in the diet. *See also* swayback, postparturient hemoglobinuria and enzootic ataxia.

**copper toxicosis** n. disease caused by ingestion of high levels of copper or the abnormal tendency to accumulate copper within the liver. Affected animals may develop abdominal pain, loss of appetite, diarrhea, weakness, increased thirst, pale or yellow mucous membranes, discolored urine, difficulty breathing and may die. Treatment can include medicines that bind copper and aid in its elimination from the body, dietary changes and supportive care.

**coprophagia** n. the tendency to eat feces, which is normal in some species (e.g., rabbits and foals) and a bad habit in others (e.g., dogs).

**copulation** n. sexual intercourse. *Also called* coitus.

**copulatory plug** n. a solid clump of the male's ejaculate that falls from the female's vagina several hours after mating in some species (e.g., guinea pigs and chinchillas).

**cor pulmonale** n. heart failure affecting primarily the right side of the heart often due to the presence of heartworms or lung disease. Affected individuals can become weak, accumulate fluid within the abdomen or chest cavity, cough and have difficulty breathing. Treatment is aimed at the underlying disease but can also include removal of abnormal fluid accumulations.

**cording up** n. *See* exertional rhabdomyolysis.

**core biopsy** n. a method of acquiring a sample of tissue (e.g., bone marrow) that retains some of its architecture, sometimes providing more information than a fine needle aspirate that removes only loose cells.

**corn** n. a hardened and painful area on the surface of the foot. Surgical removal, treatment for secondary infections and addressing any underlying causes (e.g., poorly fitting horseshoes) can be curative.

**cornea** n. the clear tissue that encloses the front of the eye and allows light to enter - **corneal** adj.

**corneal dystrophy** n. any of several diseases, often with a genetic component, that can lead to an animal having a cornea that is predisposed to developing opaque areas, inflammation and/or ulcers. Topical treatment with medicines to decrease swelling or inflammation and heal ulcers can control the condition.

**corneal edema** n. retention of fluid within the cornea that leads to an abnormal, white discoloration. Corneal edema can develop for many reasons, including wounds, infections and immune disorders. Treatment is aimed at any underlying causes and can also involve topical medications that remove fluid from the cornea.

**corneal reflex** n. the natural tendency to blink when the cornea is touched.

**corneal sequestrum** n. an abnormal dark mass on the surface of the cornea most frequently seen in cats that have chronic corneal inflammation and ulcers. The sequestrum can be removed, but the underlying disorder must also be addressed to prevent its return.

**corneal stromal abscess** n. an abscess that develops within the cornea, which is most often seen in horses recovering from a corneal ulcer. Treatment can include antibacterial, antifungal and anti-inflammatory medicines and surgery.

**corneal ulcer** n. the loss of layers of corneal tissue due to trauma, abnormal anatomy, poor tear production or genetics. Corneal ulcers cause a red, painful eye that often drains a clear fluid, mucus or pus. Some cases can be treated with topical antibiotics and pain relief while more severe ulcers may also require oral antibiotics and surgery to prevent loss of the eye. Any underlying problems must be addressed to prevent the rapid return of the ulcer.

**corneal vascularization** n. the abnormal presence of blood vessels within the cornea. Corneal vascularization can occur because of chronic injury, irritation or other problems affecting the cornea.

**cornification** n. a toughening or hardening of the surface of a tissue - **cornified** adj.

**coronary artery** n. one of the vessels that carries blood to the muscles of the heart.

**coronary band** n. the fleshy ring around the top of a hoof. *Also called* coronet.

**coronavirus** n. one of a group of related viruses that can cause various diseases depending on the specific virus and animal infected. *See also* canine and feline corona virus and feline infectious peritonitis.

**corpora nigra** n. the normal structures that look like masses along the edge of a horse's or ruminant's irises. *Also called* granula iridica.

**corpus luteum** n. an ovarian structure that develops after ovulation and secretes progesterone - **luteal** adj.

**corrected reticulocyte count** n. a measurement of the number of immature red blood cells in circulation that takes into account the total red blood cell count. A high corrected reticulocyte count is a good indication of bone marrow response to anemia.

**corrosive** adj. describes the tendency of a substance to irritate and/or damage tissue that it contacts.

**cortex** n. the outer layer of an organ or tissue - **cortical** adj. *Compare* medulla.

**cortical bone** n. *See* compact bone.

**corticosteroid** n. substances made by the adrenal glands or a manufactured drug, both of which affect many body functions (e.g., stress, inflammation and fluid and electrolyte balance). The term corticosteroid often refers to drugs used to decrease inflammation or to treat autoimmune disease and some types of cancer. Prednisone is a commonly used corticosteroid. *See also* glucocorticoid and mineralocorticoid.

**corticosterone** n. a hormone released by the adrenal glands with glucocorticoid and mineralocorticoid functions.

**corticotropin** n. *See* adrenocorticotrophic hormone.

**cortisol** n. a hormone produced by the adrenal glands with glucocorticoid activity. Also refers to a synthetically manufactured drug (i.e., hydrocortisone) often used to decrease inflammation.

**cortisol:creatinine ratio** n. a urine test that aids in the diagnosis of Cushing's disease.

**coryza** n. profuse discharge from the nose. *See also* infectious coryza.

**costal** adj. pertaining to the rib or ribs.

**costochondral** adj. pertaining to the rib and its associated cartilage.

**cough** n. a sudden forcing of air out of the lungs and through the mouth often to clear foreign material from within the airways. Coughing can be a sign of disease affecting the lungs or heart.

**counterconditioning** n. a method of behavioral modification that involves teaching an animal to perform an activity that prevents its previous, undesirable response to a stimulus. For example, a dog can be taught to sit and relax when people arrive at the front door so that it will no longer jump up on visitors.

**coupage** n. the repeated striking of the chest wall with a cupped hand to loosen respiratory secretions and encourage the animal to cough them up.

**cover** v. to breed.

**cow hocked** adj. describes a conformational flaw of horses and dogs in which the hocks are rotated inward when the animal is viewed from the rear.

**cow kick** v. to kick forward with a hind leg.

**coxofemoral joint** n. the connecting joint between the rear leg and the pelvis. Commonly called the hip.

**cracked heel** n. *See* scratches.

**crackles** n. abnormal sounds heard when listening to the lungs with a stethoscope that often indicate the presence of excess fluid within lung tissue.

**cranial** adj. pertaining to or directed towards the front end of an animal. *Compare* caudal.

**cranial cruciate ligament rupture** n. damage to the cranial cruciate ligament of the knee that results in joint instability and pain. Cranial cruciate ligament ruptures may occur due to traumatic injury (often a twisting motion), obesity, poor conformation and/or genetics. If the rupture is complete, surgery often is necessary to stabilize the joint and prevent the rapid development of severe osteoarthritis. Other cases may respond adequately to rest, anti-inflammatories, physical therapy and weight loss.

**cranial nerves** n. the peripheral nerves that leave the brain without entering the spinal cord. The health of cranial nerves and the region of the brain to which they are connected often can be determined by examination of the eyes, ears, mouth and the muscles of the face.

**craniomandibular osteopathy (CMO)** n. a suspected genetic disorder of growing dogs that causes abnormal bone growth most often affecting the lower jaw and areas of the skull. Affected individuals can be in pain and develop a fever, poor appetite and weight loss. Treatment involves pain relief and supportive care until the period of bone growth and discomfort ends.

**cranioschisis** n. an opening in the top of the head due to abnormal development of the skull.

**craniotomy** n. a surgical incision through the skull.

**cranium** n. the skull.

**crash cart** n. a moveable storage space for the supplies and medications necessary for the emergency treatment of an animal in critical condition.

**crate training** n. the use of a cage to aid in the housetraining of dogs. Crate training takes advantage of the dog's natural inhibition to urinate and defecate where it sleeps, which allows people to be present when the animal eliminates and to praise or scold appropriately.

**creatine kinase (CK)** n. a protein measured in blood samples the levels of which rise with muscle damage. *Also called* creatinine phosphokinase (CPK).

**creatinine** n. a substance usually measured in the blood the levels of which rise with kidney disease. Creatinine may also be measured in the urine to help determine the significance of other substances (e.g., protein) excreted by the kidneys.

**creatinine clearance test** n. a laboratory test that assesses kidney function by measuring the organs' ability to eliminate creatinine from the body.

**creep ration** n. a supplemental food that is available only to young animals. Often a barrier is erected that allows the young to eat the food but prevents access by larger animals.

**crepitus** n. an abnormal, crackling feeling when a part of the body is palpated. The term can be used to describe the feeling of the edges of broken bones rubbing together, the roughness of a joint affected by osteoarthritis or the feel of air under the surface of the skin.

**cribbing** n. an undesirable habit of horses during which they grasp an object with their teeth, flex their neck and swallow air. Boredom or anxiety is thought to initiate many cases of cribbing, and the resulting release of natural endorphins promotes its continuation. Treatment can include devices that make it uncomfortable for the horse to crib, relieving boredom, dietary changes, medications to block the effect of endorphins and surgery. *Also called* windsucking.

**cricopharyngeal achalasia** n. a disorder of dogs caused by the inability of a muscle in the neck to relax and allow normal swallowing. Affected individuals gag, regurgitate and can develop aspiration pneumonia. Surgery to cut the cricopharyngeal muscle can be curative.

**critical care** n. veterinary medicine that is focused on the needs of very sick or severely injured animals.

**crop** n. a dilated area of the esophagus in birds that serves as a site for storage and initial digestion of food. 2. v. to surgically remove a portion of an animal's ear, often for reasons of appearance only.

**crop burn** n. an injury to a bird's crop caused by hand-feeding formulas that are too hot. Treatment can include antibacterial and antifungal medications, surgery and supportive care.

**crop impaction** n. distension of a bird's crop with food or foreign material that is unable to move through the digestive tract. Treatment can include fluid therapy, manual removal of the material from the crop, antibiotic and antifungal medications and surgery.

**crop mycosis** n. infection of a bird's crop with the fungus *Candida albicans* that may be due to crop impaction, antibiotic use, inappropriate feeding or unsanitary conditions. Treatment can include addressing any underlying problems and antifungal medications. *Also called* thrush, candidiasis and sour crop.

**crop stasis** n. abnormally slow movement of food through a bird's crop and into the rest of the digestive tract. *See also* crop impaction.

**cross match** n. a laboratory test used to determine whether a blood transfusion is appropriate for a particular patient and to prevent transfusion reactions.

**crossed extensor reflex** n. an abnormal reaction to flexion of a hind leg that causes extension of the opposite hind leg and indicates the presence of neurologic disease.

**crown** n. the portion of a tooth that extends beyond the gums and into the oral cavity.

**crutching** n. shearing of wool from a sheep's hind end to prevent maggot infestations.

**cryoepilation** n. the use of extreme cold to destroy hair follicles and prevent unwanted hair growth.

**cryosurgery** n. the use of extreme cold to destroy and remove unwanted tissue (e.g., small, benign skin tumors).

**cryptococcosis** n. a disease caused by the fungus *Cryptococcus neoformans*. Affected individuals can develop infections of the respiratory tract, nervous system, eyes, skin or other organs and have clinical signs that differ with the site of infection. Cats are prone to develop infections of the nasal cavity, which cause sneezing, nasal discharge and swellings around the bridge of the nose. Treatment with antifungal medications is often successful.

**cryptorchid** adj. describes a male animal in which both testicles are not present in the scrotum. One or both malpositioned testicles can be in the abdomen or inguinal area. *Also called* ridgling and rig. *Compare* anorchid and monorchid.

**cryptosporidiosis** n. disease caused by infection of the gastrointestinal tract with the microscopic parasite *Cryptosporidium parvum*. Calves are most commonly affected, but many species, including humans, are susceptible. Diarrhea is the most common clinical sign and usually resolves with supportive care unless the patient is immunocompromised. There is no specific treatment for the parasite.

**crystalloid fluid** n. the most commonly used type of intravenous fluid given to animals that require rehydration, diuresis or circulatory support. Lactated Ringers solution is a commonly used crystalloid fluid. *Compare* colloidal fluid.

**crystalluria** n. the presence of crystals within the urine. Crystals come in several different forms and may be associated with infection, urinary stones, antifreeze poisoning, organ dysfunction, genetic disease or can be normal in some species or situations.

**cud** n. the wad of food that is regurgitated and rechewed by ruminants.

***Culicoides* hypersensitivity** n. a reaction to the bite of *Culicoides* midges, very small flying insects often active during warm months in damp areas. Affected animals can become agitated due to the presence of the insects and develop itchy skin lesions when bitten. Various insecticides and repellents can be helpful. *Also called* sweet, summer and Queensland itch.

**cull** v. to remove an individual from the herd.

**culture** v. to grow microorganisms or other cells in the lab.

**culture and sensitivity** n. the growth and identification of microorganisms in the lab derived from a sample (e.g., blood, urine or pus) taken from a patient. Several antibiotics are then applied to the culture to determine which is most effective.

**curb** n. a thickening and enlargement of the area on the back of a horse's hind leg below the hock due to ligament strain. Acute cases can be painful and respond to treatment including rest, cold packs and anti-inflammatories. Chronic cases are usually no longer painful and require no treatment.

**cure** v. to successfully treat a disease or injury and eliminate its effects - **curative** adj.

**curettage** n. the scraping and removal of unwanted material from a body surface or cavity.

**curette** n. an instrument used to scrape and remove unwanted material from a body surface or cavity.

**Cushing's disease** n. a disease in which the body over-secretes adrenal hormones, most notably cortisol. Affected animals often have ravenous appetites, drink and urinate more than normal, have poor quality coats and are "pot-bellied" in appearance. Horses may grow long, thick coats that fail to shed normally and sweat excessively. Cushing's disease develops because of pituitary or adrenal tumors or overuse of corticosteroid drugs. Treatment can include drugs that suppress adrenal function or help control clinical signs, surgery for adrenal tumors, radiation therapy for large pituitary tumors and slowly weaning the animal off corticosteroid drugs. *Also called* hyperadrenocorticism.

**cutaneous** adj. pertaining to the skin.

**cutaneous asthenia** n. *See* hyperelastosis cutis.

**cutaneous ichthyoses** n. a genetic disease causing animals to have skin that can flake extensively or peel off in large sheets. The condition can be improved but not cured through the use of medicated shampoos and other topical treatments.

**cutaneous mucinosis** n. a genetic disease of Shar-Pei dogs that leads to the development of skin that contains mucus pockets and is excessively folded, even for this breed. Treatment can include anti-inflammatories and supportive care.

**cuterebriasis** n. *See* warble.

**cuticle** n. 1. the fleshy area between the skin and the hoof or nail. 2. the outermost surface of hair, fur or wool.

**cyanide poisoning** n. ingestion of sufficient quantities of cyanide to cause disease. Cases can involve livestock that eat plants containing high levels of cyanide or poisoning with chemicals containing the substance. Affected individuals become excited, breath rapidly and with difficulty, drool, tear, urinate, defecate, vomit, develop muscle tremors and may quickly die. Treatment can include medicines that reverse the effects of cyanide, oxygen therapy and supportive care.

**cyanobacteria** n. a group of bacteria found in warm, often stagnant water that when ingested in large enough amounts cause algal poisoning. *Also called* blue-green algae.

**cyanocobalamine** n. *See* vitamin $B_{12}$.

**cyanosis** n. a blue tinge to the mucous membranes and the skin that is seen when blood oxygen levels are very low - **cyanotic** adj.

**cyclic hematopoiesis** n. a genetic disease of gray-colored Collies that causes intermittent, low white blood cell counts, recurrent infections and bleeding. The animals usually die at a young age. *Also called* Gray Collie Syndrome and cyclic neutropenia.

**cyclopia** n. a birth defect in which only one eye develops, sometimes in association with other facial deformities.

**cylindruria** n. the abnormal presence of casts within a urine sample, which usually indicates kidney disease.

**cyst** n. a hollow structure that is filled with a liquid or other substance.

**cystadenoma** n. a cystic tumor that is most often associated with the liver, kidneys or ovaries. In some cases, surgical removal can be curative. *See also* dermatofibrosis.

**cystectomy** n. the surgical removal of a cyst or the urinary bladder.

**cystic** adj. pertaining to a cyst or the urinary bladder.

**cystic calculus** n. *See* bladder stone.

**cystic ovaries** n. the abnormal presence of fluid-filled structures on the ovary, which disrupt the normal estrous cycle. Affected individuals may fail to come into heat, have frequent, abnormal heat cycles, develop masculine behavior and have vaginal discharge. Treatment can include manual rupture of the cyst or hormone therapy. *See also* follicular cysts and luteal cysts.

**cystine urolith** n. a type of bladder stone seen in dogs that have a genetic tendency to excrete more cystine than normal into their urine. The stones must be physically removed through surgery or urohydropulsion, but medications and dietary changes can help prevent their return.

**cystitis** n. inflammation of the urinary bladder, which is often associated with an infection. *See also* urinary tract infection.

**cystocentesis** n. insertion of a hollow needle into the urinary bladder, usually to withdraw a sample of urine for analysis.

**cystogram** n. a radiograph that is taken after the urinary bladder has been filled with a contrast agent. Cystograms are performed when a plain radiograph cannot reveal a suspected abnormality.

**cystoscope** n. a tubular instrument including a light source and a viewing device that is placed into the urinary bladder through the urethra allowing the veterinarian to see the inside of the structures and take tissue samples.

**cystotomy** n. a surgical incision into the urinary bladder.

**cystourethrogram** n. a radiograph that is taken of the urinary bladder and urethra after administration of a contrast agent that highlights these structures.

**cytauxzoonosis** n. disease caused by infection with *Cytauxzoon* parasites usually transmitted by tick bites. Cats can contract *Cytauxzoon felis*, which causes fever or low body temperature, weakness, depression, difficulty breathing, pale or yellow mucous membranes and usually death. Treatment is difficult.

**cytology** n. the science and study of cells, often describing the microscopic examination of a sample taken from a patient and applied to a glass slide.

**cytoplasm** n. the part of a cell that surrounds the nucleus and contains many of the structures and substances necessary for the cell's metabolism - **cytoplasmic** adj.

**cytotoxic** adj. having a tendency to damage cells.


# D

**dacryocystitis** n. inflammation of the sac that collects tears as they drain from the eye. The pathway for drainage of tears can become blocked leading to pooling of tears and inflammation. Treatment can include flushing the pathway to remove debris and antibiotics.

**dam** n. a female parent.

**dancing Doberman disease** n. a disorder with an unknown cause seen in Doberman Pinschers. Affected individuals intermittently flex one or both hind legs when standing. There is no treatment, but the condition rarely becomes severe enough to adversely affect the dog's quality of life.

**dazzle reflex** n. the normal, involuntary reaction to having a bright light shone into the eyes, which can consist of blinking, retraction of the eye, protrusion of the third eyelid and moving the head away from the light source. A normal dazzle reflex is a good indication that some degree of sight is present.

**dead space** n. a pocket that is formed in tissue by a wound or surgical incision. The formation of dead space can predispose an animal to developing fluid-filled areas that delay healing.

**deaf** adj. lacking the sense of hearing. Deafness can occur because of disorders affecting the ear or the nerves and parts of the brain that receive input from the ear - **deafness** n.

**debark** v. to remove a dog's vocal cords to reduce the sounds associated with barking.

**debeak** v. to surgically remove the front part of a bird's beak to reduce the damage that the animals can inflict on one another when housed in close confinement.

**debilitated** adj. describes the general state of an animal that is weak or otherwise adversely affected by illness or injury.

**debride** v. to remove foreign material and diseased or damaged tissue from a wound to prevent or treat infection and promote healing.

**decerebrate rigidity** n. an abnormal body position consisting of rigid extension of the legs and the head being arched back. Decerebrate rigidity indicates severe brain damage.

**deciduous teeth** n. the first teeth that erupt in a young animal, which should later be replaced by the permanent, adult teeth. *Also called* milk teeth and primary teeth.

**declawing** n. *See* onychectomy.

**decompensated** adj. describes the situation in which the body is no longer able to adjust to a problem, and clinical signs that were previously absent are now developing.

**decompress** v. to relieve pressure, often by removing an abnormal buildup of fluid or gas - **decompression** n.

**decongestant** n. a medicine that reduces the production of fluid and mucus in the respiratory tract, especially the nasal cavities.

**decontaminate** v. to remove unwanted microorganisms or other substances from a surface or wound.

**decubital ulcer** n. injury and loss of skin over a protruding part of the body. Decubital ulcers often develop when an animal lies in one position for an extended period of time. Treatment can include frequently changing an animal's body position, padding the animal's environment, antibiotics for secondary infections and surgery. *Also called* pressure sore.

**deep** adj. located towards the center of the body or other structure. *Compare* superficial.

**deep pain** n. a normal reaction to a painful stimulus, which is often tested by vigorously squeezing a clamp placed on a toe. The absence of deep pain indicates more severe damage to the spinal cord and a poorer prognosis than if deep pain is present.

**deer tick** n. a small tick that can attach to animals and people and transmit Lyme disease.

**defecate** v. to pass feces from the body - **defecation** n.

**defibrillation** n. the emergency

application of an electrical shock to the heart in an attempt to reestablish a normal heart rhythm.

**deficiency** n. the lack of sufficient quantities of a substance in the diet or body, which can lead to illness.

**definitive diagnosis** n. the determination of the exact disease or condition that is the cause of an animal's clinical signs.

**degeneration** n. changes that occur in cells, tissues and organs and lead to a progressive loss of function. Degeneration can occur because of aging or disease - **degenerative** adj.

**degenerative disk disease (DDD)** n. *See* intervertebral disk disease.

**degenerative joint disease (DJD)** n. *See* osteoarthritis.

**degenerative myelopathy** n. a deterioration of the spinal cord seen most commonly in German Shepherds. Affected individuals have progressively more hind leg weakness, difficulty walking and eventually become paralyzed. The cause of the disorder is unknown, and treatment is generally unrewarding.

**degenerative valve disease** n. *See* endocardiosis.

**degloving injury** n. a wound that is characterized by skin being peeled from its attachments to the body.

**deglutition** n. the act of swallowing.

**dehiscence** n. an unwanted splitting open of a wound or incision that was previously closed - **dehisce** v.

**dehorning** n. the removal of an animal's horns, which is usually performed to prevent injury to people or other animals.

**dehydration** n. a lower than normal amount of water within the body. Dehydration can occur because of increased loss of fluid from the body (e.g., vomiting, diarrhea, increased urination or sweating) or because of inadequate water intake. Treatment involves fluid therapy and addressing any underlying disorders.

**dementia** n. a progressive loss of mental ability that is often associated with aging or diseases affecting the brain. Affected animals can demonstrate a loss of training and changes in their personality or behavior.

**demodicosis** n. a disease caused by *Demodex* mites, which are normally found in the skin in small numbers but may overgrow and cause hair loss and promote skin infections, especially in young or immunosuppressed animals. Treatment can include medications to kill the mite and antibiotics. *Also called* demodectic mange and follicular mange.

**demyelinating disease** n. any of a number of disorders in which myelin, the protective coating of nerves, degenerates over time. Affected individuals develop tremors that are especially apparent when the animal is excited or eating, weakness and difficulty walking. There is no treatment.

**dendritic ulcer** n. an ulcer most commonly seen affecting the eyes of cats infected with a herpesvirus (i.e., feline viral rhinotracheitis). The ulcer is difficult to see but causes pain and drainage from the eye. Treatment can include medicines that help the body suppress the virus and antibiotics if a secondary bacterial infection develops.

**denervation** n. loss of the normal nerve supply to a tissue.

**dens** n. a bony projection from the front of the second vertebrae in the neck. In some animals, the dens does not develop normally, which can lead to spinal instability, neck pain, weakness and paralysis. *See also* atlantoaxial subluxation.

**dental** adj. pertaining to the teeth.

**dental elevator** n. an instrument used to loosen teeth prior to their removal by disrupting the ligaments that connect teeth to their sockets within the jaw.

**dental impaction** n. failure of a tooth to erupt through the gums and into its normal position.

**dental prophylaxis** n. removal of plaque and tartar from all surfaces of the teeth, polishing, a thorough oral exam and sometimes other procedures all aimed at preventing the development or worsening of dental disease. *Also called* dental cleaning.

**dental star** n. dark marks on the chewing surface of a horse's incisors that change with tooth wear and can be used to estimate the age of the individual.

**dentigerous cyst** n. a swelling in the jaw that is most frequently seen in young horses and ruminants and contains portions of a tooth that has developed abnormally. Surgical removal is curative.

**dentin** n. the hard substance that lies between the pulp cavity and outerlayers of a tooth. *Also called* dentine.

**dentition** n. the number, type and alignment of erupted teeth within the mouth of an individual animal.

**deoxyribonucleic acid (DNA)** n. the genetic material that is located primarily within the chromosomes of cells and is the blueprint for the development, maintenance and reproduction of an organism.

**dependent** adj. pertaining to the lower parts of the body or another structure. For example, dependent edema is fluid that accumulates in the legs or under the jaw or belly because of the effects of gravity.

**depigmentation** n. a fading of normal coloration that was previously present.

**depraved appetite** n. *See* pica.

**depression** n. 1. a state of mind leading to dullness and a reduced level of activity and interest in the surrounding environment. Other emotional signs of depression as are described in human psychology are difficult to assess in animals. 2. a state that is physically or functionally lower than normal.

**dermal** adj. pertaining to the skin.

**dermatitis** n. inflammation of the skin.

**dermatofibrosarcoma** n. *See* malignant fibrous histiocytoma.

**dermatofibrosis** n. a genetic disease most frequently seen in German Shepherds. Affected individuals develop multiple firm skin masses and sometimes cancer of the kidneys, uterus and vagina. *Also called* nodular dermatofibrosis.

**dermatophilosis** n. a disease caused by infection of the skin with the bacteria *Dermatophilus congolensis*. Infection is promoted by any factor that disrupts the normal, protective characteristics of skin (e.g., prolonged dampness). Lesions often consist of a crust or scab with a matted tuft of hair that easily pulls out of the skin. Treatment can include improving environmental conditions, antibiotics and medicated shampoos or dips. *Also called* streptothricosis, lumpy wool, rain rot and strawberry footrot.

**dermatophyte test media (DTM)** n. a type of agar that aids in the growth and identification of the fungus that causes ringworm.

**dermatophytosis** n. *See* ringworm.

**dermatosis** n. any disorder that affects the skin.

**dermatosparaxis** n. *See* hyperelastosis cutis.

**dermis** n. the portion of the skin that lies under the epidermis and contains blood vessels, hair follicles, nerves and other structures.

**dermoid cyst** n. *See* teratoma.

**dermoid sinus** n. a mass in the skin that is most frequently seen in Rhodesian Ridgebacks. Abnormal skin development leads to these cavities that contain hair, skin cells and other material. Some dermoid sinuses may connect to deeper structures, including the spinal canal in which case

treatment can be difficult. Otherwise, surgical removal is curative. *Also called* pilonidal sinus.

**descemetocele** n. a deep, corneal ulcer or wound that has penetrated all of the way down to Descemet's membrane, the last intact structure before the eye perforates. Treatment can include antibacterial and/or antifungal medications, pain relief and surgery to support the eye as it heals.

**Descemet's membrane** n. the inner layer of the cornea.

**descenting** n. a surgery performed to remove glands (e.g., those on the top of the head of a male goat) that produce an odor unpleasant to people.

**desensitization** n. 1. a method of behavioral modification that involves teaching an animal to relax while gradually exposing it to increasing levels of a stimulus that previously provoked an unwanted reaction. 2. repeatedly administering increasing doses of an allergen to an animal to reduce its immune response.

**desiccate** v. to dry out.

**desmitis** n. inflammation of a ligament.

**desmoid** n. a tumor arising from fibrous connective tissue associated with muscles and tendons. Desmoids do not spread to other parts of the body but can invade local tissues and be difficult to remove completely. *Also called* fibromatosis.

**desmotomy** n. the surgical cutting of a ligament.

**detail** n. the sharpness and clarity of different structures visible on a radiograph.

**detrusor atony** n. weakness of the muscle responsible for squeezing urine from the bladder. Overdistention of the bladder is a common cause of detrusor atony. Treatment can include keeping the bladder empty and medications that stimulate muscular contractions in the bladder.

**developmental orthopedic disease** n. one of several disorders of cartilage and bone maturation seen in young animals. *See also* osteochondrosis, panosteitis, physitis, angular limb deformity, flexural limb deformity, craniomandibular osteopathy, hypertrophic osteodystrophy and multiple cartilaginous exostoses.

**devitalized** adj. lacking adequate blood supply or other support necessary for tissue function and survival.

**dew claw** n. the nail and its supporting structures that is present on the inner aspect of the front or rear legs of some animals. The dew claw does not come into contact with the ground.

**dewlap** n. a loose flap of skin that is present under the jaw and neck of some breeds of animals.

**deworming** n. the administration of a medicine that kills or otherwise aids in the elimination of parasites from the body.

**dexamethasone suppression test** n. a laboratory test that measures the body's response to the administration of dexamethasone and is often used to help diagnose Cushing's disease. *See*

*also* high dose dexamethasone suppression test and low dose dexamethasone suppression test.

**dextrose** n. *See* glucose.

**diabetes insipidus** n. in central diabetes insipidus (CDI), the pituitary gland does not produce adequate amounts of antidiuretic hormone. Nephrogenic diabetes insipidus (NDI) develops when the kidneys do not respond normally to antidiuretic hormone. In either case, the body cannot resorb water from urine before it is eliminated from the body causing excessive drinking and urination. Treatment can include administration of synthetic antidiuretic hormone (CDI), medications to reduce urine output (NDI) and diet changes.

**diabetes mellitus** n. a lack of normal production or response to insulin that leads to high blood sugar concentrations. Type I diabetics do not manufacture enough insulin and are said to be insulin dependent. Type II diabetics do not respond to what should be an adequate amount of insulin secreted by the pancreas and are said to be non insulin dependent or insulin resistant. Affected individuals can drink and urinate excessively, have an excessive appetite, lose weight, develop cataracts, become weak and contract infections. Treatment may include dietary changes, weight loss, insulin injections and oral medications that can lower blood sugar levels.

**diabetic ketoacidosis (DKA)** n. a complication of severe and uncontrolled diabetes mellitus that is caused by a buildup of ketones in the body and may lead to dehydration, electrolyte disturbances and death. Treatment includes fluid therapy, electrolyte supplementation and insulin injections. *See also* diabetes mellitus.

**diabetic neuropathy** n. a disorder of nerves seen in diabetic animals. Affected individuals can walk with the back of their lower hind leg on the ground and are very sensitive to touch and pain. Some cases will resolve when their diabetes is treated and controlled.

**diabetic retinopathy** n. changes in the retina of diabetic animals, which can lead to blindness.

**diagnosis** n. a determination of which disease or condition is the cause of an animal's clinical signs. Arriving at a diagnosis can be difficult if the individual has vague symptoms or if laboratory testing is inconclusive - **diagnostic** adj., **diagnose** v.

**diagnostic imaging** n. procedures such as ultrasonography, radiography, CT scans and MRIs that allow visualization of structures within the body.

**dialysis** n. a procedure during which unwanted substances (e.g., toxins or waste products) are removed from the body. *See also* peritoneal dialysis and hemodialysis.

**diaphragm** n. the muscular structure that separates the chest cavity from the abdomen and helps move air in and out of the lungs - **diaphragmatic** adj.

**diaphragmatic flutter** n. *See* synchronous diaphragmatic flutter.

**diaphragmatic hernia** n. an abnormal opening in the diaphragm that allows abdominal contents to enter the chest cavity. Diaphragmatic hernias are caused by injury or birth defects. Affected individuals can have difficulty breathing, pain and gastrointestinal problems. Treatment involves surgery to replace the abdominal contents and repair the hernia.

**diaphysis** n. the shaft located in the middle of a long bone.

**diarrhea** n. abnormally soft or watery stool often associated with frequent or large bowel movements. Diarrhea has many causes and can lead to dehydration and electrolyte disturbances.

**diastole** n. the period of time during which the heart is relaxed and filling with blood - **diastolic** adj. *Compare* systole.

**dicumarol poisoning** n. a disease caused by the ingestion of sufficient quantities of spoiled sweet clover to produce bleeding. Affected animals may be lame, bleed from the nose or mouth, bruise easily, have blood in their feces or die suddenly. Treatment can include blood transfusions and vitamin K supplements. *Also called* sweet clover poisoning.

**diestrus** n. a normal period of time between heat cycles when the female is not receptive to being bred. *Compare* anestrus and estrus.

**dietary indiscretion** n. ingestion of things that may cause problems when eaten (e.g., carcasses, spoiled food, feces and sticks). Dietary indiscretion is a common cause of vomiting and diarrhea, especially in dogs.

**differential cell count** n. a method of determining the numbers of different types of white blood cells present in a blood sample by examining a stained slide under the microscope. A differential cell count can help diagnose infections, some types of cancer, bone marrow disease and many other problems.

**differential diagnosis** n. a list of diseases that are possible causes for an animal's clinical signs. Additional testing will often allow the list to be narrowed.

**Diff-quick**® n. a commercially available series of stains that easily prepares a slide to be viewed under the microscope.

**diffuse** adj. widespread.

**Difil-Test**® n. a laboratory test used to determine if larval forms of heartworms are present in the blood.

**digestion** n. the process by which ingested food is broken down into substances that can be absorbed and utilized by the body. Digestion is partially mechanical (e.g., chewing) and partly chemical (e.g., enzymes secreted by the pancreas) - **digestive** adj.

**digestive tract** n. *See* gastrointestinal tract.

**digit** n. a finger, toe, claw or hoof - **digital** adj.

**digital dermatitis** n. a disease of cattle caused by a variety of factors, including contagious bacteria and dirty conditions. Affected individuals develop erosions and/or growths on the back of the foot. Treatment can include antibiotic footbaths, dressings and improved sanitation. *Also called* hairy warts.

**digoxin level** n. a laboratory test used to determine if an animal taking digoxin for the treatment of heart disease is receiving the correct amount of the drug.

**dilated cardiomyopathy** n. a disorder in which the heart muscle becomes thin and unable to contract normally, and the heart enlarges. Genetics, infections, toxins and dietary insufficiencies (e.g., taurine) may play a role in the development of dilated cardiomyopathy. Affected individuals can cough, have difficulty breathing, accumulate fluid in the chest or abdomen, develop abnormal heart rhythms, become weak, collapse and die. Treatment may include dietary changes, addressing any underlying disorders and medications to remove excess fluid from the body, strengthen the heart's contractions, normalize heart rhythms and dilate blood vessels.

**dilute** v. to lessen the strength of a substance often by adding water or another substance to it - **dilution** n.

**dip** n. a liquid applied to the surface of an animal usually to kill parasites or other organisms.

**dirofilariasis** n. disease caused by a *Dirofilaria* worm. *See also* heartworm disease.

**disbud** v. to surgically remove the newly erupting horns from a young ruminant.

**discharge** n. 1. an abnormal fluid that is leaking from a tissue or organ. 2. v. to release from the hospital.

**discoid lupus erythematosus (DLE)** n. an autoimmune disease of dogs caused by the body's abnormal reaction to cells within the skin. Affected individuals develop varying degrees of red, flaky skin, erosions and other lesions on the bridge of the nose, around the lips and sometimes in other areas. Treatment includes protection from the sun, vitamin E and medications that lessen the abnormal immune response. *Compare* systemic lupus erythematosus.

**disease** n. any condition that disrupts the normal form or function of the body.

**disinfectant** n. a substance that reduces the number of microorganisms on surfaces - **disinfect** v.

**disk** n. *See* intervertebral disk.

**diskospondylitis** n. inflammation usually associated with infection, of spinal vertebrae and intervertebral disks. Affected individuals can develop pain, a fever and neurologic abnormalities. Prolonged use of antibiotics can eliminate diskospondylitis caused by infections.

**dislocation** n. an injury that allows movement of a bone out of its normal position within a joint. Treatment can include pain relief, manipulating the bone back into the joint, bandaging and surgery. *Also called* luxation.

**disorder** n. any condition that disrupts the normal form or function of the body.

**disorientation** n. the inability of an animal to assess and appropriately respond to its surroundings.

**displaced** adj. found in an abnormal location - **displacement** n.

**displaced abomasum (DA)** n. a disorder affecting cattle in which the abomasum is shifted to the left or right side of the abdomen and distended with gas. A displaced abomasum may be related to feeding a diet rich in concentrates, recent pregnancy or an underlying disease and causes affected individuals to lose their appetites. Treatment may include surgery, rolling the animal, supportive therapy and relieving any underlying conditions. *See also* abomasal torsion.

**dissect** v. to separate or cut tissues.

**disseminated intravascular coagulation (DIC)** n. a disorder of blood clotting that occurs as a complication to many other serious diseases. Small blood clots can form inappropriately and disrupt blood flow throughout the body, and/or blood may not clot when it should leading to bleeding. Treatment is often unsuccessful but can include plasma transfusions, medications to decrease the formation of clots, fluid therapy and relieving any underlying conditions.

**distal** adj. situated towards the end of a structure (e.g., down the leg towards the foot). *Compare* proximal.

**distal polyneuropathy** n. a disease of Rottweilers the cause of which is unknown. Affected individuals develop weakness and muscle atrophy that starts in the hind legs but eventually progresses to all four legs. Corticosteroids may help initially, but there is no effective long term treatment.

**distemper** n. a term that refers to different infectious diseases that affect several species. *See also* canine, feline and dryland distemper.

**distended** adj. stretched out by a greater than normal accumulation of gas, fluid or other materials within a structure - **distention** n.

**distichia** n. the presence of a double row of eyelashes, which often rub on the surface of the eye causing corneal wounds and infections. Removal or destruction of the follicles that produce the eyelashes is necessary to prevent their return.

**distraction index** n. a specific way of measuring the looseness of a dog's hips when stress is placed on the joints. A higher than normal distraction index is associated with hip dysplasia.

**ditch fever** n. *See* Potomac horse fever.

**diuresis** n. increased production of urine. Diuresis can occur because of disease (e.g., diabetes mellitus), behavior (e.g., excessive drinking) or through the administration of fluids or medicines. Diuresis through fluid therapy can be used to treat kidney failure and increase the excretion of waste materials or toxins from the body.

**diuretic drug** n. a type of medicine that increases the production of urine and removes water from the body. Furosemide is a commonly used diuretic.

**diurnal** adj. pertaining to or active during the daytime. *Compare* nocturnal.

**diverticulum** n. an outpouching in the wall of a hollow structure.

**dock** v. to surgically remove a portion of an animal's tail, often for reasons of appearance only.

**doctor of veterinary medicine (DVM)** n. a person who has been trained and has received an advanced degree in the medical and surgical treatment of animals.

**doe** n. an adult female goat, rabbit or deer.

**dolicocephalic** adj. describes a facial structure that consists of an extremely long snout and narrow head (e.g., a Collie). *Compare* brachycephalic.

**doll's eye reflex** n. *See* oculocephalic reflex.

**domestic longhair (DLH)** n. a mixed breed, longhaired cat.

**domestic shorthair (DSH)** n. a mixed breed, shorthaired cat.

**dominance aggression** n. inappropriate attacks or related behaviors (e.g., growling, hissing or snapping) that are initiated by an animal attempting to assert itself as the individual with control over the actions of other animals or people. Treatment can include avoidance of situations that incite aggression and behavior modifying protocols and drugs.

**dominant gene** n. one of two paired genes that will produce its version of a trait regardless of what the other gene expresses. *Compare* recessive gene.

**donor** n. an animal that provides blood or organs to another individual.

**dopamine** n. a compound that transmits signals from one cell to another in the central nervous system or can be administered as a drug to increase blood pressure.

**Doppler ultrasonography** n. a type of ultrasonography that can be used to measure movement, such as the flow of blood or the muscular contractions of a beating heart.

**dorsal** adj. situated towards the top side of the body - **dorsum** n. *Compare* ventral.

**dorsal displacement of the soft palate (DDSP)** n. a disorder of young horses in which the soft palate moves into an abnormal position over the epiglottis and hinders breathing. Affected animals often make harsh sounds when exhaling and are not able to exercise to their fullest potential. DDSP may be initiated by inflammation, exercise, infections or anatomic abnormalities. Treatment can include rest, anti-inflammatories, antibiotics, tying the tongue to the lower jaw and surgery.

**dose** n. the quantity of medicine or radiation given at one time.

**double contrast radiography** n. the taking of radiographs after the injection of a contrast agent and air into a hollow organ (e.g., bladder or stomach) to better outline any unusual contents.

**downer** n. an animal that cannot stand and walk because of injury or disease.

**drain** n. a device placed into a wound or other cavity that prevents the buildup of pus, blood or other unwanted fluids.

**drainage** n. the leakage or removal of fluid (e.g., pus) that has built up within a cavity or tissue - **drain** v.

**drape** n. a piece of sterile material that is attached to the skin surrounding the site of an incision or wound and helps prevent contamination of the area.

**drawer sign** n. an abnormal knee movement that can be palpated after rupture of the cranial cruciate ligament. Some animals require sedation before the presence of a drawer sign can be ruled in or out.

**drench** v. to orally administer a liquid medicine to an animal.

**dressing** n. a material applied to cover a wound.

**drip rate** n. a method of measuring the amount of an intravenous fluid given to an animal over a period of time.

**drool** n. saliva that falls from the mouth. Drooling can occur because of anatomy, increased production of saliva, difficulty swallowing or lesions in the mouth.

**dropped hock** n. an injury that causes lameness and a tendency to place the entirety of the back of the lower hind leg on the ground because of damage to the Achilles tendon. Treatment includes surgical repair of the tendon and the use of splints or other devices to prevent joint movement as healing progresses.

**dropsy** n. *See* hydrops.

**Drug Enforcement Agency (DEA)** n. the U.S. federal, regulatory agency concerned with the enforcement of laws regarding drugs with a potential for abuse.

**drug eruption** n. any skin lesion that develops because of the administration of a medicine. In most cases, stopping the drug is curative.

**drug residue** n. the unwanted presence of a medicine or its breakdown products in the tissues after administration of the drug.

**dry cow** n. a cow that is not producing milk.

**dry eye** n. *See* keratoconjunctivitis sicca and xerophthalmia.

**dry matter** n. what is left after a sample of food or another substance has had all of its moisture removed. Assessing the nutrient content of foods on a dry matter basis helps take into account the varying amount of water present in different types of feed.

**dryland distemper** n. *See* pigeon breast.

**dubbing** n. the surgical removal of the comb in very young chickens.

**duct** n. a tubular structure that carries fluid.

**ductus deferens** n. the tube that connects the epididymis to the urethra and carries sperm. *Also called* vas deferens.

**dummy foal** n. a newborn foal that did not have adequate oxygen delivered to its brain during the birthing process. *See also* neonatal maladjustment syndrome.

**duodenitis-jejunitis** n. *See* anterior enteritis.

**duodenostomy tube** n. a feeding tube that is surgically placed into the initial part of the small intestine allowing an animal to be fed while bypassing the stomach.

**duodenum** n. the initial part of the small intestine into which bile and pancreatic digestive enzymes are secreted.

**dust mite** n. a microscopic insect that lives inside homes and can cause allergies.

**dwarf** n. an animal that grows abnormally and matures to be small in stature. Genetics, poor nutrition or hormonal imbalances can play a role. *See also* pituitary dwarfism.

**dysautonomia** n. dysfunction of the autonomic nervous system. *See also* feline, canine and equine dysautonomia.

**dyschezia** n. difficult and/or painful defecation.

**dyschondroplasia** n. abnormal cartilage development affecting one or more joints in a young animal. *See also* osteochondrosis.

**dyscoria** n. abnormally shaped pupils or an abnormal pupillary response to light.

**dyscrasia** n. any abnormality affecting the condition of the blood or the rest of the body.

**dysecdysis** n. incomplete skin shedding seen in reptiles that are housed in dry or cold conditions, undernourished or otherwise stressed. Treatment can include soaking in a warm water bath, applying ointments to retained eye caps and relieving any underlying conditions.

**dysentery** n. any of a number of diseases that tend to cause diarrhea, sometimes with blood and mucus, straining to defecate and abdominal pain. *See also* lamb dysentery.

**dysmature** adj. describes a fetus that has not fully developed as would be appropriate for its gestational age. Dysmaturity can result from infections, birth defects, hormonal changes, poor nutrition, stress and disorders affecting the placenta.

**dysmetria** n. difficulty controlling movement, which can be seen with cerebellar disease.

**dysmyelinogenesis** n. any of a number of disorders in which myelin, the protective coating of nerves, fails to develop normally. Causes include genetics, poor nutrition or infections acquired during pregnancy. Affected individuals are young and develop tremors that are especially apparent when the animal is excited or eating, weakness and difficulty walking. There is no treatment, but in some cases the clinical signs resolve with time.

**dysphagia** n. difficulty swallowing - **dysphagic** adj.

**dysphoria** n. agitation and unrest, which can be seen in animals recovering from anesthesia or sedation - **dysphoric** adj.

**dysplasia** n. any abnormality of development - **dysplastic** adj. See the specific type of dysplasia for details (e.g., tricuspid valve dysplasia and hip dysplasia).

**dyspnea** n. difficulty breathing - **dyspneic** adj.

**dysrhythmia** n. *See* arrhythmia.

**dyssynergia** n. difficulty coordinating muscular contractions.

**dystocia** n. difficulty giving birth. Causes of dystocia include a large or abnormally shaped fetus, a small birth canal or abnormal fetal position. Treatment can include lubrication of the birth canal, repositioning the fetus, fetotomy if the fetus is dead, medications to stimulate strong uterine contractions and cesarian section.

**dystrophy** n. any abnormality that results from poor nutrition, either of the individual as a whole or of only a specific tissue due to abnormal physiology. *See also* corneal dystrophy, muscular dystrophy, neuraxonal dystrophy and osteodystrophy.

**dysuria** n. difficult or painful urination.

# E

**E. Collar** n. *See* Elizabethan collar.

**eardrum** n. *See* tympanic membrane.

**ear mange** n. a disease of goats caused by infestation with the mite *Psoroptes cuniculi*. Itching and skin lesions usually start around the ears but can spread to other parts of the body. Medications to kill the mite are generally effective. *Also called* psoroptic mange.

**ear mite** n. a type of small insect that infests the ear canals and surrounding skin. Affected animals can develop head shaking, scratching at the ears and skin lesions. Treatment includes removing debris from the ear canals and medications to kill the mites.

**ear notching** n. a method of marking animals in which portions of the pinna are removed in a unique pattern that can be used to identify individual animals.

**ear papillomas** n. *See* aural plaque.

**ear tag** n. a marker affixed to the ear displaying information that can be used to identify individual animals. Some ear tags also contain insecticides to help with fly control.

**ear tick** n. *See* spinose ear tick.

**Eastern equine encephalomyelitis (EEE)** n. a viral disease of horses that is transmitted by the bite of infected mosquitos. Affected individuals can develop fever, depression, difficulty walking and swallowing, head pressing, circling, wandering, weakness, seizures and may die. There is no specific treatment for the virus, but supportive care is essential. Vaccination and mosquito control can help prevent the disease. Birds are also susceptible to the virus and may develop neurologic abnormalities.

**ecchymosis** n. a large area of purple discoloration resulting from blood pooling under the skin. *Also called* bruise and contusion.

**ecdysis** n. shedding of the outer layers of the skin as is seen in reptiles.

**echinococcosis** n. *See* hydatid disease.

**echocardiography (echo)** n. the ultrasonographic examination of the heart, which allows close examination of its muscles, structures and chambers and the monitoring of heart movement and blood flow.

**eclampsia** n. a disease of females that are heavily pregnant, giving birth or lactating. Affected individuals have low blood calcium levels and can develop panting, restlessness, trouble giving birth, muscle tremors, difficulty walking, stiffness, behavioral changes, seizures and may die. Treatment includes calcium supplementation, supportive care and weaning, if appropriate. *See also* puerperal tetany and lactation tetany.

**ectoparasite** n. a parasitic organism that lives on the outside of the animal (e.g., fleas, ticks and mites). *Compare* endoparasite.

**ectopic** adj. the quality of being found in an abnormal place.

**ectopic cilia** n. an eyelash that grows towards the cornea and rubs against the surface of the eye. Removal or destruction of the follicle that produces the eyelash is necessary to prevent its return.

**ectopic ureter** n. a condition in which one or both of the tubes that normally carry urine from the kidneys to the bladder drain into an abnormal location in the lower urinary tract. Affected individuals often dribble urine and develop recurrent urinary tract infections. Surgery is usually necessary to address the abnormality.

**ectropion** n. an outward rolling of the eyelids that predisposes an animal to eye irritation and infections. Many cases of ectropion are due to anatomical abnormalities often associated with a specific breed. Treatment can include topical medications to relieve irritation and to treat or prevent infections or surgery. *Compare* entropion.

**eczema** n. any inflammation of the superficial layers of the skin that causes redness, itching, crusting or other lesions. *See also* facial eczema.

**edema** n. abnormal accumulation of a watery fluid within a tissue or body cavity. Edema can be seen with injury, inflammation, low blood protein levels or diseases affecting the function of the heart or other organs. Clinical signs depend on where the fluid accumulates (e.g., edema of the lungs causes difficulty breathing) - **edematous** adj.

**edrophonium test** n. *See* Tensilon® test.

**EDTA** n. a type of anticoagulant used to prevent blood samples from clotting and sometimes to treat lead poisoning or other disorders.

**efficacy** n. the ability to provide the desired response - **efficacious** adj.

**effusion** n. abnormal fluid accumulation within a body cavity. *See also* joint, pericardial, pleural and abdominal effusion.

**egg binding** n. a disorder of birds and reptiles involving the inability to expel a mature egg from the body, which can be associated with large eggs, anatomic abnormalities, obesity, weakness or low blood calcium levels. Treatment can include lubrication, medications to increase contractions or manual removal of the egg.

**egg peritonitis** n. a disease caused by the abnormal presence of the contents of an egg loose within the abdomen, which leads to inflammation. Affected individuals can develop a swollen abdomen, loss of appetite, weight loss and difficulty breathing. Treatment may include antibiotics, anti-inflammatories, supportive care and surgery.

**Ehlers-Danlos syndrome** n. *See* hyperelastosis cutis.

**Ehmer sling** n. a type of bandage that is placed around a hind leg, prevents weight bearing and pushes the head of the femur into the hip socket. An Ehmer sling may be used after a dislocated hip has been put back into its proper position.

**ehrlichiosis** n. a disease caused by infection with *Ehrlichia* bacteria that are transmitted through the bites of ticks. Affected dogs may develop fever, lethargy, enlarged lymph nodes, bleeding and bruising. Treatment can include medications to kill the bacteria, blood transfusions and supportive care. Tick control helps to prevent the disease. *See also* Potomac horse fever and equine granulocytic ehrlichiosis.

**ejaculate** n. the fluid that is forcibly expelled from the penis during sexual intercourse and contains sperm and other substances - **ejaculate** v.

**elaeophorosis** n. a disease caused by infestation of sheep, goats and some other species with the parasite *Elaeophora schneideri*. Affected individuals can develop blindness, difficulty walking, circling, seizures and may die. If they survive, months later the larvae of the parasites cause bloody skin lesions on the head or other parts of the body. Treatment of the skin lesions with a medication that kills the larvae is effective. No treatment exists for the other forms of the disease. *Also called* filarial dermatosis, sorehead and clear-eyed blindness.

**elastrator** n. an instrument used for castration and tail docking that places a band of rubber around the scrotum or tail to cut off the blood supply and cause the structures to fall off.

**elbow dysplasia** n. abnormal development of the elbow, which causes pain and predisposes the individual to develop osteoarthritis. *See also* ununited anconeal process, fragmented coronoid process and osteochondrosis.

**elective** adj. describes a procedure that could be delayed without harm to the patient.

**electrical alternans** n. an abnormal finding on an electrocardiogram in which the size of the wave pattern alternates between being large and being small. Electrical alternans can indicate the presence of fluid between the heart and the membrane that surrounds it.

**electrocardiogram (ECG, EKG)** n. a tracing that records the electrical activity of the heart through sensors attached to various parts of the body. An ECG can help with the diagnosis of arrhythmias or other forms of heart disease.

**electrocautery** n. a way to stop some types of surgical blood loss, which involves touching a piece of metal heated by an electrical current to small blood vessels. *Also called* **electrocoagulation**.

**electroejaculator** n. a device used to collect semen that is inserted into an animal's rectum and delivers electrical stimulation to nerves leading to ejaculation.

**electroencephalogram (EEG)** n. a tracing that records the brain's electrical activity through sensors attached to the head. An EEG can help diagnose epilepsy or other types of brain disease.

**electrolyte** n. a substance in the body that has the ability to conduct electrical current. Proper concentrations of these chemicals (e.g., potassium, calcium, sodium and chloride) are essential to normal body function.

**electromagnet therapy** n. *See* pulsed electromagnetic field therapy.

**electromechanical disassociation** n. a rapidly fatal disorder in which the muscles of the heart do not respond to the electrical activity that should stimulate contractions. Treatment can include medications to stimulate heart muscles and cardiopulmonary resuscitation.

**electromyography (EMG)** n. a tracing that records the electrical activity of moving skeletal muscle tissue. An EMG can help diagnose some types of nerve or muscle disease.

**electroretinogram (ERG)** n. a tracing that records the electrical activity of the retina in response to a flashing light. An ERG can help diagnose some types of retinal disease and assess whether an animal is blind.

**electrosurgery** n. a surgical technique utilizing a piece of metal heated by an electrical current to cut or destroy tissue or stop bleeding from small blood vessels.

**elimination** n. urination and defecation.

**Elizabethan collar** n. a device that is placed around the neck and acts as a shield to prevent licking and chewing of the body or scratching at the head. *Also called* E. collar.

**Elokomin fluke fever** n. a disease most commonly seen in dogs that is caused by ingestion of fish infested with a parasite carrying the bacteria *Neorickettsia elokominica*. Affected individuals may develop enlarged lymph nodes, fever, depression, loss of appetite, vomiting, diarrhea, discharge from the eyes and nose and sometimes death. Treatment includes antibiotics and supportive care.

**Elso heel** n. *See* spastic paresis.

**emaciation** n. extreme loss of fat and muscle tissue due to inadequate nutrition or disease.

**emasculator** n. an instrument used to castrate large animals that simultaneously cuts and crushes tissues to prevent bleeding. *Also called* **emasculatome**.

**embolism** n. blockage of a blood vessel with an embolus that prevents normal blood flow.

**embolus** n. a blood clot or other substance that travels through the circulatory system and becomes lodged in a blood vessel thereby disrupting blood flow - **emboli** pl. *Compare* thrombus.

**embryo** n. the fertilized egg in its early stages of development.

**embryo transfer** n. the removal of a fertilized egg from the reproductive tract of its biological mother, and its placement into the uterus of a surrogate mother for continued development and birth.

**emesis** n. the act of vomiting - **emetic** adj.

**emphysema** n. an abnormal collection of air within a tissue, which can result from injury to the skin or respiratory tract or from an infection with gas-producing bacteria - **emphysematous** adj. *See also* pulmonary emphysema.

**empiric treatment** n. therapeutic decisions that are based solely on practical observations of a patient's condition.

**empyema** n. an accumulation of pus within a body cavity.

**enamel** n. the extremely hard substance that covers and protects the crowns of teeth.

**enamel hypoplasia** n. a lack of normal enamel production in young animals leading to the development of weak and easily damaged or diseased teeth. Fevers, infections (especially canine distemper virus) and some chemicals can cause enamel hypoplasia.

**enamel points** n. sharp projections off teeth that are most commonly seen in horses and can cause oral pain and wounds. Routine floating to remove these points can be a necessary procedure in some horses.

**en-bloc resection** n. the complete removal of a structure (e.g., tumor) as a single, intact object.

**encapsulated** adj. completely encased by a membrane or other material.

**encephalitis** n. inflammation of the brain that can lead to muscle tremors, bizarre behavior, seizures, weakness, paralysis and death. Many cases of encephalitis are caused by viruses, and treatment for these patients is generally symptomatic and supportive - **encephalitides** pl. *See also* caprine arthritis-encephalitis, old dog encephalitis and pug dog encephalitis.

**encephalomalacia** n. a degeneration of the brain that can lead to depression, difficulty walking, bizarre behavior and death. *See also* polioencephalomalacia and leukoencephalomalacia.

**encephalomyelitis** n. inflammation of the brain and spinal cord that can lead to muscle tremors, bizarre behavior, seizures, weakness, paralysis and death. Many cases of encephalomyelitis are caused by viruses, and treatment for these patients is generally symptomatic and supportive. See the specific type of encephalomyelitis (e.g., West Nile encephalomyelitis) for details.

**encephalomyelopathy** n. any disease affecting the brain and spinal cord. *See also* leukoencephalomyelopathy and equine degenerative encephalomyelopathy.

**encephalopathy** n. any disorder affecting the brain. See the specific type of encephalopathy (e.g., bovine spongiform encephalopathy) for details.

**endemic** adj. describes any disease or other occurrence that is consistently present at a low level in a particular location.

**endocardial fibroelastosis** n. a disease with an unknown origin (possible genetic in some cases) that causes thickening of the lining of various parts of the heart in young animals and leads to congestive heart failure. Symptomatic treatment can be helpful, but no definitive therapy for the underlying condition exists.

**endocardiosis** n. a thickening of the tissues of one or more heart valves. Affected individuals develop a heart murmur and if the valves fail to work adequately, congestive heart failure. No effective therapy for the thickened valve exists, but treatments that improve heart function and remove excess fluid can be very helpful if symptoms develop. *Also called* degenerative valve disease and chronic valvular fibrosis.

**endocarditis** n. infection of the heart's inner lining, often involving one or more valves. Infections may originate or spread elsewhere in the body so clinical signs can vary, but fever, a heart murmur and congestive heart failure may develop. Treatment includes long-term antibiotic use, medications to remove excess fluid and improve heart function and supportive care.

**endocrine system** n. the network of organs and tissues producing hormones. These substances travel through the bloodstream to other parts of the body to exert their effect. The endocrine system plays a major role in regulating many body functions, including growth, reproduction and metabolism.

**endocrinopathy** n. any disorder affecting a part of the endocrine system.

**endodontic disease** n. any disease (e.g., infection) that affects a tooth's pulp cavity, root or nearby tissues.

**endogenous** adj. emanating from within the body. *Compare* exogenous.

**endometritis** n. inflammation of the endometrium, which is often associated with infection. Endometritis adversely affects the female's ability to become pregnant and maintain a pregnancy. Treatment can include antibiotics, antimicrobial medications infused into the uterus and hormones to induce a heat cycle or uterine contractions.

**endometrium** n. the inner lining of the uterus - **endometrial** adj.

**endoparasite** n. a parasitic organism that lives inside an animal (e.g., roundworms and lungworms). *Compare* ectoparasite.

**endorphin** n. a chemical produced by the body that relieves pain and provides a feeling of well-being.

**endoscope** n. a tubular instrument including a light source and viewing device that can be placed into hollow organs (e.g., the stomach) allowing the veterinarian to see inside of these structures and sometimes take samples or remove foreign objects.

**endoskeleton** n. hard tissues (e.g., bone and cartilage) within the body that provide structural support. *Compare* exoskeleton.

**endothelial dystrophy** n. a disorder, often genetic in origin, affecting the inner lining of the cornea, which may lead to corneal swelling and ulceration. Treatment can include medications to remove fluid from the cornea and surgeries or procedures to hasten healing of ulcers. **Endothelial degeneration** is a similar disorder that is seen in animals as they age.

**endothelium** n. the tissues lining the inside of the cornea, heart, blood vessels or other structures.

**endotoxemia** n. the presence in the bloodstream of toxins that are released from bacteria when they die or are damaged. Affected individuals can develop a fever, lethargy, low blood pressure and may die without prompt and aggressive treatment. *Also called* blood poisoning.

**endotoxin** n. a suvstance that can be released from bacteria when they are damaged or killed and cause illness in animals. *See also* endotoxemia.

**endotracheal tube (ET tube)** n. a hollow tube that is usually placed through the mouth and into the trachea. An endotracheal tube may be used to maintain and protect an airway and deliver oxygen and anesthetic gasses.

**end-stage** adj. describes a body part that is almost non-functional due to disease or a disorder that has advanced to the point where little can be done to improve the patient's condition.

**enema** n. placement of a liquid into the large intestine through the anus, usually to loosen and lubricate feces and encourage defecation. Other types of enemas can be used to administer medications or aid in diagnosis.

**enophthalmos** n. eyes that are more sunken into their sockets than is normal. *Compare* exophthalmos.

**entamebiasis** n. *See* amebiasis.

**enteral** adj. pertaining to the intestines. *Also called* **enteric**.

**enteral nutrition** n. food and water that is placed directly into the gastrointestinal tract through a feeding tube or taken in by mouth. *Compare* parenteral nutrition.

**enteritis** n. inflammation of the intestinal tract that may be caused by infection, parasites, immune disease, dietary indiscretion, drugs or allergies. Affected individuals develop diarrhea and sometimes vomiting and dehydration. Treatment can include supportive care, antidiarrheal and antinausea medications and addressing the underlying cause.

**enterocolitis** n. inflammation of the small and large intestine that may be caused by infection, parasites, immune disease, dietary indiscretion, drugs or allergies. Affected individuals develop diarrhea and sometimes vomiting and dehydration. Treatment can include supportive care, antidiarrheal and antinausea medications and addressing the underlying cause.

**enterohepatic circulation** n. the recirculation of blood between the small intestine and liver. Enterohepatic circulation can delay the elimination of some toxic substances from the body.

**enterolith** n. an accumulation of minerals and other materials that form a hard object within the intestinal tract capable of obstructing the normal flow of ingesta. Seen most frequently in horses, enteroliths can cause intermittent episodes of colic. Surgical removal is curative.

**enteropathy** n. any disorder affecting the intestinal tract, often resulting in diarrhea.

**enterostomy tube** n. a feeding tube that is surgically placed into the small intestine and allows an animal to be fed while bypassing the stomach and parts of the small intestine.

**enterotomy** n. a surgical incision into the intestines.

**enterotoxemia** n. a disease caused by infection of the intestinal tract with *Clostridium perfringens*. The bacteria can damage the lining of the intestines, which may lead to diarrhea (often bloody), collapse and death. Treatment can include antibiotics, antitoxin injections, antiserum and supportive care but maybe unsuccessful in severe cases. Preventive vaccination is very helpful in some species. *See also* lamb dysentery and overeating disease.

**enterotoxin** n. a harmful substance produced by some bacteria that infect an animal's intestinal tract.

**enthesiophyte** n. abnormal mineralization of a ligament or other fibrous structure where it attaches to a bone.

**entropion** n. an inward rolling of the eyelids that causes eyelashes or fur to rub on the surface of the eye leading to wounds and infections of the cornea. Entropion may be a primary problem caused by anatomic abnormalities, in which case surgery is required to correct the situation. Secondary entropion is caused by disorders that produce eye pain. Treatment of the primary problem plus pain relief and topical antibiotics can be curative in these cases. *Compare* ectropion.

**enucleation** n. the surgical removal of an entire structure, usually referring to the eyeball.

**enzootic** adj. describes any disease or other occurrence that is consistently present at a low level in animals in a particular location.

**enzootic abortion** n. a disease of sheep and goats characterized by late-term abortions and caused by infection with *Chlamydophila abortus* bacteria. Females rarely abort more than once but can shed the bacteria for the rest of their lives. Other animals in the herd may be infected and can have lameness, eye infections and pneumonia. Isolation, vaccines and antibiotics can help control herd outbreaks. *Chlamydophila abortus* can cause disease in pregnant women. *Also called* chlamydiosis.

**enzootic ataxia** n. a disorder of young animals caused by a deficiency of copper in the diet. Affected individuals can exhibit depression, diarrhea, blindness, deafness, tremors, trouble walking and paralysis. Copper supplementation can improve the condition of animals that are not too severely affected. *See also* swayback.

**enzootic balanoposthitis** n. *See* pizzle rot.

**enzootic hematuria** n. ingestion of sufficient quantities of the bracken fern plant to cause disease and sometimes death in cattle and sheep. Affected animals have intermittent bouts of blood in the urine and may develop anemia and bladder tumors. Treatment is difficult. *See also* bracken fern poisoning.

**enzyme** n. a protein that speeds up a chemical reaction in which it is involved - **enzymatic** adj.

**enzyme-linked immunosorbent assay (ELISA)** n. a type of laboratory test that is used to determine if an antigen or specific antibodies are present in a sample. For example, an ELISA test for the presence of feline leukemia virus in the blood of cats is commonly run in veterinary hospitals.

**eosinopenia** n. lower than normal numbers of eosinophils in the blood. The condition is most commonly seen with stress or corticosteroid use.

**eosinophil** n. a specific type of white blood cell that plays a role in fighting off parasites and in allergic reactions - **eosinophilic** adj.

**eosinophilia** n. higher than normal numbers of eosinophils in the blood.

**eosinophilic gastroenteritis and colitis** n. inflammation that infiltrates a part of the gastrointestinal tract and is predominantly composed of eosinophils. Parasitism and allergies to food or bacteria may play a role in some cases. Affected individuals can develop loss of appetite, weight loss, vomiting and diarrhea. Treatment may include a diet change, medications to kill parasites and immunosuppressive drugs. *See also* inflammatory bowel disease.

**eosinophilic granuloma** n. a skin lesion associated with allergic reactions, bacterial infections or a genetic predisposition. Affected areas of skin may be raised, hairless, pink and itchy although their appearance can vary. Treatment can include antibiotics, corticosteroids and surgery. *Also called* eosinophilic plaque.

**eosinophilic keratitis** n. a disease of cats with an unknown cause. Affected individuals develop an elevated pink or white lesion on the surface of the eye, which often recurs intermittently throughout the life of the animal. Treatment includes topical or systemic immunosuppressive drugs.

**eosinophilic ulcer** n. a pink lesion that usually affects the upper lip next to a canine tooth and is associated with allergies, infections or genetics in cats. Treatment can include antibiotics, corticosteroids and surgery. *Also called* rodent ulcer and indolent ulcer.

**epaxial muscles** n. the muscles that run down the length of the back on either side of the spine.

**eperythrozoonosis** n. disease caused by infection with *Eperythrozoon* bacteria, which are usually transmitted through insect bites. Affected individuals may develop anemia and have loss of appetite and weight, fever, depression and pale mucous membranes. Treatment can include blood transfusions and antibiotics.

**epidemic** n. an outbreak of disease that is spreading more rapidly than is normally seen in a particular location. *Also called* epizootic.

**epidemiology** n. the science and study of diseases within a population, including their causes, prevalence, spread, prevention and treatment.

**epidermal collarette** n. a skin lesion consisting of a ring of flaky skin, which often occurs as another type of skin lesion (e.g., a pustule) is resolving.

**epidermal inclusion cyst** n. a benign skin mass inside of which is a thick, "cheesy" material. The cysts can rup-ture and become inflamed and infected. Surgical removal is curative. *Also called* sebaceous cyst, infundibular follicular cyst and epidermoid cyst.

**epidermis** n. the outermost layer of skin - **epidermal** adj.

**epidermolysis bullosa** n. a group of similar, genetic disorders that cause a weak attachment between the epidermis and dermis. Affected animals are young and develop erosions on the surface of the skin or mucous membranes and can slough hooves, claws or footpads. Most cases are fatal.

**epididymis** n. the coiled tube that is attached to the testicle and stores and transports maturing sperm - **epididymides** pl.

**epididymitis** n. inflammation of one or both epididymides, which is usually associated with infection.

**epidural analgesia** n. a method of providing pain relief to the back end of an animal that involves injecting a drug into one of the spaces surrounding the spinal cord.

**epiglottic entrapment** n. a disorder that causes horses to have difficult and noisy breathing and an inability to exercise to their fullest potential. The epiglottis becomes stuck behind a fold of mucous membrane. Surgery to cut the tissue away from the epiglottis is usually curative.

**epiglottis** n. a flap of cartilage covered with mucous membrane that is located at the back of the mouth. The epiglottis prevents material from entering the windpipe when an animal eats or drinks and allows free flow of air during breathing.

**epilate** v. to pull out hair by the roots - **epilation** n.

**epilepsy** n. abnormal and uncontrolled electrical activity in the brain, which leads to recurring seizures. Epilepsy may be a primary disorder for which no underlying cause can be found (i.e., idiopathic epilepsy) or secondary to a brain injury, tumor or biochemical abnormalities. Treatment for mild epilepsy may not be necessary. If seizures are frequent or of long enough duration to become dangerous, anticonvulsant medications will usually reduce their occurrence and severity.

**epinephrine** n. a hormone that is produced by the adrenal glands and increases heart rate, blood pressure and blood sugar levels. It is often secreted in response to fear, excitement or sudden stress. Epinephrine can also be administered as a drug to stimulate heart contractions, open airways and treat anaphylaxis. *Also called* adrenaline.

**epiphora** n. the excessive flow of tears from an eye.

**epiphysis** n. either end of a long bone.

**epiphysitis** n. a disease that causes lameness and bony abnormalities of the legs. *See also* bent leg (goats) and physitis (horses).

**episclera** n. the tissue that is loosely connected to the outer surface of the eye's sclera - **episcleral** adj.

**episcleritis** n. inflammation of the episclera.

**epispadias** n. an abnormal urethral opening most commonly seen in males. The penis has a hole on its upper side through which urine can flow. Treatment includes surgical repair.

**epistaxis** n. bleeding from the nose.

**epithelialization** n. the process by which epithelium returns to cover a surface from which it has been lost.

**epitheliogenesis imperfecta** n. a congenital disorder characterized by the development of skin that fails to cover the entire body. Small areas can be surgically repaired, but if extensive the condition is fatal. *Also called* aplasia cutis.

**epitheliotropic lymphosarcoma** n. a type of cancer that most commonly affects dogs and cats. Individuals can develop hair loss, patches of red, flaky, sometimes raised skin or skin tumors. Treatment with corticosteroids or chemotherapeutic drugs can be helpful, but the disease is eventually fatal. *Also called* mycosis fungoides.

**epithelium** n. the layer of cells that covers the outside of skin, mucous membranes and other body surfaces or that lines the inside of hollow organs (e.g., the bladder) - **epithelial** adj.

**epizootic** n. an outbreak of disease that is spreading more rapidly in animals than is normally seen in a particular location. *Also called* epidemic.

**epizootic catarrhal enteritis (ECE)** n. a contagious, viral disease of ferrets causing vomiting, diarrhea, dehydration and loss of appetite, weight and energy. Treatment can include fluid therapy, antibiotics, medications that protect the gastrointestinal tract and supportive care. *Also called* green slime disease.

**epulis** n. a benign tumor of the gums most commonly seen in dogs. Most cause few problems, and surgical removal is usually curative. Some types (e.g., acanthomatous epulis) can grow aggressively into local tissues and be difficult to remove - **epulides** pl.

**equine** adj. pertaining to horses.

**equine adenovirus** n. a virus that can cause pneumonia in Arabian foals suffering from combined immunodeficiency disease and diarrhea in other young foals.

**equine collagenolytic granuloma** n. *See* nodular necrobiosis.

**equine degenerative encephalomyelopathy** n. a disease of young horses caused by vitamin E deficiency and/or genetics. Affected individuals have difficulty walking, are weak and tend to get worse with time. Vitamin E supplements can be helpful.

**equine dysautonomia** n. a disease with an unknown cause that disrupts the autonomic nervous system and can lead to high heart rates, colic, sweating, muscle tremors, weight loss, difficulty eating, drooling, third eyelid elevation, drooping upper eyelids, dry mucous membranes and death. There is no treatment. *Also called* grass sickness.

**equine ehrlichial colitis** n. *See* Potomac horse fever.

**equine granulocytic anaplasmosis** n. a disease of horses caused by *Anaplasma phagocytophila* bacteria (previously called *Ehrlichia equi*) transmitted through tick bites. Affected individuals may develop a fever, leg swelling, difficulty walking, jaundice and bruising. Treatment

with appropriate antibiotics is usually successful. Tick control can help prevent the disease. *Also called* **equine ehrlichiosis** and granulocytic ehrlichiosis.

**equine herpes myeloencephalitis** n. a contagious disease of horses caused by a type of herpesvirus. Affected individuals can have difficulty walking, weakness, problems with urination and defecation and may collapse. There is no specific treatment for the virus, but supportive care is essential. Equine herpesvirus vaccines do not protect against this form of the infection.

**equine herpesvirus (EHV)** n. a group of related viruses that can cause equine herpes myeloencephalitis, coital exanthema, equine rhinopneumonitis or abortion depending on which virus is contracted and where the infection localizes.

**equine infectious anemia (EIA)** n. a contagious, viral disease of horses transmitted through the bites of insects. Affected animals may develop a fever, bruising, anemia, weight loss and limb swelling. Cases of EIA must be reported to appropriate regulatory agencies. Euthanasia is recommended to prevent spread of the disease. *Also called* swamp fever.

**equine influenza** n. a contagious, viral disease of horses that can cause high fever, nasal discharge, coughing, weakness and swollen lymph nodes. Treatment includes rest, antibiotics for secondary bacterial infections and supportive care. Preventative vaccines exist.

**equine metabolic syndrome** n. a disease usually diagnosed in overweight horses that are fed a lot of grain and have limited opportunities to exercise. Affected individuals can develop laminitis, a long, curly coat that does not shed normally and other problems. Treatment includes weight loss and reducing or eliminating the amount of grain in the diet. *Also called* peripheral Cushing's disease.

**equine monocytic ehrlichiosis** n. *See* Potomac horse fever.

**equine motor neuron disease** n. a disease of horses that may be associated with vitamin E deficiency. Affected individuals become weak, tremble and lose muscle mass. There is no effective treatment, but some cases will partially improve with time.

**equine protozoal myeloencephalitis (EPM)** n. a disease of horses caused by ingestion of the parasite *Sarcocystis neurona* that is found in opossum feces. Affected individuals can develop difficulty walking, weakness, muscle wasting and other neurologic disorders. Treatment includes medications to kill the parasite and supportive care. A preventative vaccine is available. Its usefulness is still being evaluated.

**equine rhinopneumonitis** n. a contagious, viral disease of horses that can cause high fever, nasal discharge, coughing, weakness and swollen lymph nodes. Treatment includes rest, antibiotics for secondary bacterial infections and supportive care. A preventative vaccine is available.

**equine venereal balanitis** n. *See* coital exanthema.

**equine viral arteritis (EVA)** n. a contagious, viral disease of horses that can cause fever, subcutaneous swelling (especially of the legs, abdomen, penis or scrotum), nasal and ocular discharge, coughing and abortion. Some cases of EVA are transmitted to mares through the sperm of a carrier stallion. Other routes of infection are also possible. Treatment can include medications to remove excess fluid from the body, anti-inflammatories and supportive care. A preventative vaccination is available. *Also called* equine typhoid.

**eradicate** v. to eliminate completely - **eradication** n.

**erection** n. enlargement and hardening of the penis caused by engorgement with blood, which permits sexual intercourse.

**ergotism** n. a disease caused by ingestion of the fungus *Claviceps purpurea* that infects rye and other grains. Affected individuals develop poor blood flow to the feet, legs, ear tips, tail and other extremities leading to tissue death and sloughing. Abortion is also possible. Treatment is difficult. *Also called* ergot poisoning.

**erosion** n. a loss of the surface of a tissue through friction, inflammation or other causes.

**eructation** n. elimination of gasses from the gastrointestinal tract through the mouth, which is especially important in ruminants to prevent the development of bloat.

**eruption** n. coming to the surface, especially the process of teeth emerging through gum tissue or the development of a skin rash.

**erysipelas** n. a disease caused by infection with the bacteria *Erysipelothrix rhusiopathiae*. Pigs can develop fever, lameness, skin lesions, abortion or die suddenly. Other species can also be infected. Treatment includes antibiotics and supportive care. Preventative vaccines are available for pigs. *See also* nonsuppurative polyarthritis of lambs.

**erythema** n. an abnormal redness of the skin that is often a result of inflammation, infection or injury - **erythematous** adj.

**erythema multiforme** n. a disease often associated with an adverse drug reaction. Erythema multiforme can cause skin lesions, fever and depression. Treatment includes stopping administration of any drug that may be a cause, supportive care and sometimes corticosteroids.

**erythrocyte** n. the cell in blood that carries oxygen. *Also called* red blood cell.

**erythrocyte parameters** n. calculations based on laboratory tests that help determine the likely cause of abnormal red blood cell counts. *Also called* erythrocyte indices and red blood cell parameters.

**erythrocytosis** n. *See* polycythemia.

**erythron** n. mature and immature red blood cells and any part of the body (e.g., the bone marrow) that contributes to their development.

**erythropoiesis** n. the process of red blood cell development and production that occurs primarily in the bone marrow and to a lesser extent the spleen.

**erythropoietic porphyria** n. a genetic disease affecting some breeds of cattle, pigs and cats causing individuals to have permanent, dark red discoloration of their teeth, bones and urine. Cattle can develop skin lesions when exposed to sunlight. There is no treatment. *Also called* osteohemochromatosis and porphyrinuria.

**erythropoietin** n. a hormone that is produced by the kidneys or administered as a drug and stimulates the bone marrow to produce red blood cells.

**eschar** n. a leathery scab that forms on top of and protects wounds during the healing process.

**esophagitis** n. inflammation of the esophagus that may be caused by an object becoming stuck in the esophagus, the use of some drugs, anesthesia, vomiting or ingestion of an irritating substance. Affected animals can regurgitate, drool, have difficulty swallowing and be in pain. Treatment may include antibiotics, pain relief, diet changes, placement of a feeding tube and medications that decrease gastric acid production, protect damaged tissues or help prevent reflux of ingesta into the esophagus.

**esophagoscopy** n. the use of a tubular instrument including a light source and viewing device placed into the esophagus through the mouth which allows the veterinarian to see abnormalities, remove foreign objects and take samples of tissue for analysis.

**esophagostomy tube** n. a feeding tube that is surgically placed into the esophagus allowing feeding of an animal that is unable or unwilling to eat on its own.

**esophagram** n. a radiograph that is taken after administration of a contrast agent that highlights the esophagus.

**esophagus** n. the muscular tube that leads from the mouth to the stomach.

**essential amino acids** n. certain molecules that combine with one another to form proteins. Essential amino acids must be included in the diet because they cannot be manufactured by the animal.

**essential fatty acids (EFA)** n. compounds that are an important component of many body structures (especially fat) and must be included in the diet because they cannot be manufactured by the animal.

**estradiol** n. a hormone that is produced primarily by the ovary and to a lesser extent the adrenal glands and is responsible for a female being receptive to mating.

**estrogen** n. a term encompassing several hormones (e.g., estradiol) that are responsible for the development of typically female characteristics and receptivity to mating. Estrogens may also be used as drugs, for example in the treatment of urinary incontinence.

**estrogen toxicity** n. a disease caused by higher than normal levels of estrogen in the body. Unspayed female ferrets can develop an enlarged vulva, thin hair and low red and white blood cell counts leading to weakness, bleeding and infections. Dogs given estrogen as a drug are also susceptible to low blood cell counts and their effects. *See also* estrogenism.

**estrogenism** n. disease caused by ingestion of moldy grain containing the toxin zearalenone. Affected individuals can develop vulvar enlargement and discharge, mammary gland enlargement, prolapse of the uterus, abnormalities in reproduction and the estrous cycle, abortion and male infertility. Animals generally return to normal once the contaminated food is removed. *See also* estrogen toxicity.

**estrous cycle** n. the recurring pattern of periods of time during which a female is receptive (i.e., estrus) and unreceptive (i.e., diestrus) to mating.

**estrus** n. the period of time during which a female is receptive to mating and is capable of becoming pregnant. *Also called* estrum and heat.

**estrus synchronization** n. a procedure that often utilizes hormone injections or implants to bring several females into heat and ovulate at the same time.

**ethmoid hematoma** n. a mass located in the nasal passages or sinuses of horses, the cause of which is unknown. Affected individuals often develop recurrent nosebleeds. Treatment can include injection of formalin into the mass or its surgical removal.

**ethylene glycol toxicosis** n. ingestion of ethylene glycol that is often contained in antifreeze and can cause vomiting, increased thirst and urination, dullness and difficulty walking. An inability to make urine, seizures and death may occur later in the course of the disease. Recovery is possible if the animal receives intravenous fluids and specific antidotes before irreversible kidney damage occurs. Dialysis is an option in advanced cases. *Also called* antifreeze toxicosis.

**etiology** n. the origins and causes of a disease - **etiologic** adj.

**eumycotic mycetoma** n. a draining mass that is caused by a fungal infection.

**euryblepharon** n. *See* macropalpebral fissure.

**eustachian tube** n. the passageway that connects the middle ear to the throat and allows equalization of pressure on both sides of the eardrum.

**euthanize** v. to cause a painless and easy death, often to relieve suffering or to deal with animal overpopulation - **euthanasia** n. *Also called* euthanatize.

**euthyroid** adj. having an appropriate amount of thyroid hormone in the body.

**euthyroid sick syndrome** n. a condition in which the thyroid gland of an animal that is suffering from a non-thyroid illness makes less thyroid hormone than does a healthy animal. Euthyroid sick syndrome should not be confused with hypothyroidism. Thyroid hormone levels will rise if the underlying condition is resolved, and treatment with a thyroid supplement is unnecessary.

**evert** v. to turn inside out - **eversion** n.

**eviscerate** v. 1. to surgically or traumatically remove organs from the abdominal cavity. 2. to remove the contents of the eyeball - **evisceration** n.

**ewe** n. an adult, female sheep.

**ewe necked** adj. describes a conformation flaw of horses in which the middle of the neck is curved downward when viewed from the side.

**examination** n. the inspection of an animal using various senses (e.g., sight, hearing, smell and touch), procedures and/or tests to aid in the diagnosis of disease or determination of health - **examine** v.

**excise** v. to remove through surgery - **excision** n.

**excisional biopsy** n. to surgically remove a structure (e.g., a tumor) in its entirety and analyze a portion of the tissue to aid in diagnosis.

**excoriation** n. a scratch involving only the surface of a tissue.

**excrete** v. to expel a substance (e.g., feces or urine) from the body - **excretion** n.

**excretory urogram** n. radiographs that are taken after an animal receives an intravenous injection that highlights the kidneys, ureters, bladder and urethra.

**exenterate** v. to remove all of the contents held within a part of the body - **exenteration** n.

**exercise intolerance** n. an inability or unwillingness to be as physically active as would be normal for a particular individual. An animal with exercise intolerance may tire quickly when exerting itself.

**exercise-induced pulmonary hemorrhage (EIPH)** n. a condition that causes some horses to bleed into their respiratory tracts during periods of extreme exertion (e.g., racing). Affected individuals may not be able to perform to their peak ability. The cause is unknown. Treatment can include medications that decrease the amount of bleeding and strips that help keep nasal passages open. *Also called* bleeder.

**exertional rhabdomyolysis** n. a disorder primarily affecting horses during or after exercise. Affected individuals become stiff and reluctant to move because of pain, sweat excessively, breathe quickly and may develop dark, discolored urine. Permanent kidney damage can occur in severe cases. Many factors are related to the development and prevention of the disorder including diet, overexertion, lack of conditioning and temperament. Treatment can include rest, fluid therapy and pain relief. *Also called* exertional myopathy, azoturia, tying up, set-fast, Monday morning disease, cording up and black water.

**exfoliate** v. to shed cells from the surface of a tissue - **exfoliation** n.

**exfoliative cytology** n. the microscopic examination of a sample of cells that are shed from the surface of a tissue.

**exhale** v. to breathe air out of the lungs - **exhalation** n. *Compare* inhale.

**exocrine pancreatic insufficiency (EPI)** n. a disease primarily affecting dogs in which the pancreas does not produce sufficient amounts of digestive enzymes. Affected individuals can lose weight despite having an increased appetite and have large amounts of soft, sometimes greasy stool. Treatment includes supplementing the diet with pancreatic enzymes. *Also called* pancreatic acinar cell atrophy.

**exogenous** adj. emanating from outside of the body. *Compare* endogenous.

**exophthalmos** n. eyes that protrude further than is normal from their sockets. *Compare* enophthalmos.

**exoskeleton** n. hard tissues (e.g., a shell) on the outside of the body of some animals that provide structural support and protection. *Compare* endoskeleton.

**exostosis** n. an abnormal but benign growth of bone or cartilage that can cause problems if it is traumatized or impinges on other tissues - **exostoses** pl. *Also called* osteophyte, bone spur or osteochondroma.

**exotic animal** n. a species of animal that is relatively infrequently kept as a pet (e.g., snakes and sugar gliders).

**exotic disease** n. a contagious disease that is not commonly found in a particular region. *Also called* foreign animal disease.

**exotic Newcastle disease (END)** n. *See* viscerotropic velogenic Newcastle disease.

**expectorant** n. a type of medication that makes it easier to cough up mucus and other respiratory secretions.

**expectorate** v. to cough up respiratory secretions - **expectoration** n.

**exploratory surgery** n. surgery, usually of the abdominal cavity, with the purpose of identifying any abnormalities followed by corrective procedures or biopsy, if appropriate.

**exposure** n. 1. increased visibility of a structure, often because of the absence or removal of overlying tissues. 2. contact with a substance or condition that may be harmful.

**express** v. to press on a structure causing liquid to be expelled.

**exsanguination** n. the loss of a large amount of blood.

**extend** v. to straighten out a joint or limb - **extension** n. *Compare* flex.

**extensor process disease** n. *See* buttress foot.

**exteriorize** v. to move an internal structure to the outside of the body.

**external fixator** n. a device the majority of which is on the outside of the body but penetrates through the skin and into bone to prevent unwanted movement of a broken bone or joint.

**extracorporeal shock wave therapy (ESWT)** n. a type of therapy that directs high pressure, low frequency sound waves into injured tissues and is most often used to treat orthopedic diseases.

**extract** v. to pull out a structure (e.g., a tooth) or to isolate a substance from within a mixture - **extraction** n.

**extra-label drug use** n. the use of medicines in a manner that has not been expressly approved by appropriate regulatory agencies. For example, treating an animal with a drug that has only been tested in humans is an extra-label use. *Also called* off-label drug use.

**extramedullary** adj. located outside of the bone marrow.

**extramedullary hematopoiesis** n. red and white blood cell and platelet production that occurs outside of the bone marrow. If the bone marrow is diseased or the body has a great demand for new blood cells, other organs (e.g., the spleen and liver) can play a larger than normal role in the production of blood cells.

**extramedullary plasmacytoma** n. a tumor that is composed of plasma cells and most commonly located in the skin or mouth of older dogs. Most cases are benign and surgical removal is curative.

**extraocular** adj. located outside of or next to the eye.

**extravasation** n. the leakage of a fluid out of a blood vessel and into surrounding tissues.

**extravascular** adj. outside of blood vessels. *Compare* intravascular.

**extremity** n. a body part that is located far from the trunk or head (e.g., leg, tail or ear flaps).

**extrinsic** adj. 1. originating from outside of the body or body part. 2. not essential. *Compare* intrinsic.

**extrinsic allergic alveolitis** n. *See* hypersensitivity pneumonitis.

**exudate** n. a liquid that has leaked from blood vessels and contains many white blood cells and a large amount of protein. Exudates can be associated with infection or inflammation. *Compare* transudate.

**eye cap** n. the outer layers of corneal tissue on the surface of a reptile's eye, which are normally shed with the rest of the skin. If the animal is housed in dry or cold conditions, undernourished or otherwise stressed, the eye caps may need to be lubricated and gently removed.

**eyeworm** n. a type of parasitic worm that is transmitted by flies and infests the eyes of many animal species. Affected individuals develop ocular inflammation and discharge. Treatment can include medications to kill the worms, their manual removal and anti-inflammatories. *Also called* thelaziasis.

# F

**face flies** n. a type of fly (*Musca autumnalis*) that ingests tears, saliva, nasal mucus or other body fluids and can be very irritating to livestock. The use of ear tags containing pesticides can be helpful.

**facet** n. a small, smooth area on a bone.

**facial eczema** n. a disease of grazing animals caused by ingestion of the toxic spores of the fungus *Pithomyces chartarum*. The fungus grows in pastures under warm, damp conditions. The toxins damage the liver, and affected animals become jaundiced, avoid the sun, develop skin lesions and may die. Treatment and prevention includes avoiding pastures during high-risk seasons, applying chemicals that kill the fungus and zinc supplements. *Also called* pithomycotoxicosis.

**facial nerve paralysis** n. a loss of function of the facial nerve that can cause drooling, a lack of facial muscle tone and movement, loss of the ability to blink and a drooping ear and lip on the affected side(s) of the face. Causes include an idiopathic disorder, trauma, ear infections, hypothyroidism and tumors. Treatment may involve addressing any underlying conditions, giving the nerve time to regenerate and supportive care.

**factor deficiency** n. one of several similar genetic diseases in which an animal does not produce enough of one of the coagulation factors necessary for blood to clot normally. Affected individuals can bleed and bruise easily. Treatment may include blood or plasma transfusions and avoidance of trauma.

**facultative** adj. having a preference but not a requirement for certain conditions.

**fading puppy and kitten syndrome** n. a disorder of newborn puppies and kittens that causes a lack of interest in nursing, sleeping separately from the litter, whining and sometimes death. The cause may be difficult to determine but can involve hypothermia, infections, anemia, low blood sugar, birth defects and exposure to toxins. Treatment includes addressing any underlying conditions and supportive care.

**Fahrenheit (°F)** n. the system for measuring temperatures in which the freezing point of water is 32° and the boiling point of water is 212°. For a conversion equation to the Celsius scale, see the appendices.

**failure** n. decreased function of a body part or process that causes significant symptoms in the animal. *Compare* insufficiency.

**failure of passive transfer** n. a disorder most often seen in newborn foals and calves caused by a lack adequate acquisition of antibodies from the mother through suckling of colostrum. Affected individuals can develop multiple infections and die. Treatment includes feeding the newborn colostrum during the first 12-24 hours of life or transfusions of serum containing antibodies.

**failure to thrive** n. a disorder of young animals that leads to poor health, growth and weight gain. The cause may be difficult to determine but can involve inadequate nutrition, infections, birth defects and exposure to toxins. Treatment includes addressing any underlying conditions and supportive care.

**faint** v. to lose consciousness for a short period of time, usually because of a lack of adequate oxygen delivered to the brain.

**fallopian tube** n. *See* uterine tube.

**false bursa** n. *See* hygroma.

**false labor** n. behavior displayed by a pregnant animal that makes it appear as if she is about to give birth but ends without delivery of the fetus. Some dogs may undergo false labor even if they are not pregnant because of normal hormonal changes that occur after each heat cycle.

**false negative** n. a diagnostic test result wrongly indicating that an animal does not have the disorder in question when it truly does. *Compare* false positive.

**false positive** n. a diagnostic test result wrongly indicating that an animal has the disorder in question when it truly does not. *Compare* false negative.

**false pregnancy** n. *See* pseudocyesis.

**false quarter** n. a vertical line of overgrown hoof on the side of a horse's foot caused by damage to the tissues that produce new hoof wall.

**false rig** n. a castrated male horse that acts like a stallion despite the complete absence of testicular tissue.

**false strangles** n. *See* pigeon breast.

**familial** adj. occurring in a group of related individuals more frequently than in the general population.

**familial dermatomyositis** n. a genetic disease that is most often seen in young Collies and Shetland Sheepdogs. Affected individuals can develop skin lesions, muscle stiffness and difficulty opening the mouth. Treatment with anti-inflammatories may be helpful in some cases.

**Fanconi's syndrome** n. a condition, sometimes genetic, that results in the loss of glucose, sodium, potassium, phosphorus, amino acids and other substances in the urine. Affected individuals can drink and urinate more than normal and lose weight. Treatment includes dietary supplements.

**far side** n. the right side of a horse's body, described as such because a person usually leads and mounts a horse from the left side. *Compare* near side.

**farrier** n. a person trained in the trimming and shoeing of horses' feet.

**farrowing** n. the process of a sow giving birth to a litter of piglets - **farrow** v.

**fascia** n. a tough, fibrous tissue that connects and supports muscles or other body parts - **fascial** adj.

**fasciculation** n. a small, localized muscle tremor.

**fasciitis** n. inflammation of a fascial tissue, which can be painful.

**fascioliasis** n. a disease caused by infestation with a *Fasciola* fluke that most commonly affects ruminants. The flukes cause liver damage and sometimes infections, anemia, bleeding, tissue swelling, fluid accumulation and death. Medications to kill the flukes are available. *See also* Black disease.

**fast** v. to withhold food for a period of time.

**fat cow syndrome** n. *See* hepatic lipidosis.

**fat necrosis** n. death and degeneration of fat cells, which often leads to the formation of a mass of abnormal tissue. Fat necrosis is caused by trauma, lack of adequate blood supply or other diseases (e.g., pancreatitis). *See also* lipomatosis.

**fatigue** n. a feeling of exhaustion and weakness.

**fat-soluble vitamins** n. vitamins A, D, E and K, which can be dissolved and stored in fat. Oversupplementation with these vitamins can sometimes lead to toxic levels being reached in the body. *Compare* water-soluble vitamins. *See also* hypervitaminosis A and D.

**fatty acid** n. a compound that is an essential part of fat and a component of many other tissues.

**fatty liver** n. *See* hepatic lipidosis.

**faucitis** n. inflammation of the structures that surround the passageway between the mouth and the pharynx.

**fear aggression** n. inappropriate attacks or related behaviors (e.g., growling, hissing or snapping) that are initiated by an animal in response to what is perceived to be a frightening situation. Punishing an animal in this situation will often make the aggression worse rather than better. Treatment can include desensitization to fearful stimuli and behavior modifying drugs.

**feather cyst** n. a mass that develops in a bird's skin because of an ingrown feather. Surgical removal of the mass and the follicle that produces the feather is curative.

**feather mite** n. a general name for different types of small insects (e.g. red mite) that can infest birds and cause itching, feather loss and anemia.

**feather picking** n. excessive grooming that results in a bird developing bald areas and/or damaged feathers. Feather picking can be related to medical disorders (e.g., parasites, infections, liver disease and allergies), poor diet and environmental or psychological conditions. Treatment is difficult but can include addressing any underlying medical problems, relieving stress or boredom, correcting nutritional deficiencies and behavior modifying medications.

**febrile** adj. having an abnormally high body temperature, which can be associated with infections, inflammation or high environmental temperatures. *Also called* pyrexic.

**fecal egg count** n. a determination of the number and types of parasite eggs in a specific amount of feces, which helps determine an individual's or herd's level of parasitism and whether and what type of deworming is needed.

**fecal examination** n. the microscopic examination of a sample of feces to identify parasite eggs or larvae and the presence of abnormal numbers or types of bacteria.

**fecal flotation** n. the placement of a sample of feces in a liquid that allows parasite eggs to rise to the surface. A glass cover slip collects the eggs and is placed on a slide to be examined under the microscope.

**fecal gram stain** n. the microscopic examination of a sample of bird droppings smeared on a slide and stained to identify the presence of abnormal numbers or types of bacteria.

**fecal impaction** n. a blockage of the large intestine with feces, which may be due to dehydration, intestinal disorders or ingestion of undigestible materials. Affected animals develop abdominal pain, reluctance to eat and straining or inability to defecate. Treatment can include fluid therapy, stool softeners, enemas and manual or surgical removal of the feces.

**fecal incontinence** n. inability to control defecation, which may be caused by diarrhea, disorders affecting the colon, rectum or anus, pain or neurologic abnormalities. Affected individuals will often lose their housetraining or have stool that seems to drop from their rectum without their knowledge.

**fecal occult blood** n. the abnormal presence of even small amounts of blood in the feces.

**fecalith** n. an extremely hard, sometimes mineralized, piece of feces that can block the intestinal tract. Affected individuals often have intermittent episodes of abdominal pain and cannot defecate. Surgical removal is often necessary.

**fecal-oral transmission** n. a method through which contagious diseases can be spread involving an individual ingesting feces of another animal that contains an infectious organism.

**feces** n. waste produced by and evacuated from an animal's gastrointestinal tract - **fecal** adj. *Also called* stool.

**feed additives** n. medicines or other supplements that are added to food, often to prevent or treat disease or increase growth rates.

**feed efficiency** n. a measure of the level of production (e.g., milk, meat or eggs) that takes into consideration the amount of food consumed by an animal or herd.

**feeding tube** n. a hollow tube placed into the gastrointestinal tract to allow feeding of an animal that is unwilling or unable to eat on its own. Feeding tubes can be placed and removed with each feeding (e.g., nasogastric tubes) or surgically inserted and left for extended periods of time (e.g., gastrotomy tubes).

**feline** adj. pertaining to cats.

**feline AIDS** n. *See* feline immunodeficiency virus (FIV).

**feline calicivirus (FCV)** n. a contagious, viral disease of cats that may cause fever, sneezing, nasal and ocular discharge, red and swollen eyes and ulcers in the mouth. Treatment can include antibiotics to treat secondary bacterial infections, medications that help the body suppress the virus and supportive care. Some cats have intermittent or chronic relapses. Preventative vaccines exist. *See also* limping syndrome.

**feline central retinal degeneration (FCRD)** n. a disease of cats that is caused by a lack of adequate amounts of taurine in the diet and leads to retinal damage and loss of some or all vision. Correcting the diet will prevent progression of the disease.

**feline chlamydiosis** n. a contagious disease of cats that is caused by infection with *Chlamydophila psittaci* bacteria and may cause fever, red and swollen eyes, ocular discharge and sneezing. Treatment can include antibiotics and supportive care. Preventative vaccines exist. *Also called* feline pneumonitis.

**feline coronavirus** n. a virus that can cause diarrhea or feline infectious peritonitis. *See also* feline enteric coronavirus and feline infectious peritonitis.

**feline distemper** n. *See* feline panleukopenia.

**feline dysautonomia** n. a disease with an unknown cause that disrupts the autonomic nervous system and can lead to dilated pupils that do not respond to light, third eyelid elevation, drooping upper eyelids, dry mucous membranes, regurgitation, constipation, slow heart rate and incontinence. Treatment is difficult. *Also called* Key-Gaskell syndrome.

**feline enteric coronavirus (FECV)** n. a contagious, viral disease that usually affects kittens and can cause fever, vomiting and diarrhea. No specific treatment for the virus is available, but supportive care is usually effective. It is thought that some cats can maintain this virus in their bodies, and it may later mutate to cause feline infectious peritonitis.

**feline gingivitis-stomatitis syndrome** n. *See* lymphocytic-plasmacytic stomatitis.

**feline herpesvirus** n. *See* feline viral rhinotracheitis.

**feline hyperesthesia syndrome** n. *See* twitchy cat disease.

**feline immunodeficiency virus (FIV)** n. a viral disease of cats that weakens the immune system and is primarily transmitted through bite wounds. Affected individuals may remain healthy for an extended period of time, but most eventually develop chronic, recurrent infections and sometimes cancer. Treatment includes supportive care and therapy aimed at any secondary diseases. A preventative vaccine exists, but its effectiveness has not yet been thoroughly investigated. *Also called* feline AIDS.

**feline infectious anemia (FIA)** n. a disease of cats caused by infection with *Haemobartonella felis* bacteria, which are usually transmitted by blood sucking insects (e.g., fleas).

Affected individuals may develop a fever, anemia, pale or yellow skin and mucous membranes, depression, weakness, difficulty breathing and weight loss. Treatment can include antibiotics, corticosteroids, oxygen therapy and blood transfusions. *Also called* hemobartonellosis.

**feline infectious peritonitis (FIP)** n. a fatal, viral disease of cats that can cause fever, depression, eye infections, neurologic abnormalities, fluid accumulations, difficulty breathing and loss of appetite and weight. Fluid accumulation in the abdomen and/or chest cavity is seen in the wet form but not the dry form of the disease. Treatment is difficult and limited to supportive care. *See also* feline enteric coronavirus.

**feline ischemic encephalopathy (FIE)** n. a disease of cats with an unknown cause that leads to inadequate oxygen delivery and tissue death affecting a portion of the brain. Affected animals can suddenly develop circling, bizarre behavior, blindness, seizures or other neurologic abnormalities. Treatment may include corticosteroids, oxygen therapy, anti-seizure medications and supportive care.

**feline leukemia virus (FELV)** n. a viral disease of cats that weakens the immune system and is primarily transmitted through bite wounds and close contact with an infected cat. Affected individuals may remain healthy for a period of time, but most eventually become sick and can develop a wide variety of disorders, including chronic, recurrent infections, cancers and anemia. Treatment includes supportive care and therapy aimed at any secondary diseases. A preventative vaccine exists. *See also* fibrosarcoma.

**feline lower urinary tract disease (FLUTD)** n. *See* feline urologic syndrome.

**feline odontoclastic resorptive lesion (FORL)** n. a disorder of cats the cause of which is unknown. Affected individuals may demonstrate oral pain, loss of appetite and drooling because of tooth enamel degeneration, holes in the teeth and inflamed gums. Extraction of damaged teeth is necessary. *Also called* neck lesion and cervical line lesion.

**feline panleukopenia** n. a contagious, viral disease of cats that can cause vomiting, diarrhea, dehydration, neurologic abnormalities, low white blood cell counts and death. Disease is most often seen in poorly vaccinated kittens. Treatment may include fluid therapy, antibiotics for secondary infections, antinausea medications and blood or plasma transfusions. Vaccination on an appropriate schedule will usually prevent disease. *Also called* feline distemper and **feline parvovirus**.

**feline pneumonitis** n. *See* feline chlamydiosis.

**feline urologic syndrome (FUS)** n. a disease of cats that leads to straining or inability to urinate and bloody urine. In some animals, the cause cannot be identified while other cases can be associated with crystals in the urine, bladder stones and sometimes infections. Treatment may include diet changes, medications to dissolve crystals or treat infections, surgery to remove bladder stones and anti-inflammatories. *Also called* feline lower urinary tract disease (FLUTD).

**feline viral rhinotracheitis (FVR)** n. a contagious, viral disease of cats that may cause fever, sneezing, nasal and ocular discharge, red and swollen eyes and ulcers affecting the eyes, mouth or skin. Treatment can include antibiotics to treat secondary bacterial infections, medications that help the body suppress the virus and supportive care. Some cats develop intermittent or chronic relapses. Preventative vaccines exist. *Also called* feline herpesvirus.

**feminization** n. the development of typically female characteristics. Feminization may be seen in a male animal with a hormonal imbalance (e.g., an estrogen secreting tumor).

**femoral head** n. the ball that is located at the top of the femur and connects with the pelvis to form the hip joint.

**femoral head ostectomy (FHO)** n. the surgical removal of the femoral head. A femoral head ostectomy may be performed when injury to or degeneration of the bones involved in the hip joint causes intractable pain. *Also called* femoral head resection.

**femoral nerve paralysis** n. a loss of function of the femoral nerve, which is most commonly seen after a difficult birth during which a calf has been pulled from the cow. Affected calves have difficulty walking and wasting of the muscles at the front of the upper hind leg. Treatment can include supportive care and anti-inflammatories.

**femoral pores** n. holes in the skin on the inside of the hind leg of some reptiles. Femoral pores are usually large in males and secrete hormones and other substances important in the behavior of the species.

**femur** n. the large, long bone in the upper leg between the hip and the knee - **femoral** adj.

**fenestrate** v. to surgically create an opening through a structure that encloses another body part - **fenestration** n.

**feral** adj. describing a domestic animal that lives without human care and develops behaviors more typical of related wild species.

**fermentation** n. the breakdown of carbohydrates into simpler molecules in the absence of oxygen. Fermentation is an important component of digestion in some species (e.g., ruminants and horses) and can also be used to preserve and store forage in the form of silage.

**fertile** adj. capable of producing offspring - **fertility** n.

**fertilization** n. the fusion of a sperm and egg to form an embryo - **fertilize** v. *Also called* conception.

**fescue** n. a type of grass that is often found in fields and hay and is a good source of nutrition but when infected by certain types of fungus can cause disease in some animals. *See also* fescue toxicosis.

**fescue foot** n. a disorder that is most commonly seen in cattle and sheep and is caused by ingestion of fescue grass or hay infected with a fungus. Affected individuals can become lame and depressed, have swelling, redness and other skin lesions on their lower legs and tail, and lose their appetite and weight. Treatment includes preventing access to infected grass or hay and supportive care.

**fescue toxicosis** n. a disease caused by ingestion of fescue grass or hay infected with a fungus. Pregnant mares may have prolonged gestational times, difficulty giving birth, abortions and fail to produce adequate amounts of milk. Cattle and sheep can develop lameness and skin lesions on their lower legs and feet, necrosis of intra-abdominal fat or decreased weight gain and other problems associated with warm weather. Treatment includes preventing access to infected grass or hay, supportive care and medications that limit the effect of the fungus (horses). *See also* fescue foot, summer slump and lipomatosis.

**fetal membranes** n. the structures that encircle, protect and support the development of the fetus inside the uterus (e.g., the allantois and amnion).

**fetal resorption** n. degeneration and absorption of a fetus within the uterus, which can be caused by infections, hormone deficiencies and abnormalities in fetal development.

**fetlock** n. the joint located on top of the narrowed area above a large animal's hoof.

**fetopelvic disproportion** n. a condition in which the fetus is relatively larger than can easily pass through the mother's pelvis during the birthing process. *Also called* fetal-maternal disproportion. *See also* dystocia.

**fetotomy** n. the process of cutting a dead fetus into pieces to aid in its removal from the birth canal.

**fetus** n. a developing animal that is still within the uterus but in the later stages of maturation - **fetal** adj.

**fever** n. an abnormally high body temperature, which can be associated with infections, inflammation or high environmental temperatures - **febrile** adj. *Also called* pyrexia.

**fever of unknown origin (FUO)** n. a disorder that causes a persistently elevated body temperature, the cause of which is uncertain. Infections, inflammation, autoimmune disease and cancer can sometimes be difficult to diagnose and may cause a fever of unknown origin. Treatment may include supportive care, medications that decrease inflammation and body temperature and antibiotics until further testing hopefully can uncover a more definitive diagnosis.

**fiber** n. 1. partially digestible or indigestible carbohydrates, which are important to normal function of the gastrointestinal tract. 2. a structure shaped like a thread.

**fibrillation** n. repeated involuntary and unsynchronized contractions of muscle fibers. *See also* atrial and ventricular fibrillation.

**fibrin** n. a protein in the blood that helps form blood clots.

**fibrin degradation products (FDPs)** n. breakdown products of fibrin and fibrinogen that inhibit the formation of blood clots. Higher than normal levels of fibrin degradation products in the blood are often associated with disseminated intravascular coagulation. *Also called* fibrin split products.

**fibrinogen** n. a protein in the blood that when broken down into fibrin helps form blood clots.

**fibrinolytic drug** n. a type of medicine that breaks down fibrin and small blood clots.

**fibroadenoma complex** n. *See* mammary gland hyperplasia.

**fibroblast** n. a cell that can mature into the cells that form connective tissue.

**fibrocartilaginous emboli (FCE)** n. a disorder that is most commonly seen in dogs and is caused by blockage of blood vessels leading to or from a part of the spinal cord with material originating from intervertebral disks. Affected individuals suddenly develop difficulty walking and sometimes other neurologic abnormalities but are not in pain. Treatment can include corticosteroids, supportive care and time to allow neurologic function to improve. *Also called* fibrocartilaginous infarct.

**fibroid** adj. 1. composed primarily of fibrous connective tissue. 2. n. a fibroma.

**fibroma** n. a benign tumor that arises from connective tissue and most commonly affects the skin of older dogs. Surgical removal is curative.

**fibromatosis** n. the presence of one or more tumors arising from connective tissue. *See also* fibroma and desmoid.

**fibromatous epulis** n. a benign tumor of the gums most commonly seen in dogs. Most cause few problems, and surgical removal is curative.

**fibroplasia** n. the development of fibrous connective tissue (e.g., the formation of scars).

**fibrosarcoma** n. an aggressive cancer of fibroblasts most commonly located in and under the skin. Fibrosarcomas do not tend to spread to distant tissues but can be very invasive at their location. Some cases of fibrosarcoma in cats have been associated with specific types of injectable vaccines (e.g., FELV). Treatment includes wide surgical excision, which can be difficult to achieve, and chemotherapy.

**fibrosis** n. the growth and development of a tough and inelastic tissue. Fibrosis may be desirable (e.g., wound healing), or it can hinder normal function of a structure or organ. For example, fibrosis of the tissues around a joint can prevent normal use of the leg - **fibrotic** adj.

**fibrotic and ossifying myopathy** n. a disorder seen in horses, usually after injury to the muscles on the back side of the upper hind leg. The affected leg is moved in a jerky manner. Treatment can include surgery to remove the abnormal tissue or to cut the ligaments of involved muscles.

**fibrotic myopathy** n. a disease with an unknown cause that is most commonly seen in dogs. The leg muscles of affected individuals degenerate and become scarred, which leads to stiffness and difficulty walking. Treatment is often unsuccessful but may include surgery to remove or cut affected tissues.

**fibrous** adj. composed of strands or fibers, often describing a type of tissue that is tough and does not bend easily.

**fibrous joint** n. 1. a normal connection between some bones that consists of fibrous connective tissue. 2. scarring around a joint that prevents normal movement.

**fibrous osteodystrophy** n. the abnormal replacement of bone with a more flexible tissue, which can be caused by a tumor that over-secretes parathyroid hormone, a deficiency of calcium and phosphorous in the diet or renal failure. Affected individuals may have bones that bend or fracture easily, be unable to close their mouths and their teeth may fall out. *See also* renal and nutritional secondary hyperparathyroidism and primary hyperparathyroidism.

**fibula** n. the thin bone that is located on the outside of the leg below the knee.

**fibular head transposition** n. a surgery that can be performed after cranial cruciate ligament rupture to reduce pain and lameness. The top of the fibula and its attached ligaments are moved forward and affixed in this new position to help stabilize the stifle joint.

**figure eight bandage** n. a bandaging technique often used to prevent unwanted motion of a joint.

**filamentous** adj. composed of long, thread-like structures.

**filaria** n. a type of parasitic worm - **filarial** adj. *Also called* filarid.

**filarial dermatitis** n. a disease of cattle caused by parasites transmitted by horn fly bites. Affected individuals develop skin lesions along the bottom of their chest and abdomen. Treatment includes medications to kill the parasites. *Also called* stephanofilariasis.

**filarial dermatosis** n. bloody skin lesions on the head or other areas of sheep, goats and some other species caused by the larvae of the parasite *Elaeophora schneideri. See also* elaeophorosis.

**filly** n. a female horse under four years of age.

**filtration angle** n. the area where the iris attaches to the wall of the eye and through which anterior chamber fluid is circulated. Disorders affecting the filtration angle can lead to glaucoma. *Also called* iridocorneal angle.

**fine needle aspirate** n. a method of obtaining cells or fluid from the body. A needle and syringe are used to withdraw a sample, which then may be placed upon a slide for microscopic examination or otherwise tested.

**first degree burn** n. a mild burn that damages only the outer layer of skin. *Compare* second and third degree burns.

**fissure** n. a deep and long groove or opening.

**fistula** n. an abnormal channel that either connects structures within the body or leads from the inside of the body through the skin. Fistulas can develop because of injury, infection, inflammation or abnormal development - **fistulous** adj.

**fistulous withers** n. a disease of horses in which fluid filled sacs at the top of the shoulders swell, rupture and drain to the surface of the skin. Trauma or infection (e.g., *Brucella* bacteria) are potential causes. Treatment can include surgical removal of affected tissues and antibiotics.

**fixator** n. a device that prevents unwanted movement of a broken bone, joint or other tissues.

**fixed and dilated pupil** n. a wide pupil that does not respond to light, which can indicate severe brain damage or blindness.

**flaccid** adj. soft and weak.

**flagellate** n. a microorganism (e.g., *Giardia*) that has a long "tail" used to propel itself.

**flail chest** n. an abnormal movement of a portion of the chest wall that is seen when an animal breathes. A flail chest indicates the presence of multiple broken ribs or other severe injuries and is often associated with difficulty breathing and pain.

**flank** n. the part of the body located in front of the hips and behind the ribs.

**flap** n. a portion of skin, mucous membrane or other tissue that is cut free from surrounding tissues but left attached at one edge. The flap can allow access to deeper structures or be pulled and sutured in place across a wound or other defect.

**flat line** n. a wave pattern seen on an electrocardiogram when the heart is not beating or when the sensors have become disconnected.

**flat puppy syndrome** n. *See* swimmer puppy.

**flatulence** n. the production of gastrointestinal gasses and their evacuation through the anus.

**flatulent colic** n. *See* gas colic.

**flatworm** n. one of several types of parasitic worms (e.g., tapeworms) that tend to be flat rather than round.

**flea** n. a small, blood-sucking insect that infests the skin and coat of many species. Their bites often cause itching and can transmit disease. Heavily infested animals may become anemic.

**flea allergy dermatitis** n. an allergic reaction to the bite of fleas, which can cause itching, skin lesions and hair loss. Therapy may include treatments that kill fleas and prevent others from reinfesting the animal, decreasing the number of fleas in the animal's environment and medications to stop itching. *Also called* flea bite hypersensitivity.

**flea dirt** n. flea feces, which can be found on the skin or in the environment of infested animals.

**fledgling** n. a young bird that is not yet fully feathered.

**fleece** n. a sheep's coat of wool, which can be sheared and removed in one piece.

**flehmen response** n. a curling of the lips and extension of the head and neck. The posture helps an animal's vomeronasal organ identify chemical signals produced by another individual.

**flex** v. to bend a joint or limb - **flexion** n. *Compare* extend.

**flexion test** n. a procedure used to reveal lameness in horses. A leg is bent and held in position for a period of time, after which the horse is immediately trotted and watched to see if it is favoring the leg. Further testing after a poor response to a flexion test is needed to determine the cause of the lameness.

**flexural limb deformity** n. a disorder in which one or more legs are continually flexed and cannot be straightened. Newborns can be born with a flexural limb deformity because of being abnormally positioned within the uterus, toxins that are ingested by the dam and genetics. Older animals may develop the problem because of pain in the affected leg. Some animals may not be able to stand, while others walk on the tips or the fronts of their hooves or develop a club foot. Treatment can include splints, casts, nutritional changes, hoof trimming, pain relief and surgery. *Also called* flexion deformity and contracted tendons.

**flight feather** n. a long, smooth feather on a bird's wing or tail that is essential to flight.

**float** v. to file down a horse's teeth to remove sharp edges or other abnormalities.

**floating rib** n. a rib that is not firmly attached to a vertebra. The condition can be normal in some situations. For example, a dog's last rib is often a floating rib.

**flooding** n. a method of behavioral modification that involves continually presenting an animal with a stimulus that previously provoked a fearful response until it no longer does so.

**flora** n. the population of microorganisms that lives on a body surface, within the gastrointestinal tract or in other locations.

**flu** n. *See* influenza.

**fluid rate** n. the amount of intravenous fluid given to a patient over a period of time.

**fluid therapy** n. the administration of liquids into the circulatory or gastrointestinal system or under the skin. Fluid therapy can be used to treat dehydration or shock, help administer drugs or other substances or enhance the excretion of toxins from the body.

**fluid wave** n. an abnormal pulse of moving liquid that can be felt when pushing or tapping on a part of the body.

**fluke** n. a type of parasitic organism that is fairly large and flat and can infest the liver, lungs, intestinal tract, blood or other tissues in a variety of species. *See also* the specific fluke (e.g., liver fluke) for details.

**fluorescein dye** n. a substance applied to the surface of the eye that highlights wounds by glowing when illuminated by a Wood's lamp.

**fluorescent antibody test (FA)** n. a laboratory test used to determine if a microorganism or other antigen is present in a sample.

**fluoride toxicosis** n. ingestion of sufficient quantities of fluoride to cause disease. Sources of fluoride include industrial waste or fumes, fertilizers, mineral supplements and toothpaste. Affected individuals can develop vomiting, diarrhea, abnormal heart rhythms, neurologic abnormalities and die if they are exposed to a large amount of fluoride at one time. Chronic ingestion of smaller amounts leads to abnormalities of bones and developing teeth, lameness and loss of appetite and weight. Treatment can include medications that bind to and aid in the excretion of fluoride and supportive care. *Also called* **fluorosis**.

**fluoroscopy** n. a method of visualizing internal structures that utilizes x-rays to produce a moving, real-time picture.

**flush** v. 1. to thoroughly irrigate a wound or cavity with a liquid to remove foreign material and microorganisms. 2. to increase the amount of food eaten by a female animal prior to breeding to increase the chances of a successful mating.

**flutter** n. repeated rapid but rhythmic movements of a muscle. *See also* atrial, ventricular and synchronous diaphragmatic flutter.

**fly strike** n. *See* myiasis.

**foal** n. a horse under one year of age.

**foal heat** n. the period of time during which a mare can be bred that usually occurs a week or two after she has given birth.

**foal heat diarrhea** n. diarrhea that tends to be seen in foals about the same time that their dam undergoes her foal heat. The cause of the diarrhea is not known, but it is usually mild and resolves on its own.

**foaling** n. the process through which a mare gives birth to a foal.

**focal** adj. limited to a small area.

**focal adnexal dysplasia** n. a benign raised skin mass caused by an abnormal collagen deposit. Surgical removal is curative. *Also called* collagenous nevi.

**focal seizure** n. *See* partial seizure.

**fog fever** n. *See* bovine atypical interstitial pneumonia.

**folate** n. a type of vitamin B that is important in the formation of proteins, DNA and other substances. A dietary deficiency can lead to anemia. *Also called* folic acid.

**Foley catheter** n. a hollow tube with an inflatable bulb on the end. Foley catheters have a variety of uses, including their surgical placement into the bladder to drain urine.

**follicle** n. a sac-like depression, particularly the structure in the skin that produces hair and the part of the ovary that contains an egg - **follicular** adj.

**follicle stimulating hormone (FSH)** n. a hormone produced by the pituitary gland or used as a drug that stimulates the maturation of eggs in the ovary or sperm production.

**follicular cyst** n. 1. a benign skin mass inside of which is a thick, "cheesy" material. *See also* epidermal inclusion cyst. 2. persistent, fluid-filled structures on the ovaries that can cause animals to fail to come into heat, have frequent, abnormal heat cycles, develop masculine behavior and have vaginal discharge. Treatment includes manual rupture of the cyst or hormone therapy.

**follicular dysplasia** n. a group of disorders, some of which are genetic, that all cause thin hair growth often involving only certain areas of skin. Treatment is difficult. *See also* color dilute alopecia and alopecia X.

**follicular mange** n. *See* demodicosis.

**folliculitis** n. inflammation of a hair follicle.

**fomite** n. a contaminated object that can pass disease from one animal to another. For example, medical instruments that are not disinfected between uses on different animals can act as fomites.

**fontanelle** n. a normal opening in the skull of a newborn, which should close as the animal matures.

**food aggression** n. inappropriate attacks or related behaviors (e.g., growling, hissing or snapping) that are initiated by an animal in the presence of food. In many cases, it is best to simply avoid this problem by keeping the animal isolated when food is available.

**food allergy** n. an allergic reaction to beef, chicken, eggs, wheat, corn or other substances present in the diet. Affected individuals can develop skin lesions, itching, ear and skin infections, vomiting and diarrhea. Treatment of a food allergy involves feeding a diet that does not contain the offending allergen. *Also called* food hypersensitivity.

**Food and Drug Administration (FDA)** n. the U. S. federal government agency responsible for regulating the safety of veterinary and human drugs, food and other products.

**food intolerance** n. an adverse reaction to components in an animal's diet that does not involve the immune system, unlike a food allergy. Affected individuals can develop vomiting, diarrhea or other symptoms that resolve when a diet not containing the offending substance is fed.

**food trial** n. feeding a diet that excludes substances suspected of inciting a food allergy or intolerance. A food trial may need to continue for up to three months before an animal's clinical signs resolve.

**food-elicited cataplexy test** n. a way of diagnosing and evaluating cataplexy and narcolepsy in dogs. Desirable foods are offered, and the excitement that results can provoke an episode.

**foot and mouth disease (FMD)** n. a contagious, viral disease of cattle, sheep, goats, pigs and some wildlife species. Animals can develop a fever, blisters affecting their mouth, feet and teats, lameness and loss of appetite, weight and milk production. Foot and mouth disease has been eradicated from many countries. Treatment should not be attempted, and suspected cases must be reported to appropriate regulatory agencies.

**foot scald** n. infection between the claws of sheep, cattle or goats caused by dampness or anything that irritates the skin in this area. Affected individuals can become lame. Treatment includes improving environmental conditions and the use of topical antiseptics or antibiotics. *See also* footrot.

**footrot** n. a severe infection that originates between the claws of cattle, sheep, goats or pigs causing lameness, sometimes to the point where the animal will kneel rather than stand. The most severe form is a contagious disease of sheep and goats caused by two types of bacteria, *Fusobacterium* *necrophorum* and *Dichelobacter nodosus*. Affected individuals develop lesions between their claws, and without treatment, the infection spreads into the hoof wall, causing it to detach from its supporting structures. Therapy includes antibiotics, hoof trimming and antiseptic footbaths. *See also* strawberry footrot and foot scald.

**forage** n. plants (e.g., grasses and alfalfa) or their hay and silage that can be the main component of a grazing animal's diet.

**forage mite** n. a small insect that can be found in hay or straw and bite animals causing them to itch. Medications to control itching can be helpful. *Also called* straw itch mite.

**forage poisoning** n. *See* botulism.

**foramen** n. a naturally occurring hole, especially in bone.

**foramen magnum** n. the hole at the back of the skull through which the spinal cord connects to the brain.

**forceps** n. a surgical instrument used to grasp tissues or other objects.

**forebrain** n. the part of the brain that is responsible for controlling many of the so called "higher" functions such as reasoning, personality, sight, hearing, smell, touch and some aspects of movement.

**foreign animal disease** n. a contagious disease that is not commonly found in a particular country. *Also called* exotic disease.

**foreign body** n. an object from the environment that is contained within the body in an abnormal manner. For example, a rock within the stomach or a piece of wood that broke off under the skin would both be considered foreign bodies.

**forelimb** n. an arm or front leg.

**forging** n. *See* overreaching.

**formaldehyde** n. a gas that when dissolved in water is a potent disinfectant and preservative.

**formalin** n. a diluted form of formaldehyde that can be used to preserve tissues and treat some diseases (e.g., footrot).

**fossa** n. a hollowed-out area.

**founder** n. *See* laminitis.

**fowl** n. certain species of birds that are commonly used for food, including chickens, turkeys, ducks and geese.

**fowl cholera** n. a contagious disease of chickens, turkeys and other birds caused by infection with *Pasteurella multocida* bacteria. Affected individuals can develop diarrhea, difficulty breathing, localized infections, or they may die suddenly. Treatment with antibiotics can be successful if started early enough. Preventative vaccines exist.

**foxtail** n. a type of grass seed that has long and sharp bristles on its surface. Foxtails can penetrate the skin and move surprising distances within the body, causing chronic infections. They can also be found under the eyelids, leading to wounds and infections on the surface of the eye.

**fracture** n. a break, especially of a bone. *See also* specific types of fractures (e.g., open, closed, comminuted and greenstick) for details.

**fragmented coronoid process** n. a developmental disorder of dogs in which a piece of bone on the inside of the elbow fails to attach to the main part of the ulna. Affected individuals can have elbow pain, lameness and develop osteoarthritis at an early age. Treatment may include surgery to remove the piece of bone and medications that decrease pain and inflammation.

**free choice feeding** n. a method of feeding animals in which food is available throughout the day, and the individual can eat when and how much it chooses. Some animals will overeat and become obese with free choice feeding. *Also called* free feeding. *Compare* meal feeding.

**free gas bloat** n. an accumulation of gas within the rumen that may be caused by lying down for prolonged periods of time and physical or physiologic abnormalities that prevent eructation. Affected animals develop abdominal distension and pain, difficulty breathing and may die. Treatment can include passage of a stomach tube or surgical procedures to dislodge any foreign bodies and release the gas from the rumen.

**free radical** n. a group of atoms containing oxygen and electrons that can alter and damage the chemical structure of cells or other compounds.

**free T$_4$ by equilibrium dialysis** n. a laboratory test that measures the amount of active thyroid hormone in circulation. This test is less affected by non-thyroid illness than are some other methods of measuring thyroid function.

**freemartin** n. a female animal affected by male hormones to which she was exposed while developing in the uterus with a male twin. The disorder is seen almost exclusively in cows. Affected individuals are infertile and may have abnormal appearing genitalia.

**fremitus** n. a vibration that can be heard or felt.

**French molt** n. a disease with an unknown cause that primarily affects young budgerigars and leads to feather breaking and loss. There is no specific treatment, but some individuals may eventually develop normal feathers. Improved nutrition, pulling broken feathers and reducing stress may improve the condition.

**frenulum** n. a fold of tissue that attaches one structure to another.

**fresh frozen plasma** n. plasma that has been handled and stored in such a way as to maintain high levels of all coagulation factors. Use of fresh frozen plasma is required when treating some types of factor deficiencies.

**freshening** n. the process of a dairy cow starting to produce large amounts of milk after giving birth.

**friable** n. easily broken into pieces.

**friction rub** n. an abnormal sound that can be heard with a stethoscope when unhealthy membranes (e.g., around the lungs or heart) rub against each other.

**frog** n. 1. a type of amphibious animal. 2. a "V" shaped, fleshy structure on the bottom of a horse's foot.

**frontal sinus** n. a hollow, normally air-filled area in the skull over the eyes.

**frostbite** n. damage to skin that is caused by exposure to cold temperatures. If severe, amputation of affected tissues may be necessary.

**frothy bloat** n. gas that has accumulated within the rumen and mixed with fluid to form foam that cannot be eructated out of the gastrointestinal tract. Access to increased amounts of certain types of feed (e.g., alfalfa, clover and grain) is associated with some cases of frothy bloat. Affected animals develop abdominal distension and pain, difficulty breathing and may die suddenly. Treatment can include passage of a stomach tube, medications that break down the foam and surgical procedures to release gas from the rumen. *Also called* pasture bloat.

**frounce** n. infection of the mucous membranes of a bird's mouth, crop and esophagus with the parasite *Trichomonas gallinae*. Affected individuals can drool and have difficulty eating. Treatment includes medications to kill the parasite. *Also called* trichomoniasis.

**fructosamine** n. a protein the levels of which can be measured in the blood to monitor diabetic control during the previous several weeks.

**full-thickness** adj. involving the entire depth of skin or another tissue. *Compare* partial thickness.

**fulminant** adj. occurring suddenly and severely.

**fumonisin toxicosis** n. *See* fusariotoxicosis.

**functional tumor** n. a tumor that secretes large amounts of a hormone or other substance that adversely affects the body.

**fundic exam** n. observation of the back of the eye with a magnifying instrument. *Also called* **fundoscopy**.

**fundus** n. the back of an organ (e.g., the eye) or that part farthest away from an opening.

**fungus** n. a group of plant-like organisms that do not contain chlorophyll. Some types of fungi can cause disease in animals - **fungal** adj., **fungi** pl.

**fur ring** n. a band of fur around a chinchilla's penis that prevents the organ from being retracted fully into its sheath. *Also called* hair ring.

**fur slip** n. the tendency of chinchillas to lose a patch of hair when traumatized or stressed.

**furcation** n. the part of a structure where a separation into branches occurs.

**furuncle** n. a painful lump in the skin consisting of a central area of dead tissue surrounded by inflammation. *Also called* boil.

**furunculosis** n. a disease characterized by multiples areas of deep infection in the skin resulting from disruption of the hair follicle, inflammation and bacterial infection. Affected individuals are often very itchy and develop nodules, ulcers, draining tracts and possibly permanent hair loss. Treatment can include long term antibiotic use and whirlpool baths.

**fusariotoxicosis** n. a disease caused by ingestion of molds that usually infect corn. Affected horses can develop depression, blindness, circling, difficulty walking and swallowing, inability to stand and jaundice. Other species can also be affected. Neurologic damage to horses is permanent. *Also called* moldy corn poisoning and fumonisin toxicosis.

**fusiform** adj. tapered at both ends.

**fusion** n. a connection between different structures (e.g., within a joint or between vertebrae) that prevents movement. Fusions may be a developmental abnormality, secondary to disease or created through surgery - **fused** adj.


# G

**gag reflex** n. the normal, involuntary response to retch when the back of the mouth is touched.

**gait** n. the manner and pattern of leg movements observable when an animal is in motion.

**galactorrhea** n. excessive production of milk and/or its leakage from the mammary glands.

**galactostasis** n. inadequate production or expression of milk from the mammary glands.

**gall** n. 1. an injury to the skin and sometimes to deeper tissues that is caused by the friction of an ill-fitting saddle, harness or other piece of equipment. Eliminating the cause of the injury is essential. Additional treatment may include antibiotics, anti-inflammatories and surgery. *Also called* saddle sore. 2. *See* bile.

**gall sickness** n. *See* anaplasmosis.

**gallbladder** n. the balloon-like structure within the liver of most species (not horses) that collects and holds bile before it is excreted into the gastrointestinal tract.

**gallop** n. 1. the fastest gait of horses during which four distinct beats or footfalls are evident. 2. an abnormal heart rhythm that sounds like a horse running because of the presence of an extra heart beat.

**gallstones** n. *See* cholelithiasis.

**Galvayne's groove** n. an indented line on a horse's outermost incisors that can be used to estimate age. On average, the groove appears at the gum line at age 10, reaches the end of the tooth by age 20 and has disappeared by age 30.

**gamete** n. the reproductive cell of a female or male animal (e.g., egg or sperm) that can form an embryo after fertilization.

**gamma globulin** n. *See* antibody.

**gamma-glutamyl-transpeptidase (GTP)** n. a substance the levels of which rise in the blood when bile flow from the liver is impeded.

**gammopathy** n. abnormally high levels of antibodies in the blood. *See also* monoclonal and polyclonal gammopathy.

**gangrene** n. tissue death that can result from an inadequate supply of blood to a part of the body. Bacteria will often infect the tissue soon after gangrene develops. Treatment can include antibiotics, oxygen therapy and surgical removal of affected tissues - **gangrenous** adj.

**gape** v. 1. to hold the mouth open. 2. n. a behavior seen in cats responding to chemical signals emitted by another individual (e.g., in the urine). Cats will keep their mouth open and sometimes lick their nose while staring into the distance. *Also called* flehmen response.

**gapeworm** n. a parasitic worm that invades the lungs and airways of birds and can cause difficulty breathing. Treatment includes medications to kill the worms.

**garbage poisoning** n. a disease caused by ingestion of decaying garbage often containing bacteria and toxins that can cause vomiting, diarrhea, abdominal pain and tremors. The problem is most frequently seen in dogs and can be treated with antibiotics, antiemetics, fluid therapy and medications and procedures to limit absorption of toxins and damage to the gastrointestinal tract.

**gas colic** n. intermittent abdominal pain in horses that is caused by an increased amount of gas produced by bacteria within the large intestine. Abrupt diet changes can precipitate an episode of gas colic. Affected individuals often are restless, repeatedly lie down, paw, look at their sides and roll. Treatment can include pain relievers and the temporary placement of a stomach tube to allow infusion of substances (e.g., mineral oil) that ease the passage of material through the intestinal tract. *Also called* flatulent colic.

**gas gangrene** n. infection of wounds or diseased tissues with bacteria that produce pus and gas. Affected individuals may be in severe pain. Treatment can include antibiotics and surgical removal of damaged tissues.

**gaskin** n. the area between the stifle and the hock in the rear leg.

**gasterophilosis** n. disease caused by the larvae (i.e., bots) of a type of fly that attaches its eggs to the hair around a horse's legs. The larvae migrate throughout the body and eventually attach themselves to the inside of a horse's stomach. Treatment includes scraping the eggs from the horse's coat and medication to kill the bots in the stomach.

**gastrectomy** n. the surgical removal of part or all of the stomach.

**gastric** adj. pertaining to the stomach.

**gastric acid** n. the chemical compounds that are produced by glands within the stomach, have a very low pH and help with the digestion of food. Overproduction of gastric acid can cause or delay the healing of gastrointestinal ulcers.

**gastric acid inhibitors** n. medications that decrease the amount of gastric acid produced by glands within the stomach and help prevent and treat gastrointestinal ulcers.

**gastric dilatation and volvulus** n. a life-threatening condition, most often seen in large, deep-chested dogs, during which the stomach becomes filled with gas and flips into an abnormal position. Symptoms include unsuccessful attempts to vomit and a very enlarged abdomen. Immediate surgery is required to replace the stomach in its normal position and release the gas before permanent damage occurs. The spleen may also have to be removed. The stomach is permanently attached to the body wall during surgery to prevent the otherwise likely recurrence of the condition.

**gastric emptying time** n. the length of time that it takes for ingested food to leave the stomach and enter the intestinal tract. Prolongation of the gastric emptying time can be seen with physical or physiological abnormalities of the gastrointestinal tract.

**gastric stasis** n. a disease of rabbits caused by the accumulation of food and/or hair within the stomach. Gastric stasis is often seen in animals fed a diet that is too low in fiber from hay. Affected individuals lose their appetite and produce fewer stools than normal. Treatment can include fluid therapy, antibiotics, medications to stimulate movement of food through the gastrointestinal tract or surgery. *Also called* wool block.

**gastrin** n. a hormone that is secreted by glands within the stomach and stimulates the production and release of gastric acid and digestive enzymes.

**gastrinoma** n. a tumor within the pancreas that secretes gastrin. Affected individuals develop gastrointestinal ulcers that often bleed, vomiting, diarrhea and weight loss. Treatment can include gastric acid inhibitors and surgery to remove the tumor(s).

**gastritis** n. inflammation of the stomach that may be caused by infection, parasites, immune disease, dietary indiscretion, drugs or allergies. Affected individuals can vomit and become dehydrated. Treatment may include fluid therapy, antiemetic medications and addressing any underlying disorders.

**gastrocnemius rupture** n. a tear in the gastrocnemius muscle that is located in the hind leg and causes lameness and a tendency to place the entirety of the back of the lower leg on the ground. Treatment is difficult.

**gastroenteritis** n. inflammation of the stomach and intestinal tract that may be caused by infection, parasites, immune disease, dietary indiscretion, drugs or allergies. Affected individuals can develop vomiting, diarrhea and dehydration. Treatment may include fluid therapy, antidiarrheal and antiemetic medications and addressing any underlying disorders.

**gastroesophageal reflux** n. a backwards flow of stomach contents into the esophagus, which may be caused by anesthesia or abnormalities associated with the sphincter between the esophagus and stomach. Stomach acids present in the material can damage the esophagus. *See also* esophagitis.

**gastrointestinal (GI) tract** n. all of the parts (e.g., mouth, esophagus, stomach, small intestine and large intestine) of the organ system primarily responsible for nutrient intake, digestion and elimination of solid waste. *Also called* digestive and alimentary tract.

**gastropexy** n. a surgery that attaches the stomach to the body wall to prevent rotation of the organ. *See also* gastric dilatation and volvulus.

**gastroscopy** n. the use of a tubular instrument including a light source and a viewing device that is placed into the stomach through the mouth to allow the veterinarian to see inside and sometimes take samples or remove foreign objects.

**gastrostomy tube** n. a feeding tube that is surgically placed into the stomach allowing feeding of an animal that is unable or unwilling to eat on its own.

**gastrotomy** n. a surgical incision into the stomach.

**gauge** n. a measure of the diameter of a hypodermic needle, catheter or other similar device. Larger numbers indicate a smaller diameter.

**gauze** n. a piece of loosely woven material with many uses, including fluid absorption and to provide support within a bandage.

**gavage** v. to forcibly feed or provide liquids to an animal through a tube passed into the gastrointestinal tract.

**gelding** n. a castrated male horse - **geld** v.

**gene** n. a portion of a chromosome that codes for the production of a single protein. Most chromosomes and therefore most genes occur in pairs. Some inherited traits are determined by a single gene pair while others are the result of the actions of many genes - **genetic** adj.

**general anesthesia** n. unconsciousness and a lack of sensation through-

out the whole body that is induced by intravenous or inhaled drugs. General anesthesia is used to prevent discomfort and movement during major procedures (e.g., abdominal surgery). *Compare* local anesthesia.

**generalized** adj. involving the whole body or body part or occurring in many situations. *Compare* localized.

**generalized seizure** n. a type of seizure during which an animal loses consciousness, cannot remain standing and may become stiff, exhibit jerking motions, urinate and defecate. Generalized seizures result from abnormal electrical activity affecting a large portion of the brain. *See also* seizure. *Also called* grand mal seizure. *Compare* partial seizure.

**generalized tremor syndrome** n. a disease with an unknown cause that leads to the development of rhythmic, involuntary muscle contractions throughout the body and sometimes other neurologic abnormalities. The syndrome is most commonly seen in young, small, white dogs. Treatment can include drugs that suppress the immune system or decrease tremor severity. *Also called* little white dog shaker syndrome.

**generic drug** n. a medication that can be made by multiple manufacturers. The active ingredients in generic drugs are identical to those found in the trade or brand name medications.

**genital horsepox** n. *See* coital exanthema.

**genitalia** n. the organs of reproduction, especially those located on the outside of the body (e.g., the penis, testes and vulva) - **genital** adj.

**genitourinary** adj. pertaining to the reproductive and urinary tracts.

**genome** n. the complete set of an animal's genes.

**geographic ulcer** n. an ulcer most commonly affecting the eye of cats infected with a herpesvirus (i.e., feline viral rhinotracheitis). A geographic ulcer can form when multiple dendritic ulcers combine into a larger area of ulceration. *See also* dendritic ulcer.

**geriatric** adj. old.

**gestation** n. the period of time during which a fertilized egg within the uterus develops into a fetus that is ready to be born. *Also called* pregnancy.

**giant cell tumor** n. *See* malignant fibrous histiocytoma.

**giardiasis** n. disease caused by infection of the intestinal tract with *Giardia* protozoal parasites, which can cause diarrhea, vomiting and weight loss. The disease is transmitted through the ingestion of *Giardia* cysts that are shed in the feces of infected animals. Treatment includes medications that kill the parasite and supportive care. A vaccine is available, which may decrease clinical signs of giardiasis in dogs and cats. Humans can be infected with *Giardia*. *Also called* giardioses, lambliasis and lambliosis.

**GIF tube** n. a long catheter that can be placed into the tissues under the skin, sutured and remain in place for an extended period of time. GIF tubes are used in some animals that require subcutaneous fluid therapy on a regular basis.

**gigantism** n. *See* acromegaly.

**Gigli wire** n. a sharp wire that can be used to saw through bone, horn or other hard structures.

**gilt** n. a young, female pig that has not given birth.

**gingiva** n. the mucous membrane that surrounds teeth - **gingival** adj.

**gingival hyperplasia** n. a non-cancerous overgrowth of gingival tissue that can be caused by an accumulation of tartar and plaque on teeth or a genetic predisposition. Treatment includes dental cleanings and sometimes the surgical removal of the abnormal tissues.

**gingivitis** n. inflammation of the gingiva. Gingivitis can be caused by an accumulation of plaque and tartar on teeth, infection of the overlying gum or a genetic predisposition. Affected animals have red gums that bleed easily and may have bad breath. Treatment includes routine dental cleanings.

**gingivoplasty** n. the surgical reconstruction of the gingiva.

**girth** n. 1. a band of material that passes under a horse's chest and holds a saddle or harness in place. 2. the part of the body encircling the chest behind the shoulders and elbows.

**girth itch** n. a ringworm infection that affects the area under a horse's girth and saddle. *See also* ringworm.

**gizzard** n. *See* ventriculus.

**gland** n. an organ that produces and releases a substance (e.g., hormones, sweat and mucus) that is needed by other parts of the body - **glandular** adj.

**glaucoma** n. higher than normal pressure within the eyeball, which may be caused by infection, inflammation, genetic predisposition, anatomical abnormalities or cancer within the eye. Affected animals develop a red, painful eye that may appear enlarged and become blind. Treatment can include medications to decrease eye pressure, addressing any underlying conditions and surgery to reduce eye pressure or to remove the eye.

**globe** n. the eyeball.

**globulin** n. any of the large proteins that circulate in the blood, including antibodies and clotting factors.

**glomerular filtration rate (GFR)** n. a measurement of kidney function. A reduced GFR is seen with kidney insufficiency and failure.

**glomerulonephritis** n. abnormal deposition of antibodies and antigens within the kidneys, which can be caused by infection or inflammation elsewhere in the body. The kidneys become less able to filter blood leading to a buildup of waste products within the body and loss of water into the urine. Affected animals may develop increased thirst and urination, low blood protein levels, abnormal fluid accumulations, weight loss, high blood pressure and blood clots. The disease may progress to chronic renal failure. Treatment can include addressing any underlying conditions, diet changes and medications to decrease fluid accumulation, protein loss, blood clotting and to suppress the immune system.

**glomerulonephropathy** n. any disease that adversely affects glomeruli.

**glomerulus** n. one of many microscopic structures within the kidneys that filter blood to remove waste products, conserve water and produce urine - **glomerular** adj., **glomeruli** pl.

**glossitis** n. inflammation of the tongue.

**glottis** n. the vocal cords and the space between them within the larynx.

**glucagon** n. a hormone that raises blood sugar levels and is produced by the pancreas or used as a drug.

**glucocorticoid** n. one of several substances that affect the body's stress and inflammatory responses and are made by the adrenal glands or manufactured as a drug. Glucocorticoids are often used to decrease inflammation or to treat autoimmune disease and some types of cancer. Prednisone is a commonly used glucocorticoid.

**glucose** n. a form of sugar that is an important source of energy for cells. *Also called* dextrose.

**glucose curve** n. a procedure that measures blood glucose levels at regular intervals throughout the day. A glucose curve can be used to help monitor the effectiveness of insulin therapy in a diabetic animal.

**glucosuria** n. the abnormal presence of glucose in the urine, which can be seen with diabetes mellitus, some types of kidney disease, stress or the use of corticosteroids.

**gluteal muscles** n. the large muscles in the upper hindquarters that move the thigh.

**glycogen** n. the molecule that stores glucose in the muscles and liver and can be quickly broken down to provide energy for cells.

**glycogen storage disease** n. one of several similar diseases, some of which are genetic, causing glycogen to accumulate in tissues throughout the body. Affected animals are young and become progressively weaker, have poor growth and eventually die. *Also called* glycogenosis.

**goiter** n. a noncancerous enlargement of the thyroid gland producing a mass in the front part of the neck. Causes of goiter include dietary iodine levels that are either too high or too low, ingestion of large amounts of some plants (e.g., soybeans) or congenital diseases.

**goitrogen** n. a substance that when ingested can induce the formation of a goiter.

**gold therapy** n. the use of substances containing the metal gold to treat autoimmune or other types of disease.

**gonad** n. an organ that produces sperm or eggs (i.e., the testes or ovaries) - **gonadal** adj.

**gonadotropin releasing hormone (Gn-RH)** n. a hormone that is produced by a part of the brain or used as a drug and stimulates estrus behavior, ovulation or testicular function.

**goniodysgenesis** n. abnormal development of the part of the eye through which anterior chamber fluid is circulated, which often leads to glaucoma.

**gonioimplants** n. a device that is surgically implanted into the eye to drain anterior chamber fluid and treat glaucoma.

**gonioscopy** n. observation of the eye's filtration angle with a magnifying instrument.

**goose-honk cough** n. a repetitive, dry cough with a characteristic, honking sound that is often heard in dogs with a collapsing trachea.

**gout** n. abnormal accumulation of uric acid crystals within the joints or abdomen, which is seen most frequently in birds and reptiles. Causes include renal failure, high protein diets and congenital abnormalities in uric acid metabolism. Affected individuals may be lame, listless or die suddenly. Treatment can include low protein diets and medications that help remove uric acid from the body.

**gown** n. a garment that can be sterilized and worn over the body during surgery to reduce contamination of the surgical field.

**graft** v. 1. *See* transplant. 2. to place a newborn with a female animal that is not the biological mother and encourage her to raise it.

**grain** n. 1. the seeds of certain plants (e.g., oats) that can be fed to animals as a source of energy and other nutrients. 2. a measurement of weight. For conversions, see the appendices.

**grain overload** n. ingestion of sufficient quantities of a carbohydrate (e.g., grain) to cause illness. Affected ruminants and horses can become weak and dehydrated, have abdominal pain and diarrhea, develop laminitis and may die. Treatment can include removal of the carbohydrate source from the rumen or stomach, fluid therapy and medicines to prevent absorption of more carbohydrates, to normalize the pH of the gastrointestinal tract and body and to prevent or treat laminitis. *Also called* carbohydrate overload, rumen impaction and lactic acidosis.

**Gram's stain** n. a staining procedure that aids in the identification of bacteria. Gram-positive bacteria appear purple, and gram-negative bacteria are a red color when viewed under the microscope. Classifying a bacterial infection as being gram negative or positive can help determine the appropriate treatment.

**grand mal seizure** n. *See* generalized seizure.

**granula iridica** n. *See* corpora nigra.

**granulation tissue** n. pink, raised, bumpy tissue that develops as an open wound heals. Granulation tissue bleeds easily but is very resistant to infection and is not painful. When a good bed of granulation tissue is in place, surgery to cover the wound with skin can be performed if necessary. *See also* proud flesh.

**granule** n. a small particle.

**granulocyte** n. a white blood cell containing granules (e.g., neutrophils and eosinophils).

**granulocytic ehrlichiosis** n. *See* equine granulocytic anaplasmosis.

**granulocytopathy syndrome** n. *See* leukocyte adhesion deficiency.

**granuloma** n. a mass that can develop because of chronic infections or inflammation and consists of inflammatory cells, connective tissue and capillaries - **granulomatous** adj.

**granulomatous meningoencephalitis (GME)** n. an inflammatory disease affecting the brains of dogs that can cause weakness, difficulty walking, neck pain, seizures or other neurologic abnormalities. Treatment includes drugs that suppress the immune system, but most cases become unmanageable with time.

**granulosa-theca cell tumor** n. a tumor of the ovary that can secrete hormones causing abnormal heat cycles, behavioral changes, uterine infections, low blood cell counts and infertility. In most cases, surgical removal of the affected ovary is curative. Cats tend to have a more aggressive form of the cancer.

**grass crack** n. a vertical fissure in a horse's hoof that starts at the bottom of the foot and travels upwards. Grass cracks can be caused by poor conformation, overgrown hooves or injury. Corrective trimming and shoeing can promote healing of the crack. *Compare* sand crack.

**grass sickness** n. *See* equine dysautonomia.

**grass staggers** n. a disease of grazing animals that eat some species of grass (e.g., rye, Bermuda and Dallis grass) infected with certain types of bacteria or fungus. Affected individuals can demonstrate tremors, incoordination, stiffness and collapse that become worse with stress. Recovery is likely if the animals can be separated from the infected forage before they have ingested too much of it. *See also* hypomagnesemic tetany.

**grass tetany** n. *See* hypomagnesemic tetany.

**gravel** n. a foot abscess in horses that originates when foreign material enters through a wound or weak area between the sole and hoof wall. Gravel causes lameness and drainage that may erupt at the top of the hoof. Treatment can include paring out diseased hoof wall, antiseptic foot soaks, antibiotics, pain relief and bandaging.

**gravid** adj. pregnant.

**Gray Collie Syndrome** n. *See* cyclic hematopoiesis.

**gray matter** n. the portion of the brain and spinal cord that is composed primarily of nerve cell bodies. *Compare* white matter.

**greasy heel** n. *See* scratches.

**green slime disease** n. *See* epizootic catarrhal enteritis.

**greenstick fracture** n. an injury in which one side of a bone is bent and the other side is broken. Greenstick fractures are primarily seen in young animals and tend to heal very quickly.

**grit** n. hard particles that are eaten by birds and help to grind up food within the ventriculus.

**gross** adj. large or visible to the naked eye.

**growth hormone (GH)** n. *See* somatotropin.

**growth hormone responsive alopecia** n. a disease of dogs in which hair that is lost or thinning regrows when the animal is treated with growth hormone. *See also* alopecia X.

**growth plate** n. *See* physis.

**growth promotant** n. any drug or other substance that causes an increase in an animal's rate of growth. Antibiotics and hormones may be used as growth promotants.

**gruel** n. a mixture of food and water that forms a slurry, which can be easily eaten or passed through a feeding tube.

**grunt test** n. a procedure used to test cattle for hardware disease. The animal is made to bend its back or otherwise move in such a way as to feel discomfort associated with the disease. An affected animal will often grunt in pain.

**guaranteed analysis** n. a statement of the percentages of certain nutrients (e.g., protein, fat and fiber) contained within a commercially prepared animal food, which must be displayed on the packaging.

**guard hairs** n. the long, slick hairs on the surface of the coat of some animals.

**guarding** n. tensing of the abdominal muscles in response to pressure applied to the belly. Animals will often guard their abdomen to prevent a worsening of pain associated with disease or injury in the area. *Also called* splinting.

**gut** n. 1. the intestines. 2. a type of suture material made from intestines.

**gut loading** n. the process of feeding insects well so that they can provide good nutrition to the reptiles and amphibians that will eat them.

**guttural pouch** n. one of the air-filled structures located on each side of a horse's head below the ears.

**guttural pouch empyema** n. infection and pus accumulation within a horse's guttural pouch, which can cause nasal discharge, difficulty eating and breathing and swelling under the ear on the affected side. Treatment includes flushing out the affected guttural pouch and antibiotics.

**guttural pouch mycosis** n. a fungal infection within a horse's guttural pouch, which may cause potentially fatal nosebleeds, difficulty eating and Horner's syndrome. Treatment can include antifungal medications given systemically and infused into the guttural pouch and the surgical occlusion of blood vessels in the area.

**guttural pouch tympany** n. a distension of a horse's guttural pouch with air, which can be caused by upper respiratory tract infections, inflammation or anatomic abnormalities. Affected individuals develop a swelling under the ear and may have difficulty breathing. Treatment can include antibiotics, anti-inflammatories and surgery to provide an opening for air to escape from the area.

**gynecomastia** n. abnormal enlargement of a male animal's mammary glands, which can be caused by an estrogen-secreting tumor.

# H

**H₂ blocker** n. *See* histamine blocker.

**habituation** n. 1. the process of an animal becoming adapted to an environment. 2. the process of an animal adapting to a stimulus to the point where it no longer responds dramatically.

**habronemiasis** n. a disease of horses caused by the larvae of stomach worms transmitted by flies. Affected individuals develop skin or eye lesions that are slow to heal. Treatment can include medications that kill the larvae. Fly control can help prevent the disease. *Also called* summer and jack sores.

**hackles** n. the areas of hair along some animals' neck, shoulders and back that can be raised if they are frightened or aggressive.

**hair ring** n. *See* fur ring.

**hairball** n. *See* trichobezoar.

**hairy shaker disease** n. *See* border disease.

**hairy warts** n. *See* digital dermatitis.

**half-life** n. the period of time required for half of a substance to be eliminated from the body or to lose half of its radioactivity.

**halitosis** n. foul smelling breath.

**hamartoma** n. a benign overgrowth of mature cells that are normally located within a tissue. Some types of hamartomas are congenital defects. Surgical removal is curative.

**hand-rearing** n. the feeding and care of a young animal by humans either because the mother is unable or unwilling to do so or to encourage the newborn to become especially bonded to people.

**hard palate** n. the bony area located towards the front of the roof of the mouth. *Compare* soft palate.

**hardpad disease** n. *See* canine distemper.

**hardware disease** n. a disease of cattle caused by ingestion of sharp metal objects that poke through the animal's reticulum. Affected individuals can develop a fever, decreased milk production, pain, reluctance to move and may grunt or groan. Sometimes the metal will enter the chest and cause difficulty breathing and heart failure. Treatment can include antibiotics, surgical removal of the metal and supportive care. Placement of a magnet into the reticulum can help treat and prevent the disease. *Also called* traumatic reticuloperitonitis and traumatic gastritis.

**harelip** n. *See* cleft lip.

**harvest mite** n. *See* chigger.

**hatchling** n. a young bird that has recently emerged from the egg.

**haws** n. a condition in which the third eyelid protrudes upward further than is normal. Haws can be caused by dehydration and anatomic or neurologic abnormalities.

**hay belly** n. an enlarged abdomen that is caused by an animal eating a lot of often poor-quality hay. A better diet will usually improve the condition.

**head gate** n. a piece of equipment used to restrain large animals for examination and minor procedures (e.g., injections).

**head nodding** n. an abnormal up and down movement of the head. Head nodding can be seen when an animal bears weight on a lame leg. Some types of neurologic disease can cause an animal to nod its head while at rest.

**head pressing** n. persistently pushing the head against an object, which can be seen with some types of brain disease.

**head shy** adj. describes a horse that resists having its head handled.

**head tilt** n. a persistent leaning of the head to one side. Head tilts can be seen with diseases affecting the ear or brain.

**headshaking** n. a disorder of horses in which affected animals will repeatedly shake or toss their heads and may become so agitated as to be difficult to handle. Causes can include improperly fitting tack, pain, flies or poor behavior. In these cases, symptoms resolve once the underlying condition is addressed. Other individuals may suffer from irritating sensations thought to arise from the trigeminal nerve. Episodes can be triggered by exposure to sunlight, pollen and other environmental factors. Treatment is difficult but can include devices that block sunlight and/or apply pressure to the nose, providing shade, riding only during low light conditions and medications that may decrease the frequency and severity of headshaking.

**health certificate** n. an official document that is completed by a veterinarian stating that an animal or herd appeared free of contagious diseases on a certain date. Many health certificates will also contain information on vaccines or diagnostic tests.

**heart** n. the organ that is responsible for pumping blood throughout the body.

**heart attack** n. *See* myocardial infarction.

**heart block** n. an irregular heart rhythm that results from a lack of normal conduction of impulses through a portion of the heart. *See also* atrioventricular (AV) block and sinoatrial node block.

**heart failure** n. the inability of the heart to adequately pump blood and meet the needs of the body, which can be caused by many types of heart disease. *See also* congestive heart failure.

**heart massage** n. *See* cardiac compressions.

**heart rate (HR)** n. the number of times a heart beats per minute.

**heartworm disease (HW)** n. a disease primarily of dogs (infrequently seen in cats, ferrets and other species) that is caused by *Dirofilaria immitis* parasites transmitted through the bites of infected mosquitos. Affected individuals can develop coughing, difficulty breathing, exercise intolerance, weight loss, abnormal fluid accumulations and may die. Treatment includes medications to kill the worms and their larvae, rest and symptomatic care. Effective heartworm preventatives are available. *Also called* dirofilariasis.

**heat** n. 1. the period of time during which a female is receptive to mating and is capable of becoming pregnant. *Also called* estrus. 2. energy that raises the temperature of an object.

**heat exhaustion** n. exposure to high environmental temperatures or excessive activity that causes weakness, rapid breathing and sweating. Treatment includes rest, fluid therapy and procedures to cool the body. *Also called* heat prostration. *See also* heatstroke.

**heat tape** n. a device that can be placed in a reptile's cage to provide warmth. Burns are possible with the inappropriate use of heat tape.

**heat tolerance** n. the ability of some breeds or species of animals to thrive under hot conditions, often because of their effective heat loss mechanisms.

**heatstroke** n. high body temperature caused by excessive activity or high environmental temperatures. Affected animals can become restless, weak, depressed, comatose and die. Treatment includes fluid therapy, procedures to cool the body and supportive care.

**heave line** n. a groove visible on the side of the abdomen of a horse affected by recurrent airway obstruction. The extra effort required to breath causes the muscles in the area to enlarge.

**heaves** n. *See* recurrent airway obstruction.

**heavy metal** n. metals such as lead, zinc, arsenic, copper, iron and mercury that when ingested can cause disease. See the particular metal poisoning for details.

**heifer** n. a young cow that has not given birth more than once.

**Heinz body** n. an abnormal structure that can form on red blood cells, particularly in cases of poisoning (e.g., acetaminophen and onion). The immune system will destroy red blood cells with Heinz bodies, leading to anemia.

**helicobacteriosis** n. disease caused by infection of the gastrointestinal tract with *Helicobacter* bacteria. Affected individuals can develop vomiting, diarrhea, weight loss and ulcers. Treatment includes combination therapy with antibiotics and medications that decrease the acidity of the stomach.

**hemacytometer** n. *See* hemocytometer.

**hemagglutination** n. a clumping together of red blood cells that can disrupt blood flow through small vessels. Causes include autoimmune disease and infections.

**hemangioma** n. a benign tumor of blood vessels that is usually located in the skin and is dark red and soft. Surgical removal is curative. *Compare* hemangiosarcoma.

**hemangiopericytoma** n. a tumor most often located in or under the skin of older dogs. Hemangiopericytomas can be locally invasive but less frequently spread to distant sites. Treatment can include surgical removal, chemotherapy and radiation therapy. *Also called* malignant fibrous histiocytoma and spindle-cell sarcoma.

**hemangiosarcoma** n. an aggressive cancer of blood vessels. Tumors are most often located in the spleen, heart or just under the skin where they may appear as a red mass or bruise. Hemangiosarcomas may bleed, causing pale mucous membranes, weakness and collapse. Treatment can include supportive care and surgical removal of the tumor, but reoccurrence at the site of surgery or spread to other organs is likely. *Compare* hemangioma.

**hemarthrosis** n. a blood-filled joint.

**hematemesis** n. vomiting of blood.

**hematinics** n. medications or nutritional supplements that increase red blood cell counts.

**hematochezia** n. red blood in the feces. *Compare* melena.

**hematocrit (HCT)** n. a measure of an animal's red blood cell count.

**hematogenous** adj. produced by the blood or carried in the bloodstream.

**hematologic** adj. pertaining to blood cells. *Also called* hematological.

**hematology** n. the science and study of blood and/or the tissues that produce it.

**hematoma** n. an accumulation of blood within a tissue, often because of damage to a vessel. *See also* aural and ethmoid hematoma.

**hematopoiesis** n. the process of red and white blood cell and platelet production that occurs primarily in the bone marrow.

**hematuria** n. the presence of blood in the urine.

**hemilaminectomy** n. the surgical removal of the bone overlying one side of a part of the spinal cord. A hemilaminectomy can be performed to relieve pressure on the spinal cord that disrupts neurologic function.

**hemimandibulectomy** n. the surgical removal of half of the lower jaw, which is usually performed because of the presence of a large or invasive tumor.

**hemiparesis** n. weakness or incomplete paralysis affecting one side of the body.

**hemiplegia** n. paralysis of one side of the body.

**hemistanding** n. a procedure used to test neurologic function. The animal is held and forced to stand on a front and back leg on the same side of its body.

**hemivertebra** n. a birth defect in which one side of a vertebra develops incompletely. Most individuals have no problems associated with a hemivertebra. Others may require surgery to relieve instability of the spine or pressure on spinal cord.

**hemiwalking** n. a procedure used to test neurologic function. The animal is held and forced to hop sideways on a front and back leg on the same side of its body.

**hemoabdomen** n. an accumulation of blood within the abdominal cavity.

**hemobartonellosis** n. *See* feline infectious anemia.

**hemochromatosis** n. a disease in which iron accumulates in and disrupts the function of organs, especially the liver. Affected animals may have ingested toxic amounts of iron or be unable to effectively metabolize and excrete it, causing weight loss, lethargy, diarrhea and a poor quality coat. Treatment is difficult. *Also called* iron storage disease. *See also* iron toxicosis.

**hemoconcentration** n. loss of water from the blood, often because of dehydration. Hemoconcentration can cause a higher than expected red blood cell count and changes in other laboratory parameters.

**hemocytometer** n. a device that can be used to estimate the number of cells present in a blood sample. *Also called* hemacytometer.

**hemodialysis** n. a procedure during which unwanted substances (e.g., toxins or waste products) are removed from the body using a machine that filters the blood.

**hemoglobin (Hgb)** n. the protein that carries oxygen and is contained within red blood cells.

**hemoglobinemia** n. the abnormal presence in the blood of hemoglobin that is not contained within cells.

**hemoglobinuria** n. the abnormal presence of hemoglobin in the urine, which can be seen with diseases that cause red blood cells to rupture.

**hemogram** n. a table or graph that portrays the number and types of cells present in a blood sample.

**hemolymphatic system** n. the organs and tissues (e.g., blood vessels, lymph nodes and bone marrow) that produce and transport blood and lymph.

**hemolysis** n. rupture of red blood cells, which can reduce the oxygen carrying capacity of blood and cause anemia. Autoimmune disease, infections, toxins, transfusion reactions and tumors can all be associated with hemolysis - **hemolytic** adj. *See also* immune mediated hemolytic anemia.

**hemonchosis** n. a disease caused by *Haemonchus* worms within the rumen of cattle, sheep and goats. The parasites can remove large quantities of blood resulting in pale mucous membranes, rapid breathing, accumulation of fluid under the skin, weight loss and sometimes death. Treatment is becoming increasingly difficult because the parasite has developed resistance to many dewormers. *Also called* barber's pole worm.

**hemophilia** n. a genetic disease that prevents production of one of the coagulation factors necessary for blood to clot normally. Affected individuals (usually male) can bleed and bruise easily and excessively. Treatment includes blood or plasma transfusions and avoidance of trauma.

**hemoptysis** n. the coughing up of blood.

**hemorrhage** n. profuse bleeding from a damaged blood vessel or heart - **hemorrhagic** adj.

**hemorrhagic gastroenteritis (HGE)** n. a disease of dogs with an unknown cause. Affected individuals can very quickly develop bloody diarrhea, vomiting, depression, shock and may die. Treatment includes fluid therapy, antibiotics, antiemetics and drugs to protect the gastrointestinal tract.

**hemorrhagic shock** n. inadequate delivery of oxygen to tissues that is caused by profuse blood loss and may result in organ failure and death. Treatment can include fluid and oxygen therapy, blood transfusions, corticosteroids, medications to increase blood pressure and stopping the loss of blood.

**hemosiderin** n. a substance containing iron that can accumulate within tissues when an animal is affected by a disease that causes red blood cells to rupture.

**hemospermia** n. the abnormal presence of blood within the ejaculate, which can decrease fertility.

**hemostasis** n. 1. the cessation of bleeding, either through the natural formation of a blood clot or assisted by medical or surgical procedures. 2. lack of normal blood flow through a vessel - **hemostatic** adj.

**hemostat** n. a surgical instrument used to clamp off a blood vessel.

**hemothorax** n. an accumulation of blood within the chest cavity.

**hepatic** adj. pertaining to the liver.

**hepatic encephalopathy** n. neurologic dysfunction that arises from liver disease causing the accumulation of harmful waste products (e.g., ammonia) within the blood. Animals can develop bizarre behavior, seizures, head pressing, difficulty walking and blindness. Treatment includes addressing the underlying disease, diet changes and medications that decrease the production and absorption of waste products from the intestinal tract. *Also called* hepatoencephalopathy.

**hepatic enzymes** n. *See* liver enzymes.

**hepatic lipidosis** n. a disease most often seen in overweight animals caused by a lack of adequate food intake. In response, body fat is mobilized and deposited in the liver where it disrupts normal function. Affected individuals can lose their appetite and weight, have yellow or pale skin and mucous membranes, become weak, vomit and have diarrhea. Treatment may include fluid therapy, glucose supplements, corticosteroids, nutritional support and addressing any underlying conditions. *Also called* fatty liver.

**hepatic portal system** n. a number of veins that drain blood away from digestive organs (e.g., the intestinal tract and pancreas) to the liver.

**hepatitis** n. inflammation of the liver, which can be caused by infections, toxins, parasites, genetic factors and drugs. *See also* cholangiohepatitis, infectious canine hepatitis, infectious necrotic hepatitis, postvaccinal hepatitis and chronic active hepatitis.

**hepatobiliary** adj. pertaining to the liver and biliary system.

**hepatocutaneous syndrome** n. a skin condition that arises because of underlying disease of the liver, pancreas or other organs. Affected individuals can develop skin lesions, lethargy and loss of appetite and weight. Treatment is difficult but can include addressing any underlying disease, medications for secondary infections, vitamin and zinc supplements, diet changes and medicated baths. *Also called* superficial necrolytic dermatitis, metabolic epidermal necrosis and necrolytic migratory erythema.

**hepatocyte** n. the primary functional cell within the liver - **hepatocellular** adj.

**hepatoid gland tumor** n. *See* perianal gland tumor.

**hepatoma** n. a tumor of the liver. Some types are benign while others are malignant. Treatment can include surgical removal of the affected part of the liver as long as spread of the tumor is not evident.

**hepatomegaly** n. enlargement of the liver.

**hepatopathy** n. any disease affecting the liver.

**hepatoportal microvascular dysplasia** n. a disease of dogs in which blood vessels within the liver do not develop normally. Mildly affected animals may not demonstrate any clinical signs while more severe abnormalities can lead to bizarre behavior, vomiting, the formation of urinary stones and seizures. Treatment includes diet changes and medications that decrease the production and absorption of waste products from the intestinal tract.

**hepatosplenomegaly** n. enlargement of the liver and spleen.

**hepatotoxic** adj. capable of damaging the liver.

**hepatozoonosis** n. a disease of dogs caused by infection with *Hepatozoon* parasites transmitted by the ingestion of ticks. Affected individuals can develop fever, depression, pain, reluctance to move, weight loss, weakness, ocular discharge and diarrhea. No treatment has been shown to eliminate the infection, but combination therapy with antibiotics, parasiticides and anti-inflammatories can help control the disease.

**herbal medicine** n. a form of alternative veterinary medicine that relies upon the use of substances derived from plants or other natural products.

**herbicide** n. a chemical used to kill plants.

**herbivore** n. an animal that normally eats only plants.

**hereditary** adj. capable of being passed from one generation to the next. *Also called* heritable.

**hereditary chondrodysplasia** n. a genetic disease of sheep causing lambs to be born with long, thin and bent legs as well as other musculoskeletal problems. No treatment exists. *Also called* spider lamb syndrome.

**hermaphrodite** n. an animal that has genitalia with characteristics of both sexes and both ovarian and testicular tissue. *Compare* pseudohermaphrodite.

**hernia** n. the abnormal protrusion of tissues or organs through an opening in a structure. Hernias can be traumatic or developmental in origin. Surgery is usually necessary to move the displaced organs and tissues back to their normal location and to close the hernia. *See also* diaphragmatic, hiatal, inguinal, perineal, peritoneopericardial, scrotal and umbilical hernia.

**herniated disk** n. protrusion of disk material into the spinal canal. *Also called* slipped disk. *See also* intervertebral disk disease.

**herniorrhaphy** n. the surgical repair of a hernia.

**herpesvirus** n. a group of related viruses that can infect many species causing a variety of diseases. *See also* the specific disease for details (e.g., canine herpesvirus, coital exanthema and feline viral rhinotracheitis).

**heterobilharziasis** n. a disease of dogs caused by the parasite *Heterobilharzia americana*, which is transmitted to dogs when they contact water containing the organism. Affected individuals can develop vomiting, diarrhea, weight loss and skin lesions. Treatment with a medication to kill the parasite is usually effective.

**heterochromia iridis** n. eyes with different color irises or an eye with a multicolored iris.

**heterophil** n. a type of white blood cell, often specifically referring to forms that occur in the blood of non-mammals (e.g., birds and reptiles).

**heterosis** n. *See* hybrid vigor.

**heterozygous** adj. having two different forms of a gene, one on each chromosome in a pair. The dominant form of the gene is usually expressed by the individual. *Compare* homozygous.

**hiatal hernia** n. protrusion of abdominal organs through a naturally occurring opening in the diaphragm (i.e., the hiatus). Causes include trauma or birth defects that enlarge the hole. Affected animals can have difficulty breathing, pain, vomiting, regurgitation and drooling. Treatment may include medications to treat any secondary disorders (e.g., esophagitis or aspiration pneumonia) and surgery to replace the abdominal organs and partially close the hiatus.

**hiatus** n. a normal opening, often specifically referring to the opening in the diaphragm that allows passage of the esophagus, trachea, blood vessels and other structures between the chest and abdominal cavities.

**hiccup** n. an involuntary, spasmodic contraction of the diaphragm. Hiccups are most commonly seen in puppies and require no treatment.

**hide box** n. an enclosed area within an animal's cage where it can retreat when stressed or wanting to avoid stimulation.

**high dose dexamethasone suppression test (HDDS)** n. a laboratory test measuring the body's response to administration of a relatively high dose of dexamethasone. A HDDS test can be used to determine if an animal has the adrenal or pituitary form of Cushing's disease.

**high mountain disease** n. a disorder most often seen in cattle living at high altitudes. Affected animals often develop lethargy, swelling around the chest and neck, diarrhea, difficulty breathing and can die when forced to exert themselves. Treatment may involve moving the individual to a lower altitude, medications to remove fluid from the body and supportive care. *Also called* brisket disease and altitude sickness.

**high-rise syndrome** n. the injuries that are seen in cats that fall from balconies or out of windows.

**hilus** n. a depression in an organ where vessels or other structures exit - **hilar** adj.

**hindbrain** n. that part of the brain that controls involuntary functions (e.g., digestion and breathing) and helps coordinate movement.

**hindgut** n. the large intestine and rectum.

**hindlimb** n. a back leg.

**hinny** n. the offspring of a mating between a male horse and a female donkey. *Compare* mule.

**hip dysplasia** n. abnormal development of the hip that causes increased looseness to the joint and primarily affects dogs. Affected individuals may be lame and develop osteoarthritis at an early age. Treatment can include medications to protect or encourage healing of cartilage, anti-inflammatories, pain relievers and surgery to correct joint laxity in early cases or alleviate pain in advanced cases.

**hirsutism** n. an abnormally profuse growth of hair, which can be seen in horses with Cushing's disease or equine metabolic syndrome. *Also called* hypertrichosis.

**histamine** n. a compound produced by the body that incites allergic reactions and inflammation. Histamine can also bind with special receptors in the stomach and increase the secretion of gastric acid.

**histamine blocker** n. a type of drug often used to prevent or treat gastric ulcers by decreasing the production of gastric acid. Cimetidine is a commonly used histamine blocker. *Also called* $H_2$ blocker.

**histiocyte** n. a type of cell that is located within tissues and is a part of

133

the immune system - **histiocytic** adj. *Also called* macrophage.

**histiocytoma** n. a benign tumor that consists primarily of histiocytes and is most frequently seen in the skin of young dogs. These tumors tend to disappear over a period of a few months, but surgical removal can be considered if they are bothersome. *See also* fibrous histiocytoma and malignant fibrous histiocytoma.

**histiocytosis** n. an abnormally high number of histiocytes within a tissue. One form causes skin plaques and nodules that tend to wax and wane. Treatment can include corticosteroids and chemotherapy, but the response is variable. A second form, called malignant histiocytosis involves internal organs and is fatal. Dogs, especially Bernese Mountain dogs, are most commonly affected by both types of histiocytosis.

**histology** n. the science and study of tissues.

**histopathology** n. the microscopic examination of tissues in order to diagnose or study disease.

**histoplasmosis** n. a disease primarily of dogs and cats caused by infection with a *Histoplasma* fungus. Affected individuals can develop fever, weight loss, diarrhea, coughing, enlarged lymph nodes, skin lesions, lameness and eye abnormalities. Treatment with antifungal medications is usually effective.

**history** n. an account of an animal's past that includes its diseases, injuries, treatments, general care and lifestyle. A thorough history can help determine the likely causes of a patient's current condition.

**hive** n. a raised, red, usually itchy area that forms in the skin often due to an allergic reaction. *Also called* wheal. *See also* urticaria.

**hoarse** adj. describes raspiness or a loss of volume to an animal's vocalizations, which can be associated with overuse or disease affecting the vocal cords.

**hob** n. a male ferret.

**hobble** n. a device placed around a horse's legs that can be used to restrict its ability to run or kick.

**hock** n. *See* tarsus.

**holistic medicine** n. therapies focussed on treating the body, mind and spirit of an animal as a whole, often using forms of alternative medicine (e.g., homeopathy and acupuncture).

**hollow wall** n. *See* seedy toe.

**holosystolic** adj. occurring throughout the entire time that the ventricles of the heart are contracted and pushing blood into circulation.

**Holter monitor** n. a device that is worn over an animal's chest and records a continuous electrocardiogram for 24 hours. Holter monitors are useful when an animal is thought to have an intermittent heart arrhythmia. A similar device can be worn for a longer period of time and will record an electrocardiogram only when a person pushes a button when clinical signs associated with the arrhythmia are evident.

**homeopathy** n. a type of alternative medicine based on the use of extremely diluted solutions of substances that incite similar symptoms to those associated with an animal's disease.

**homeostasis** n. a balanced state that develops within the body or another system through continuous, small adjustments.

**homozygous** adj. having identical forms of a gene, one on each chromosome in a pair. *Compare* heterozygous.

**hoof tester** n. a device that applies pressure to parts of the hoof and helps localize a source of pain.

**hooks** n. pointed areas that develop on some horse's teeth with wear and can cause pain and difficulty eating. Treatment includes routine floating (i.e., filing) of the teeth.

**hookworm** n. a type of parasite that attaches to the intestinal wall, often causing vomiting, diarrhea and blood loss. Larval forms can migrate throughout the body. Animals are infected through the ingestion of eggs in the environment, the penetration of larvae through the skin or from suckling milk from an infected dam. Some types of dewormers can kill the parasites.

**hordeolum** n. inflammation of one of the glands within an eyelid, which is often associated with infection. A pus-filled cyst can develop necessitating treatment with warm compresses and antibiotics.

**horizontal transmission** n. any method of passing disease from an infected to an uninfected animal, except for that associated with a dam trans-

mitting disease-causing microorganisms or other pathogens to her young during pregnancy, birth or lactation. *Compare* vertical transmission.

**hormone** n. a substance produced in one part of the body that is secreted into the bloodstream and transported to another area to exert an effect.

**hormone-responsive incontinence** n. a disorder most commonly affecting spayed female dogs characterized by leakage of urine, especially when the animal is relaxed or sleeping. Treatment can include medications to tighten the sphincters that hold urine in the bladder or estrogen.

**horn flies** n. a type of fly that tends to congregate around the horns, shoulders, back and sides of cattle. They can be very irritating and cause individuals to lose weight and develop skin lesions. Treatment includes the use of pesticides or other substances that reduce fly populations.

**Horner's syndrome** n. a neurologic disorder that can be caused by trauma, tumors, infection, idiopathic disease or other lesions affecting nerves that run through the brain, ear and parts of the spinal cord. Affected individuals develop a narrowed pupil, drooping upper eyelid and elevation of the third eyelid. Treatment is directed towards the underlying disease.

**horse flies** n. large flies that can bite and draw blood from animals, transmit disease and cause extreme agitation. Control of horse flies can be difficult because high doses of pesticides are often required.

**hospice care** n. medical treatment that is aimed at relieving pain and providing comfort rather than curing disease in an animal nearing the end of its life.

**host** n. an animal in which another organism (e.g., parasite) lives.

**hot rock** n. a device that can be placed in a reptile's cage to provide warmth. Burns are possible with the inappropriate use of a hot rock.

**hot spot** n. *See* moist dermatitis.

**Hotz-Celsus procedure** n. a surgery used to repair entropion that involves removing a portion of the eyelid and suturing the incised skin edges together.

**humerus** n. the large bone in the upper forelimb located just below the shoulder.

**humoral immunity** n. resistance to disease that is conferred through antibodies. *Compare* cell mediated immunity.

**hunter's bump** n. an abnormally elevated part of the pelvis on one or both sides of a horse's lower back that is caused by injury to the connection between the spine and pelvis. Some cases are painful and lead to lameness while others may have healed and are asymptomatic. Treatment can include rest and anti-inflammatories. *Also called* jumper's bump.

**husbandry** n. the feeding, housing and general care of an animal.

**hutch burn** n. a disease of rabbits caused by the irritation of wet and dirty hutch floors. Individuals develop skin lesions, especially around their anus and genitalia. Treatment can include cleaning the affected skin, antibiotics and improving the animal's environment.

**hybrid** adj. describes an animal with parents of different breeds or varieties.

**hybrid vigor** n. the improved health that is seen in some mixed-breed animals. The increased genetic diversity of these individuals is often responsible for a lower incidence of disease. *Also called* heterosis.

**hydatid disease** n. a disease caused by cysts containing the larvae of *Echinococcus* tapeworms that can form in the liver, lungs, brain or other tissues. Clinical signs depend on the location of the cyst, and treatment can include its surgical removal. *Also called* echinococcosis.

**hydranencephaly** n. a birth defect often caused by viral infections contracted during pregnancy. The brain develops with less tissue than normal, and the resulting space is filled with cerebrospinal fluid. Affected individuals can be blind, circle, head press and have other neurologic abnormalities. There is no treatment.

**hydration status** n. the amount of fluid within the body. *See also* dehydration and overhydration.

**hydrocephalus** n. a birth defect in which the pressure exerted by abnormal accumulations of cerebrospinal fluid damages brain tissues. Affected individuals may be blind, have abnormal behavior and other neurologic abnormalities. Treatment can include corticosteroids or surgery to provide a path for drainage of cerebrospinal fluid.

**hydrometra** n. a uterus that is filled with a watery fluid. Treatment can include surgical removal of the uterus or hormones that stimulate expulsion of the fluid.

**hydromyelia** n. an abnormal accumulation of cerebrospinal fluid within the central canal of the spinal cord, which can be caused by trauma, tumors, inflammation or birth defects (e.g., Chiari type malformation). Affected individuals may have difficulty walking, weakness and pain. Treatment can include corticosteroids, surgery and addressing any underlying causes.

**hydronephrosis** n. dilation of the central part of the kidney, which is often a result of a blocked ureter causing urine to back up into the kidney. Treatment can include surgery to relieve any blockages or to remove the kidney.

**hydrophilic** adj. attracting or easily dissolved in water. *Compare* hydrophobic and lipophilic.

**hydrophobic** adj. repelling or afraid of water. *Compare* hydrophilic.

**hydrops** n. the abnormal accumulation of a watery fluid within a cavity or a tissue. *Also called* dropsy.

**hydrotherapy** n. treatments that involve running water over a body part to remove debris or decrease inflammation. Hydrotherapy can also refer to physical therapy that involves baths or swimming.

**hydrothorax** n. an accumulation of watery fluid around the lungs. *See also* pleural effusion.

**hygiene** n. cleanliness of the body or the environment as it relates to health.

**hygroma** n. a fluid-filled sac that develops to protect an area (e.g., a joint) from continued irritation and trauma. It may be drained if unsightly or bothersome but will often recur unless the source of irritation is removed. *Also called* false bursa and acquired bursa.

**hymen** n. a piece of tissue that can span the vagina in some female animals and is normally broken down during mating.

**hyoid apparatus** n. the bones and associated tissues that support the larynx and back of the tongue.

**hypalgesia** n. a decreased or low sensitivity to pain.

**hyperadrenocorticism** n. *See* Cushing's disease.

**hyperbilirubinemia** n. the presence of higher than normal levels of bilirubin in the blood, which can be seen with liver disease or increased destruction of red blood cells.

**hypercalcemia** n. abnormally high levels of calcium in the blood, which can be associated with hormonal disorders, some types of poisons, cancer and disease of the kidneys or bones.

**hypercalciuria** n. abnormally large amounts of calcium in the urine, which can lead to the formation of stones within the urinary tract.

**hypercapnia** n. excessively high levels of carbon dioxide in the blood, which can be caused by decreased respiratory function. *Also called* hypercarbia.

**hypercholesterolemia** n. abnormally large amounts of cholesterol in the blood, which can be associated with a recent meal, hypothyroidism or other metabolic disorders.

**hypercoagulability** n. an increased tendency to form blood clots.

**hyperelastosis cutis** n. a genetic disease causing animals to produce abnormal collagen, leading to the development of loose, stretchy skin that tears easily, a tendency to bruise or bleed and other disorders. No treatment is available. *Also called* dermatosparaxis, cutaneous asthenia and Ehlers-Danlos syndrome.

**hyperemia** n. an abnormal reddening of a tissue caused by the presence of larger than normal amounts of blood - **hyperemic** adj.

**hyperesthesia** n. an increased sensitivity to stimuli, especially touch or pain.

**hyperextension** n. to straighten a joint and continue the movement past the normal point, which can lead to pain and tissue damage.

**hyperflexion** n. to bend a joint and continue the movement past the normal point, which can lead to pain and tissue damage.

**hyperglycemia** n. greater than normal amount of glucose in the blood, which is usually associated with diabetes mellitus or stress.

**hyperimmune serum** n. the non-cellular portion of blood collected from an animal that has been stimulated to produce antibodies to particular diseases. Hyperimmune serum can be given to animals in need of immediate protection from those same diseases.

**hyperinsulinemia** n. higher than normal levels of insulin in the blood, which causes low blood sugar levels and can be associated with some types of pancreatic tumors.

**hyperkalemia** n. abnormally high levels of potassium in the blood, which can be caused by kidney disease, diabetes mellitus or Addison's disease. Hyperkalemia can lead to slow heart rates and death.

**hyperkalemic periodic paralysis (HYPP)** n. a genetic disease of Quarter Horses and related breeds that causes high blood potassium levels, muscle tremors, weakness and sometimes inability to stand and difficulty breathing. Treatment includes diet changes and medications that lower blood potassium levels.

**hyperkeratosis** n. a thickening of the skin's outer layer.

**hyperlipidemia** n. *See* lipemia.

**hypermature cataract** n. a cataract containing lens proteins that have begun to liquify, which can cause the cataract to shrink and/or induce eye inflammation. *See also* cataract and uveitis.

**hypermetria** n. exaggerated stepping motions (e.g., marching) displayed by animals with some types of neurologic disease.

**hypermotility** n. abnormally fast movement of ingesta through the intestinal tract or excessive gut contractions.

**hypernatremia** n. higher than normal levels of sodium in the blood, which can be seen with dehydration.

**hyperparathyroidism** n. a disease caused by abnormally high levels of parathyroid hormone in the body. *See also* primary hyperparathyroidism and renal and nutritional secondary hyperparathyroidism.

**hyperpathia** n. an exaggerated response to pain.

**hyperphosphatemia** n. a higher than normal level of phosphorous in the blood, which is often associated with kidney disease.

**hyperpigmentation** n. a darker color than is normally seen.

**hyperplasia** n. an increase in the number of normal cells present in a tissue or organ causing an enlargement or thickening - **hyperplastic** adj.

**hyperpnea** n. rapid or deep breathing.

**hyperproteinemia** n. a higher than normal concentration of protein within the blood, which can be seen with infections, dehydration, some types of cancer and other diseases.

**hyperreflexia** n. an exaggerated reflex response.

**hypersegmented neutrophil** n. a neutrophil with a greater number of lobes to its nucleus than is typically seen. Hypersegmented neutrophils can be associated with stress or the use of corticosteroids.

**hypersensitivity** n. an exaggerated immune response. *See also* allergy and anaphylaxis.

**hypersensitivity pneumonitis** n. a disease of cattle caused by an allergic reaction to inhaled mold spores found in contaminated hay or other feed. Affected individuals may develop difficulty breathing, coughing, loss of appetite and weight and low milk production. Treatment can include corticosteroids and preventing access to moldy feed. *Also called* extrinsic allergic alveolitis.

**hypersialism** n. overproduction of saliva, which often results in drooling. *Also called* hypersialosis.

**hypersomatotropism** n. *See* acromegaly.

**hypersplenism** n. any condition that causes the spleen to enlarge and results in a decreased number of one or more types of blood cells in circulation.

**hypersthenuria** n. highly concentrated urine, which can be seen with dehydration and indicates that the kidneys are functioning well. *Compare* isosthenuria and hyposthenuria.

**hypertension** n. high blood pressure, which is usually caused by another disease (e.g., kidney failure) in animals. Prolonged hypertension can damage many organs within the body, including the eye and the brain.

**hypertensive retinopathy** n. damage to the retina that is caused by high blood pressure and can lead to blindness. Medications that decrease inflammation and lower blood pressure can restore sight in some cases.

**hyperthermia** n. a higher than normal body temperature.

**hyperthyroidism** n. a disease most commonly seen in cats that is usually caused by a benign tumor secreting large amounts of thyroid hormone. Affected individuals can develop a ravenous appetite, vomiting, diarrhea, increased thirst and urination, weight loss and heart disease. Treatment may include medications, surgery or administration of radioactive iodine to decrease thyroid hormone levels. *Also called* thyrotoxicosis.

**hypertonic saline** n. an intravenous fluid that contains large amounts of salt, which can be used to quickly draw fluid into the circulatory system.

**hypertrichosis** n. *See* hirsutism.

**hypertriglyceridemia** n. a greater than normal level of triglycerides within the blood, which can be associated with a recent meal, hypothyroidism or other metabolic disorders.

**hypertrophic cardiomyopathy** n. a disease most frequently seen in cats that is caused by a thickening of the muscular walls of the heart's left ventricle. Some cases are due to primary heart disease while others are associated with hormonal disorders (e.g., hyperthyroidism). Affected individuals may develop difficulty breathing, collapse and lose use of their hind legs. Treatment can include addressing any underlying disorders and medications that improve heart function, decrease fluid accumulations and help prevent the formation of abnormal blood clots.

**hypertrophic osteodystrophy (HOD)** n. a disease most often affecting young, large-breed dogs that may be caused by nutritional imbalances, infections or other disorders. Individuals can develop fever, loss of appetite, lameness and swellings usually located in the lower front legs. Treatment includes pain relief and supportive care until the condition ends when the animal stops growing.

**hypertrophic osteopathy** n. a disorder causing enlargement and pain in the bones of animals with cancer or other lesions in their abdomen or chest. Treatment can include addressing the underlying disease and pain relief.

**hypertrophy** n. an increase in the size of cells that are normally present in a tissue or organ, which causes an enlargement or thickening - **hypertrophic** adj.

**hyperventilation** n. 1. abnormally rapid or deep breathing. 2. an increased amount of air within the lungs.

**hyperviscosity syndrome** n. an increased thickness to the blood, which adversely affects organ function and can be seen with cancers (i.e., myelomas) that secrete antibodies.

**hypervitaminosis A** n. a disease seen most frequently in cats fed a diet consisting almost exclusively liver. Hypervitaminosis A causes bony abnormalities in the spine and pain.

**hypervitaminosis D** n. a disease caused by overuse of supplements or medications containing vitamin D, which can cause abnormal tissue calcification and kidney failure.

**hyphema** n. blood within the aqueous humor of the eye.

**hypoadrenocorticism** n. *See* Addison's disease.

**hypoalbuminemia** n. low blood albumin levels, which can be caused by diseases affecting the intestines, kidneys or liver and may result in abnormal fluid accumulations throughout the body.

**hypoallergenic** adj. having a decreased tendency to incite allergic reactions.

**hypocalcemia** n. a decreased amount of calcium in the blood. Hypocalcemia can cause muscle tremors, weakness, stiffness, paralysis, bloat (ruminants), easily fractured bones and sudden death. *See also* parturient paresis, transport tetany and eclampsia.

**hypocapnia** n. a lower than normal amount of carbon dioxide in the blood, which can be caused by hyperventilation. *Also called* hypocarbia.

**hypochloremia** n. a decreased amount of chloride in the blood, which can be seen with vomiting and diarrhea.

**hypodermosis** n. *See* warble.

**hypofibrinogenemia** n. a lower than normal amount of fibrinogen in the blood, which can be caused by genetic disorders, liver disease and disseminated intravascular coagulation. Affected individuals have a tendency to bleed and bruise easily.

**hypogammaglobulinemia** n. a deficiency of antibodies in the blood, which can lead to an increased susceptibility to infections. Newborn foals and calves can be affected if they fail to quickly ingest or absorb colostrum. Other causes include genetic disorders, some types of cancer (e.g., myelomas), loss of antibodies through the gastrointestinal tract and viral infections that damage tissues responsible for producing antibodies.

**hypoglycemia** n. abnormally low levels of glucose in the blood, which can be seen with insulin secreting tumors, insulin overdose, poor diet, gastrointestinal disease, severe infections and liver failure. Affected individuals can have weakness, lethargy, muscle tremors and seizures.

**hypokalemia** n. a low blood potassium level, which is often associated with a displaced abomasum, kidney disease, diabetes mellitus, vomiting or diarrhea. Clinical signs can include weakness, loss of appetite and coma.

**hypokalemic polymyopathy** n. a disorder affecting cats caused by low blood potassium levels due to inadequate dietary intake or excessive loss through the kidneys or gastrointestinal tract. Affected individuals are weak, bend their head and neck towards their feet and can lose their appetite and have muscle pain. Treatment with a potassium supplement is usually successful.

**hypomagnesemic tetany** n. a disease caused by low blood magnesium levels seen in young calves with diarrhea or those fed only milk after about two months of age and also in lactating ruminants that are fed lush, green forage. Affected animals can develop abnormal behavior, muscle tremors, seizures or die suddenly. Treatment includes magnesium and calcium supplements and diet changes. *Also called* grass tetany, grass staggers and milk tetany.

**hypomyelinogenesis** n. any of a number of disorders in which myelin, the protective coating of nerves, fails to develop normally. Causes include genetics, poor nutrition or infections acquired during pregnancy. Affected individuals are young and develop tremors that are especially apparent when the animal is excited or eating, weakness and difficulty walking. There is no treatment, but in some cases the clinical signs resolve with time.

**hyponatremia** n. a decreased amount of sodium in the blood, which can be caused by diarrhea.

**hypoparathyroidism** n. disease caused by abnormally low levels of parathyroid hormone in the body, which may result from damage to or surgical removal of the parathyroid glands. Affected individuals develop low calcium and high phosphorous levels in the blood. Treatment can include calcium and vitamin D supplements.

**hypophosphatemia** n. a lower than normal amount of phosphorous in the blood most commonly associated with inadequate dietary intake. Affected animals can develop easily fractured bones, lameness, organ disfunction and poor growth and coat quality. *See also* primary hyperparathyroidism and postparturient hemoglobinuria.

**hypophysis** n. the pituitary gland - **hypophyseal** adj.

**hypopigmentation** n. a lighter color than is normally seen.

**hypopituitarism** n. *See* panhypopituitarism.

**hypoplasia** n. incomplete development of a structure - **hypoplastic** adj.

**hypoproteinemia** n. lower than normal levels of protein in the blood. *See also* hypoalbuminemia and hypogammaglobulinemia.

**hypopyon** n. the presence of pus in the anterior chamber of the eye.

**hyporeflexia** n. a diminished reflex response.

**hyposensitization** n. repeated injections of increasing doses of an allergen, which make an animal less susceptible to its effects.

**hypospadia** n. an abnormal urethral opening most commonly seen in males. The penis has a hole on its lower side through which urine can flow. Treatment involves surgical repair.

**hypostatic pneumonia** n. a disease caused by pooling of blood in the lungs because of an animal spending prolonged periods of time lying down in one position. Bacteria will often infect the tissues. Individuals may have difficulty breathing and cough. Treatment can include frequently changing an animal's position, antibiotics and supportive care.

**hyposthenuria** n. extremely dilute urine, which can be seen with kidney infections and some hormonal diseases. *Compare* isosthenuria and hypersthenuria.

**hypotension** n. low blood pressure, which may be seen with blood loss, heart failure or shock. Prolonged hypotension can damage many organs within the body.

**hypothermia** n. a lower than normal body temperature.

**hypothyroidism** n. a disease caused by destruction or improper development of the thyroid gland leading to an under-secretion of thyroid hormone. Affected individuals can develop lethargy, weight gain, hair loss, intolerance to cold temperatures, poor growth and neurologic abnormalities. Treatment with a thyroid supplement is generally very successful.

**hypotonic** adj. having decreased strength or muscle tone - hypotonia n.

**hypotrichosis** n. *See* alopecia.

**hypoventilation** n. 1. abnormally slow breathing. 2. a decreased amount of air within the lungs.

**hypovolemia** n. a decreased amount of fluid in the circulatory system, which may be caused by bleeding or dehydration - **hypovolemic** adj.

**hypovolemic shock** n. inadequate delivery of oxygen to tissues caused by profuse blood or fluid loss, which may result in organ failure and death. Treatment can include fluid and oxygen therapy, blood transfusions, corticosteroids, stopping the loss of fluid or blood and medications to increase blood pressure.

**hypoxemia** n. a decreased amount of oxygen carried within the blood. *See also* hypoxia.

**hypoxia** n. a lower than normal level of oxygen within the body that is most often caused by disorders of the lungs or heart. Affected animals often breathe quickly or deeply and have a rapid heart rate and blue-tinged mucous membranes. Treatment can include oxygen therapy and addressing any underlying disorders - **hypoxic** adj. *Also called* anoxia.

**hypoxic ischemic encephalopathy** n. *See* neonatal maladjustment syndrome.

**hysterectomy** n. the surgical removal of the uterus.

# I

**iatrogenic** adj. caused by medical treatment, procedures or personnel. For example, overuse of corticosteroid drugs can cause iatrogenic Cushing's disease.

**ictal** adj. pertaining to the period during which an animal has seizures. *Compare* preictal and postictal.

**icterus** n. *See* jaundice.

**idiopathic** adj. having an unknown cause.

**idiopathic acute hepatic disease** n. *See* Theiler's disease.

**idiopathic polyradiculoneuritis** n. an immune mediated disease most often seen in dogs that causes weakness progressing to paralysis. Some cases develop after the animal is bitten or scratched by a raccoon or after vaccination. Affected individuals remain alert and able to eat, drink, urinate, defecate and wag their tails but are otherwise paralyzed. Treatment is limited to supportive care, and most animals recover over a period of weeks to months if their respiratory muscles remain unaffected. *Also called* coonhound paralysis.

**idiopathic thrombocytopenic purpura** n. *See* immune mediated thrombocytopenia.

**ileocecal** adj. pertaining to the area where the ileum and the cecum join.

**ileocolonic agangliosis** n. a disease resulting in colic and death of white foals born to two Overo Paint Horse parents. The fetus fails to develop normal nerve cells in the colon, and there is no treatment. *Also called* lethal white syndrome and Overo lethal white disorder.

**ileum** n. the final section of the small intestine that is closest to the colon - **ileal** adj.

**ileus** n. failure of ingesta to move through the intestines, which can be seen with blockage of the intestinal tract or diseases that reduce intestinal contractions (e.g., peritonitis).

**imaging** n. the production of visual representations of internal body structures (e.g., radiography and ultrasonography).

**imbricate** v. to fold and surgically attach tissue in a pleated pattern to limit the ability of the structure to move or stretch.

**immature** adj. not yet fully developed. *Compare* mature.

**immature cataract** n. a cataract that is in the process of becoming bigger and more opaque.

**immune complex** n. an antibody that has bound to an antigen. Immune complexes can circulate in the blood and become lodged in various organs (e.g., the kidneys) where they damage tissues and disrupt normal function.

**immune mediated** adj. caused by the immune system.

**immune mediated arthritis** n. inflammation of joints that is caused by the deposition of immune complexes. Affected individuals can develop lameness, swollen joints, fever, lethargy and loss of appetite. Treatment includes addressing the underlying cause of the immune reaction and medications to decrease inflammation and suppress the immune system.

**immune mediated hemolytic anemia (IMHA)** n. a disease in which the immune system destroys the body's red blood cells resulting in a potentially life-threatening anemia. The disorder can be initiated by infections, medications or vaccines, but many cases seem to have no underlying cause. Affected animals can have pale or yellow mucous membranes, breathe rapidly and be very weak. Treatment may include drugs to suppress the activity of the immune system, supportive care, blood transfusions and addressing any underlying conditions. *Also called* autoimmune hemolytic anemia.

**immune mediated thrombocytopenia** n. a disease in which the immune system destroys the body's platelets. The disorder may be initiated by infections, medications or vaccines, but many cases seem to have no underlying cause. Affected animals can bleed and have extensive areas of bruising. Treatment may include drugs to suppress the immune system, supportive care and addressing any underlying conditions. *Also called* idiopathic thrombocytopenic purpura and autoimmune thrombocytopenia.

**immune system** n. the organs, tissues and cells that are responsible for identifying and removing potentially harmful organisms or other substances (e.g., cancerous or damaged cells) from the body. White blood cells, antibodies, lymph nodes, the thymus and bone marrow are all parts of the immune system.

**immunity** n. protection against disease provided by the immune system.

**immunization** n. *See* vaccination.

**immunocompetence** n. the presence of a well-functioning immune system that can protect an individual from many infections or diseases.

**immunocompromised** adj. *See* immunosuppressed.

**immunodeficient** adj. *See* immunosuppressed.

**immunoglobulin** n. *See* antibody.

**immunoglobulin A (IgA)** n. a type of antibody that provides immunity on the surface of mucous membranes (e.g., the lining of the intestinal tract).

**immunoglobulin E (IgE)** n. a type of antibody that plays an important role in allergic reactions.

**immunoglobulin G (IgG)** n. a type of antibody that is important in fighting infections. IgG levels tend to rise later in the course of disease.

**immunoglobulin M (IgM)** n. a type of antibody that is important in fighting infections. IgM levels tend to rise in the early stages of disease.

**immunomodulator** n. a type of drug that modifies the function of the immune system. For example, prednisone is commonly used to decrease immune reactions.

**immunostimulant** n. a drug that enhances the function of the immune system.

**immunosuppressed** adj. having an immune system that is not functioning adequately. Immunosuppression can be caused by genetic disorders, drugs and diseases that hinder the immune system or can be intentionally induced to treat disease (e.g., autoimmune disorders). *Also called* immunocompromised and immunodeficient.

**immunotherapy** n. treatments that are aimed at either increasing or decreasing the function of the immune system.

**impaction** n. a disorder caused by a material (e.g., feces) or body part (e.g., tooth) that is incapable of moving past a particular point. *See also* dental, fecal, meconium, rumen, cecal and crop impaction.

**imperforate** adj. lacking a normal opening.

**implant** n. an object placed and retained within the body for a prolonged period of time.

**impotent** adj. unable to maintain an erection sufficient for breeding.

**impression smear** n. a procedure in which tissue is pressed onto a glass slide so that the cells left behind can be studied under the microscope. *Also called* touch prep.

**imprinting** n. the process of a young animal becoming attached to a certain individual or learning basic behaviors.

**in situ** adj. at the original site.

**in utero** adj. within the uterus.

**in vitro** adj. outside of the body (e.g., in the laboratory setting).

**in vivo** adj. within the body.

**inactivated vaccine** n. *See* killed vaccine.

**inappetent** adj. having a reduced appetite for food.

**inbreeding** n. the mating of individuals that are closely related to one-another, which increases the chances of producing offspring with genetic abnormalities. *Compare* outbreeding.

**incarcerated** adj. trapped and unable to move out of a certain location.

**incipient cataract** n. a cataract that is just beginning to develop.

**incise** v. to cut - **incision** n.

**incisional biopsy** n. to surgically remove a sample of tissue from a larger structure (e.g., a tumor) for subsequent analysis to aid in diagnosis.

**incisor teeth** n. the teeth located in front of the canine teeth.

**incompetent** adj. describes an anatomic structure that is not functioning adequately - **incompetence** n.

**incomplete fracture** n. a break that does not involve the entire circumference of the bone.

**incontinence** n. *See* urinary and fecal incontinence.

**incoordination** n. the inability to produce smooth and synchronized movements.

**incubation** n. 1. the development of an embryo within the egg of some animals (e.g., birds and reptiles). 2. the period of time between becoming infected with and displaying clinical signs of a disease. 3. conditions provided to ensure the growth of microorganisms or immature animals.

**indication** n. a finding that calls for a particular diagnosis, prognosis or treatment. For example, the presence of parasite eggs in a fecal sample is an indication to prescribe deworming medications.

**indolent ulcer** n. *See* eosinophilic ulcer.

**induce** v. to cause a process or procedure (e.g., anesthesia or labor) to begin - **induction** n.

**induced ovulation** n. a characteristic of some species (e.g., cats) in which females do not ovulate until bred.

**indwelling** adj. left in place for a prolonged period of time.

**infanticide** n. the killing of a newborn animal, often by its dam or other members of the herd.

**infarct** n. an area within a tissue that is damaged because of a blocked blood supply.

**infection** n. the abnormal presence in an animal of microorganisms capable of causing disease - **infectious** adj.

**infectious arthritis** n. *See* septic arthritis.

**infectious bovine rhinotracheitis (IBR)** n. a disease of cattle caused by infection with a herpesvirus. Affected individuals can develop fever, depression, cough, nasal and ocular discharge and difficulty breathing. Antibiotics can help control secondary bacterial infections, but no specific treatment for the virus exists. Preventative vaccines are available. The same virus can cause abortion and infections of the reproductive tract, eyes, brain and mammary glands.

**infectious bronchitis** n. a contagious, viral disease of chickens that can cause coughing, sneezing, difficulty breathing, reduced growth, low egg production and death. Treatment is limited to supportive care and antibiotics for secondary bacterial infections. Preventative vaccines exist.

**infectious canine hepatitis (ICH)** n. a contagious, viral disease of dogs and some wildlife species. Affected individuals often develop a fever, low white blood cell counts, lethargy, loss of appetite, red eyes and nasal and ocular discharge. Treatment can include supportive care, antibiotics for secondary infections and blood transfusions. Upon recovery, some animals may develop a blue-white discoloration of the cornea. Preventative vaccines are available. *See also* blue eye.

**infectious coryza** n. a contagious disease of chickens caused by infection with *Haemophilus paragallinarum* bacteria. Affected individuals can develop nasal discharge, sneezing, facial swelling and diarrhea. Treatment includes antibiotics and supportive care. Preventative vaccines are available.

**infectious keratoconjunctivitis** n. a contagious, bacterial infection of the eyes of cattle, sheep and goats, which can cause squinting, corneal ulcers, drainage and redness. Environmental irritants and stress may predispose animals to the disease. Treatment can include antibiotics, shade, anti-inflammatories and surgery to speed the healing of corneal lesions. Preventative vaccines can help reduce the severity of the disease. *Also called* pinkeye.

**infectious laryngotracheitis** n. a contagious, viral disease of chickens that can cause coughing, difficulty breathing, ocular discharge and death. Treatment may include supportive care, expectorants and antibiotics for secondary bacterial infections. Preventative vaccines are available.

**infectious necrotic hepatitis** n. *See* Black disease.

**infectious stomatitis** n. a disease of reptiles caused by infection of the mouth with bacteria or other microorganisms. Affected individuals develop oral lesions and lose their appetite. Poor nutrition, parasites, trauma and other stressors may predispose an animal to the disease. Treatment can include antibiotics, topical antiseptics, surgical removal of damaged tissues and debris, addressing any underlying issues and supportive care. *Also called* mouth rot.

**inferior** adj. below. *Compare* superior.

**infertile** adj. unable to produce offspring - **infertility** n.

**infestation** n. the abnormal presence of parasitic organisms (e.g., fleas or worms) within or on an animal's body.

**infiltration** n. the movement or injection of substances (e.g., cells or fluids) into a tissue where they are not typically located - **infiltrative** adj.

**inflammation** n. pain, heat, swelling and redness of a tissue that develops in response to a wide variety of insults, including infection, allergies, trauma and immune disorders.

**inflammatory bowel disease (IBD)** n. a disorder in which inflammatory cells (e.g., lymphocytes or eosinophils) infiltrate sections of the intestinal tract as part of an abnormal immune reaction. Affected individuals may develop vomiting, diarrhea and loss of appetite and weight. Treatment can include diet changes and medications that suppress the immune system or decrease inflammation within the gastrointestinal tract. If the disease affects only a small section of bowel, surgery to remove that area can be considered.

**influenza** n. a contagious virus that usually infects the respiratory system causing fever, sneezing, coughing, loss of appetite and nasal and ocular discharge. Occasionally, an influenza virus that infects one species will mutate and gain the ability to infect a new species creating the possibility for a widespread epidemic. Treatment may include antiviral medications, antibiotics for secondary infections, anti-inflammatories and supportive care. *See also* equine and avian influenza.

**informed consent** n. a legal term indicating that the owner of an animal has given permission for a procedure or treatment after being made aware of the potential risks and any other pertinent information.

**infraspinatus contracture** n. a disorder in which a muscle in the shoulder scars and shortens, often because of trauma to the area. Individuals will hold and swing a front leg out to the side at an awkward angle. Surgery can be curative.

**infundibular follicular cyst** n. *See* epidermal inclusion cyst.

**infundibular keratinizing acanthoma** n. *See* keratoacanthoma.

**infusion** n. the slow administration of a liquid into the circulatory system or other part of the body.

**ingesta** n. food, water and other materials that enter the body through the mouth and travel through the gastrointestinal tract.

**ingluvitis** n. inflammation of a bird's crop.

**inguinal** adj. pertaining to the area between the thigh and abdomen (i.e., the groin).

**inguinal hernia** n. protrusion of abdominal contents through a hole in the inguinal region. Causes include trauma or birth defects that enlarge a normal passageway in this area. Affected animals can have abdominal pain and a swelling in the inguinal region or scrotum. Surgical repair is necessary if abdominal organs have or are likely to become trapped in the hernia.

**inhalant dermatitis** n. inflammation of the skin that is a result of allergic reactions to inhaled substances (e.g., pollen). *See also* atopic dermatitis.

**inhalation pneumonia** n. *See* aspiration pneumonia.

**inhalational anesthesia** n. unconsciousness and a lack of sensation throughout the whole body that is induced by drugs inhaled into the lungs. *See also* general anesthesia.

**inhale** v. to breathe air or other substances into the lungs - **inhalation** n. *Compare* exhale.

**inherit** v. to acquire a trait through the genetic material passed on by a parent - **inheritance** n.

**inhibit** v. to prevent or lessen a process or response - **inhibition** n.

**inject** v. to force a liquid into the body or another object, often using a syringe and needle - **injectable** adj., **injection** n.

**injected** adj. 1. introduced into a tissue using a needle and syringe. 2. having an abnormal buildup of blood within vessels, which makes them more red and prominent - **injection** n.

**inner ear** n. the portion of the ear that contains the nerves that transmit auditory signals to the brain and structures that play an important role in balance. *See also* middle and outer ear.

**innervation** n. all of the nerves that serve a part of the body - **innervate** v.

**innocent murmur** n. a murmur that is heard in a young animal but is not caused by a heart defect and does not adversely affect the individual. Most innocent murmurs will disappear as the animal matures.

**inoculate** v. 1. to introduce a substance (e.g., killed bacteria) into the body to induce a protective immune response. 2. to place microorganisms into a material used to promote their growth - **inoculation** n.

**inotrope** n. a drug that increases (i.e., positive inotrope) or decreases (i.e., negative inotrope) the force of the heart's contractions. Digitalis is a commonly used positive inotrope - **inotropic** adj.

**insect growth regulator** n. a chemical that prevents external parasites (e.g., fleas) from maturing and reproducing.

**insecticide** n. a chemical that kills insects.

**insectivore** n. an animal that eats primarily insects.

**inseminate** v. to introduce sperm into a female's reproductive tract, either through natural breeding or with instruments.

**insoluble** adj. incapable of being dissolved by a liquid. *Compare* soluble.

**inspissate** v. to thicken, often because of evaporation of water - **inspissated** adj.

**insufficiency** n. decreased function of a body part or process that causes only mild symptoms in the animal. Organ insufficiency can progress to failure.

**insufflation** n. to blow a substance (e.g., a gas containing aerosolized drugs) into a body part.

**insulin dependent** adj. describes a diabetic animal that requires insulin injections to control the disease adequately. *Compare* insulin independent.

**insulin independent** adj. describes an animal with diabetes that can be controlled through the use of diet changes, weight loss and drugs other than insulin. *Compare* insulin dependent.

**insulin resistant** adj. describes a diabetic animal with blood sugar levels that do not fall as expected with insulin therapy. Insulin resistance can be seen in animals suffering from other diseases in addition to their diabetes.

**insulin shock** n. over-administration or production of insulin (e.g., by a tumor) that lowers blood sugar levels to the point of inducing seizures, unconsciousness and sometimes death.

**insulin:glucose ratio** n. a laboratory test that can help diagnose the presence of an insulin-secreting tumor.

**insulinoma** n. a pancreatic tumor that secretes insulin and sometimes other hormones and can cause low blood sugar levels, weakness, difficulty walking, changes in behavior, seizures and collapse. Treatment may include surgical removal of the tumor, changes in diet and feeding schedules and drugs that raise blood sugar levels. *Also called* islet cell tumor.

**intact** adj. not neutered.

**integument** n. the skin.

**intensive care unit (ICU)** n. a part of the veterinary hospital staffed and equipped to take care of severely sick or injured animals.

**intention tremor** n. trembling, usually of the head, that gets worse when an animal concentrates on something (e.g., food) and attempts to move. Intention tremors can be an indication of a lesion affecting the cerebellum.

**intercostal** adj. between ribs.

**interdigital** adj. between fingers or toes.

**interferon** n. a substance produced by the body or used as a drug that can stimulate the immune system to fight infection.

**intersex** adj. having behavioral or physical characteristics of both sexes. *See also* hermaphrodite and pseudohermaphrodite.

**interstitial** adj. within the spaces between cells or body parts.

**interstitial pattern** n. a finding on a chest radiograph indicating that the tissues surrounding the alveoli in the lung are thickened.

**intertrigo** n. infection and inflammation of skin folds. The moist environment is an ideal site for recurrent bacterial infections. Treatment can include topical antiseptic and drying solutions, antibiotics and surgery.

**intervertebral disk disease (IVDD)** n. deterioration of or injury to the disks located between spinal vertebrae. Disk material bulges or ruptures into the spinal column resulting in pain, difficulty walking or paralysis. Chondrodystrophic breeds of dogs (e.g., Dachshunds) are commonly affected.

Treatment can include pain relief, rest, anti-inflammatories and surgery to relieve pressure on the spinal cord. *Also called* degenerative disk disease.

**intestine** n. the part of the gastrointestinal tract between the stomach and anus that plays a major role in digestion and absorption of nutrients - **intestinal** adj. *See also* small and large intestine.

**intolerance** n. the inability to maintain normal function in the presence of a certain substance (e.g., a drug or type of food) or in a particular situation - **intolerant** adj.

**intoxication** n. the condition of being poisoned.

**intra-articular** adj. within a joint.

**intracameral** adj. within the anterior chamber of the eye.

**intracardiac (IC)** adj. within the heart.

**intracellular** adj. within cells.

**intracranial** adj. within the skull.

**intracranial pressure** n. the pressure within the space between the brain and skull. Sustained increases in intracranial pressure are often caused by bleeding or swelling and can lead to brain damage.

**intractable** adj. difficult to manage, improve or cure.

**intradermal** adj. within the skin.

**intradermal skin test** n. a procedure involving multiple injections of potential allergens into the skin. The animal responds by forming red, raised areas around the antigens to which it is allergic. Knowing what substances incite an allergic reaction helps determine appropriate treatment.

**intramammary infusion** n. the administration of liquid medications into the mammary gland through the teat opening.

**intramedullary** adj. 1. within the space containing marrow at the center of bones. 2. within the spinal cord.

**intramural** adj. within the wall of a hollow organ.

**intramuscular (IM)** adj. within a muscle.

**intranasal (IN)** adj. within the nose.

**intraocular** adj. within the eye.

**intraocular pressure (IOP)** n. the pressure within the eye. Changes in intraocular pressure can be seen with various diseases. *See also* glaucoma.

**intraosseous** adj. within a bone, sometimes referring specifically to the space at the center of bones that contains marrow.

**intraperitoneal (IP)** adj. within the peritoneal cavity.

**intravascular** adj. within blood vessels. *Compare* extravascular.

**intravenous (IV)** adj. within a vein.

**intravenous pyelogram (IVP)** n. a procedure in which a contrast agent is injected into a vein to highlight the kidneys and ureters when radiographs are taken. *Also called* intravenous urography.

**intravitreal** adj. within the vitreous chamber of the eye.

**intrinsic** adj. 1. originating from inside the body or body part. 2. essential. *Compare* extrinsic.

**intromission** n. the insertion of one structure into another (e.g., penis into vagina).

**intubation** n. the placement of a tube into a body part. *See also* endotracheal and nasogastric tube and orogastric intubation.

**intussusception** n. an abnormal telescoping or swallowing of a part of the gastrointestinal tract by an adjacent section, which blocks the movement of ingesta and causes vomiting and abdominal pain. Many intussusceptions are caused by disorders that alter intestinal contractions (e.g., prolonged diarrhea). Surgery is necessary to normalize the alignment of or removal of the affected structures.

**invasive** adj. 1. tending to spread. 2. penetrating the skin.

**involuntary muscle** n. *See* smooth muscle.

**involution** n. 1. a normal decrease in size of an organ that can occur after some of its functions have been completed. For example, the uterus will involute to its prepregnancy size after birth has occurred. 2. a normal degeneration or shrinking of tissues that occurs with age.

**iodine** n. an element the correct dietary levels of which are essential to the normal function of the thyroid gland. Iodine containing solutions can also be used as antiseptics.

**iodine deficiency** n. inadequate amounts of iodine in the diet that can lead to enlargement of the thyroid gland (i.e., goiter) and hypothyroidism in severe cases. Improving the diet will usually reverse the condition unless permanent damage has occurred.

**iodine toxicosis** n. disease caused by ingestion of too much iodine, which can cause thyroid enlargement (i.e., goiter), flaky skin, hair abnormalities, weakness, loss of appetite and other problems. Most clinical signs will resolve with time and removal of the source of iodine.

**iodine-131** n. a radioactive form of iodine that is a safe and effective way to treat hyperthyroidism in cats. After injection, iodine-131 accumulates in and destroys parts of the thyroid gland.

**ionized calcium** n. the portion of calcium in the bloodstream that is not bound to protein and is free to engage in metabolic reactions. Assessing ionized calcium may be necessary when other factors (e.g., low blood albumin levels) make total calcium measurements unreliable.

**ipsilateral** adj. on the same side. *Compare* contralateral.

**iridectomy** n. the surgical removal of a part of the iris.

**iridic cyst** n. a benign, fluid-filled structure that can be attached to the iris or float in the anterior chamber of the eye. Multiple cysts can affect a single eye. Most cases require no treatment, but if bothersome or responsible for secondary diseases (e.g., glaucoma) the cysts can be surgically deflated or removed.

**iridocorneal angle** n. *See* filtration angle.

**iridocyclitis** n. *See* anterior uveitis.

**iris** n. the muscular structure that surrounds and determines the size of an eye's pupil - **iridal, iridial, iridic** adj.

**iris atrophy** n. a degeneration of the iris that can occur with age. Affected individuals can still see well but have an iris that is enlarged, misshapen, does not constrict normally when exposed to light or has holes in it. Treatment is not necessary.

**iris prolapse** n. protrusion of the iris through a perforation in the cornea. Surgery is necessary to return the iris to its normal position and repair the cornea or to remove the eye.

**iritis** n. inflammation of the iris. *See also* anterior uveitis.

**iron** n. an element that is an important part of the diet to ensure normal development and function of red blood cells.

**iron deficiency anemia** n. anemia caused by a lack of adequate amounts of iron in the diet, which is needed to make new red blood cells. Treatment includes iron supplements and addressing any underlying conditions (e.g., blood loss).

**iron storage disease** n. *See* hemochromatosis.

**iron toxicosis** n. a disease caused by ingestion of too much iron. Affected individuals can develop lethargy, vomiting, diarrhea, trembling, infections, tissue calcification, liver failure, neurologic abnormalities, a poor quality coat, weight loss and may die. Treatment is difficult but can include repeated blood withdrawals, fluid therapy and medications that bind and aid in the excretion of iron.

**irrigate** v. to thoroughly wash a wound or cavity by flushing it with a liquid to remove foreign material and microorganisms - **irrigation** n.

**irritable bowel syndrome** n. a condition in which stress causes an animal to develop diarrhea. Treatment can include reducing stress, a bland diet and medications that reduce diarrhea.

**ischemia** n. a lack of adequate blood delivery to a body part, which can be caused by a blocked blood vessel and result in tissue damage and loss of function - **ischemic** adj.

**ischiatic paralysis** n. *See* calving paralysis.

**islet cell tumor** n. *See* insulinoma.

**isoenzyme testing** n. *See* alkaline phosphatase isoenzyme test.

**isolate** v. 1. to keep an animal apart from other animals, often to prevent transmission of disease. 2. to separate a structure from nearby tissues in surgery.

**isosporosis** n. disease caused by a type of *Coccidia* parasite. *See also* coccidiosis.

**isosthenuria** n. dilute urine, which can indicate that the kidneys are not functioning normally. *Compare* hypersthenuria and hyposthenuria.

# J

**Jaagsiekte** n. *See* pulmonary adenomatosis.

**jack** n. a male donkey.

**jack sores** n. *See* habronemiasis.

**Jacobson's organ** n. *See* vomeronasal organ.

**Jamshidi needle** n. an instrument that can be used to sample marrow from within a bone.

**jaundice** n. yellow discoloration of the skin, eyes, mucous membranes and other tissues caused by abnormally high levels of bilirubin in the blood. Jaundice can be a sign of disease affecting the liver or red blood cells. *Also called* icterus.

**jejunostomy tube** n. a feeding tube that is surgically placed into the middle part of the small intestine allowing an animal to be fed while bypassing the preceding sections of the gastrointestinal tract.

**jejunum** n. the middle and longest section of the small intestine.

**jenny** n. a female donkey.

**jill** n. a female ferret.

**Johne's disease** n. *See* paratuberculosis.

**joint** n. a structure that connects bones and often consists of bone, cartilage, ligaments, fibrous tissue, membranes and joint fluid. Most joints allow motion while still providing stability.

**joint capsule** n. the fibrous and membranous structure that surrounds a joint space and contains joint fluid.

**joint effusion** n. the presence of an increased amount of fluid within a joint.

**joint fluid** n. the slippery fluid that lubricates, absorbs shock and nourishes cartilage within a joint. *Also called* synovial fluid.

**joint ill** n. *See* septic arthritis.

**joint mice** n. pieces of bone or cartilage that float in joint fluid and can cause pain and arthritis. Treatment can include surgery to remove the joint mice and anti-inflammatories.

**jugular groove** n. a vertical depression on both sides of the neck in which a jugular vein normally lies.

**jugular pulse** n. a rush of blood that is visible in the jugular vein. An abnormally strong jugular pulse can be associated with heart disease.

**jugular vein** n. one of two blood vessels that lie on either side of the neck and drain blood from the head back to the heart.

**jumper's bump** n. *See* hunter's bump.

**juvenile cataract** n. a cataract that develops in a young animal usually because of genetic factors.

**juvenile cellulitis** n. *See* puppy strangles.

**juvenile onset** adj. describes a condition that develops in a young animal. *Compare* adult onset.

**juvenile vaginitis** n. *See* puppy vaginitis.

# K

**keel** n. the bony ridge that runs down the midline of a bird's chest. *Also called* carina.

**keel bursitis** n. *See* breast blister.

**kennel cough (KC)** n. a term used to describe a contagious respiratory disease that produces a dry, persistent cough in dogs and can be caused by a number of bacteria or viruses. In rare cases, some susceptible individuals may develop pneumonia. Therapy can include antibiotics, cough suppressants and supportive care. Vaccination helps to prevent some forms of the disease.

**keratectomy** n. the surgical removal of a portion of the cornea.

**keratic precipitates** n. particles that become attached to the inside of the cornea, usually because of infection within the eye.

**keratin** n. the protein that can be found in and toughens nails, hooves, hair and the outer layer of the skin.

**keratinization** n. the process of keratin being deposited in tissues making them harder - **keratinized** adj.

**keratitis** n. inflammation of the cornea. *See also* chronic superficial keratitis and eosinophilic keratitis.

**keratoacanthoma** n. a benign skin tumor of dogs that sometimes has a central area of hard tissue. Surgical excision is curative. Some individuals develop a form of the disease in which multiple tumors arise in the skin. These cases may be improved with medications. *Also called* infundibular keratinizing acanthoma.

**keratoconjunctivitis sicca (KCS)** n. a lack of tear production that is often associated with an autoimmune disease of the tear glands in dogs, but injuries, infections, drug treatment and genetics can also be to blame. Affected individuals may develop recurrent eye infections, discharge from the eyes and corneal ulcers and pigmentation. Treatment can include medications to control the immune disorder and stimulate tear production, artificial tear and antibiotic solutions and surgery to move ducts carrying saliva to the eye. *Also called* dry eye.

**keratolytic** adj. having properties that break down keratin. Keratolytic substances are often added to shampoos to help decrease the formation of skin flakes and treat some types of skin disease.

**keratoma** n. *See* keratosis.

**keratopathy** n. any disease affecting the cornea, excluding those associated with inflammation. *See also* stromal lipid keratopathy.

**keratoplasty** n. the surgical reconstruction of the cornea.

**keratosis** n. an overgrowth of the layer of skin containing keratin that causes areas of thickened and hard skin. *See also* actinic keratosis.

**keratotomy** n. a surgical incision into the cornea.

**ketoacidosis** n. a lowering of the body's pH caused by fat breakdown and the production of ketones. *See also* diabetic ketoacidosis, bovine ketosis and pregnancy toxemia.

**ketone** n. a breakdown product of fat metabolism. *Also called* ketone body.

**ketonemia** n. the presence of abnormally large amounts of ketones in the blood. *See also* diabetes ketoacidosis, bovine ketosis and pregnancy toxemia.

**ketonuria** n. the abnormal presence of ketones in the urine.

**ketosis** n. *See* ketoacidosis.

**Key-Gaskell syndrome** n. *See* feline dysautonomia.

**kidding** n. the process through which a doe gives birth to a newborn goat.

**kidney** n. one of a pair of organs in the body that filter blood, conserve water and excrete waste products in the form of urine.

**kidney failure** n. *See* renal failure.

**kidney stone** n. an accumulation of minerals and other substances within the kidney that form hard objects of varying sizes. Individuals may develop bloody urine and be in pain. Treatment can include medications or foods that dissolve some types of stones and surgery to remove the stone or kidney. Treatment may not be necessary if the effects of the kidney stones are minimal. *Also called* nephrolith.

**killed vaccine** n. a type of vaccine containing killed microorganisms. Killed vaccines generally are not as effective as modified live vaccines but can be safer in some situations (e.g. during pregnancy). *Also called* inactivated vaccine.

**kilocalorie (kcal)** n. one thousand calories, a unit of measurement used to quantify the energy content of food or energy expended by an animal.

**kindling** n. the process through which a doe gives birth to newborn rabbits.

**kissing spines syndrome** n. a disorder of horses in which the tops of the spinal vertebrae in the back touch one another causing bony lesions and back pain. Treatment can include rest, physical therapy and surgery to remove the tops of one or more of the affected vertebrae. *Also called* overriding dorsal spinous processes.

**kitten mortality complex (KMC)** n. *See* fading puppy and kitten syndrome.

**knee** n. in small animals, the joint in the rear leg between the hip and the hock. *Also called* stifle. In large animals, the joint in the front leg between the elbow and the fetlock. *Also called* carpus.

**knock kneed** adj. describes a conformation fault in which the carpi are closer together and the feet further apart than is normal.

**knocked down hip** n. a fracture of the front part of the pelvis that causes one hip to appear lower than the other. The fracture will usually heal adequately with rest, but the affected animal may no longer be able to perform to its peak ability.

**Knott's test** n. a laboratory test used to determine if larval forms of heartworms are present in the blood.

**knuckling** n. standing or walking on the tip or top side of the foot or hoof. Knuckling indicates disease or injury to the nervous or musculoskeletal system. *See also* flexural limb deformity.

**kunkers** n. masses under the skin of horses suffering from pythiosis.

**kyphosis** n. an abnormal upward curvature to the back when the animal is viewed from the side. *Compare* lordosis.

# L

**labial** adj. 1. pertaining to or situated towards the lips. 2. pertaining to the folds of tissue that surround the vulva.

**labile** adj. having a tendency to change or move.

**labor** n. the process of giving birth, which occurs in three stages. The first stage of labor is the time during which the cervix dilates and uterine contractions become increasingly frequent; the second stage involves the birth of the fetus; and the third stage consists of the delivery of the placenta. *Also called* parturition.

**laceration** n. a tear in the surface of a tissue - **lacerate** v.

**lacrimation** n. the process of producing tears - **lacrimal** adj.

**lactation** n. the process of producing and secreting milk.

**lactation tetany** n. a disease that is associated with low blood calcium levels during lactation. Affected individuals can develop muscle tremors, difficulty walking, stiffness, behavioral changes, seizures and may die. Treatment includes calcium supplementation and supportive care. *Also called* eclampsia.

**lactic acid** n. a chemical that is produced through the breakdown of carbohydrates.

**lactic acidosis** n. *See* grain overload.

**lactose intolerance** n. vomiting, diarrhea and/or abdominal discomfort that develop when an animal is fed milk or other dairy products. The cause is a deficiency of the enzyme lactase within the intestinal tract.

**lagophthalmos** n. an inability to fully close the eyelids usually because of anatomy (e.g., brachycephalic animals) or disorders affecting nerves running to the eyelids. Affected individuals may develop corneal ulcers, pigmentation and scarring. Treatment can include topical medications to protect the eye and surgery to allow full closure of the eyelids.

**lamb dysentery** n. a disease of young lambs caused by infection of the intestinal tract with *Clostridium perfringens* type B and C bacteria. The infection severely damages the lining of the intestines, which may lead to diarrhea (often bloody), collapse and death. Treatment can include antibiotics, antitoxin injections, antiserum and supportive care but is often unsuccessful. Vaccination of the pregnant ewe can help protect her lambs. *Also called* enterotoxemia.

**lambing jug** n. a small pen in which a ewe and her recently born lamb(s) can be placed for a few days to encourage good bonding with and care of the newborns.

**lambliasis** n. *See* giardiasis. *Also called* lambliosis.

**lameness** n. an alteration of the way an animal moves its legs during locomotion, which is often caused by a painful injury or disease.

**lamina** n. a thin structure or layer, often referring specifically to the sensitive and insensitive laminae within hooves that mesh to connect the hoof wall with the deeper tissues of the foot - **laminae** pl. *See also* laminitis.

**laminectomy** n. the surgical removal of bone overlying a part of the spinal cord. A laminectomy can be performed to relieve pressure on the spinal cord that disrupts neurologic function.

**laminitis** n. inflammation and degeneration of the connection between the layers that connect the hoof wall with the deeper tissues of the foot. Potential causes include overeating of grain, sudden diet changes, infections, use of corticosteroids, uneven weight bearing, and overwork on hard surfaces. Affected individuals can develop reluctance to walk or stand, lameness and abnormal hoof growth. In severe cases, the bone incased by the hoof may rotate and protrude through the sole of the foot. Treatment can include medications that decrease pain and inflammation and improve blood flow to the damaged tissues and therapeutic hoof trimming and shoeing. *Also called* founder.

**lance** v. to puncture a fluid-filled structure (e.g., abscess) to allow the drainage of the enclosed material.

**laparoscope** n. a tubular instrument consisting of a light source and viewing device that is placed into the abdominal cavity allowing the veterinarian to see inside, take samples and perform some types of surgery.

**laparotomy** n. a surgical incision into the abdominal cavity. *Also called* celiotomy.

**large intestine** n. *See* colon.

**large strongyle** n. an intestinal worm of horses that can cause anemia, diarrhea and weight loss. The immature forms of the worm may block blood vessels leading to the intestinal tract causing colic. Many dewormers are effective. *Also called* blood worm.

**larva** n. an immature form of some types of animals and insects (e.g., parasites) - **larval** adj., **larvae** pl.

**larval migrans** n. disease caused by the movement of larval forms of some parasitic organisms (e.g., roundworms and hookworms) throughout parts of the body. Treatment can include medications to kill the parasites and decrease inflammation.

**laryngeal chondropathy** n. inflammation, infection, ulcers and tissue death involving the mucous membranes and cartilage in parts of the larynx. Affected individuals develop difficult and noisy breathing and exercise intolerance. Treatment can include antibiotics, anti-inflammatories and surgery to remove or bypass the abnormal tissues.

**laryngeal hemiplegia** n. a loss of the ability to fully open the larynx, which may be caused by genetic factors, trauma and toxins. Affected individuals develop difficult and noisy breathing and exercise intolerance. Treatment includes surgery to widen the passageway into the trachea. *Also called* roaring.

**laryngeal paralysis** n. a disease that is caused by an inability to fully open the larynx and produces noisy and difficult breathing, voice changes and a cough. Some cases are associated with hypothyroidism or other disorders but most have no known underlying cause. Treatment can include medications to decrease inflammation and anxiety and surgery to widen the passageway into the trachea.

**laryngeal saccule eversion** n. an abnormal outpouching of tissues on either side of the larynx that can lead to noisy and difficulty breathing. *See also* brachycephalic airway syndrome.

**laryngitis** n. inflammation of the larynx, which can be caused by infection, irritation (e.g., excessive barking), tumors and trauma. Laryngitis will often lead to changes in the sound of an animal's vocalizations.

**laryngoplasty** n. the surgical reconstruction of the larynx.

**laryngoscope** n. an instrument that allows visualization of the larynx through the mouth and the performance of certain procedures (e.g., placement of an endotracheal tube).

**laryngospasm** n. an involuntary closure of the larynx that can be associated with allergic reactions or a reflex when tissues in the area are touched or irritated. Prolonged laryngospasm can prevent breathing.

**larynx** n. the box-like structure between the back of the mouth and throat that regulates the passage of air into and out of the trachea and allows vocalization - **laryngeal** adj. *Also called* voice box.

**laser** n. a beam of light that has been focussed and modified allowing it to cut through or destroy tissue.

**latent** adj. not yet fully developed but having the potential to emerge.

**lateral** adj. situated to the side of the body. *Compare* medial.

**lateral ear canal resection** n. a surgery that removes the outer part of the ear canal and provides an opening into the deeper structures. A lateral ear canal resection is often performed to treat chronic disorders (e.g., infections) that have not responded adequately to medical treatment but do not significantly involve the deep parts of the ear canal. *Compare* total ear canal ablation.

**lavage** v. to thoroughly wash out a wound or cavity by flushing it with a liquid to remove foreign material and/or microorganisms.

**lavender foal** n. *See* Arabian fading syndrome.

**laxative** n. a medication taken to loosen and/or lubricate feces or otherwise promote defecation.

**laxity** n. an abnormal looseness.

**lead** n. 1. an element that can be used to block radiation. *See also* lead poisoning. 2. a wire that transmits electrical activity from within the body to a recording device (e.g., electrocardiogram). 3. the front leg that hits the ground furthest forward when an animal is cantering or galloping.

**lead poisoning** n. a disease caused by ingestion of toxic amounts of lead, which can cause vomiting, diarrhea, abdominal pain, anemia, weakness, blindness, bizarre behavior, seizures and other neurologic abnormalities. Treatment includes medications and procedures that remove lead from the body, supplements to help decrease the effects of lead and supportive and symptomatic care.

**left displaced abomasum (LDA)** n. *See* displaced abomasum.

**left dorsal displacement of the colon** n. abnormal movement of a part of a horse's large intestine and its entrapment between the spleen and left kidney causing abdominal pain. Treatment can include fasting, sedating and rolling the animal, administration of a medication that causes the spleen to contract and forcing the horse to trot, or surgery. *Also called* nephrosplenic entrapment

**left shift** n. the presence of abnormally large numbers of immature neutrophils (i.e., bands) in the blood, which indicates the presence of infection within the body.

**leg mange** n. *See* chorioptic mange.

**Legg-Calvé-Perthes disease** n. a disease of young, small breed dogs in which blood flow to the top of the femur is disrupted leading to destruction of the bone. Affected individuals usually limp on one or both hind legs and are in pain. Treatment involves surgical removal of the femoral head. *Also called* aseptic necrosis of the femoral head.

**leiomyoma** n. a benign tumor of smooth muscle most often located in the uterus, bladder or gastrointestinal tract. Treatment includes surgical removal of the tumor.

**leiomyosarcoma** n. a malignant tumor of smooth muscle that most commonly affects the gastrointestinal tract. Treatment includes surgical removal of the tumor.

**leishmaniasis** n. a disease that is most commonly seen in dogs and is caused by infection with *Leishmania* parasites transmitted through the bites of sandflies. Affected individuals can develop loss of appetite and weight, skin lesions, swollen lymph nodes, nose bleeds, lameness, renal failure and ocular abnormalities. Treatment is difficult but can include medications that help the body eliminate the parasite. Humans can be infected with *Leishmania* organisms.

**lens** n. a transparent structure (e.g., within the eye or a microscope) that focusses light.

**lens luxation** n. movement of an eye's lens out of its normal position, which is most frequently caused by trauma or genetic factors. The misplaced lens often leads to the development of glaucoma. Treatment involves lowering eye pressure, if necessary and then surgically removing the lens.

**lenticular sclerosis** n. a normal, aging change of the eyes' lenses that leads to a blue-white discoloration but does not significantly affect vision. *Also called* nuclear sclerosis. *Compare* cataract.

**lentigo** n. a benign proliferation of melanin and melanin producing cells in the skin (i.e., a freckle).

**leprosy** n. a disease of cats caused by infection with *Mycobacterium lepraemurium* bacteria, which may be transmitted by insects or through the bite of an infected rodent. Affected individuals develop raised, sometimes ulcerated skin lesions. Treatment can include surgical excision of the masses and medications to kill the bacteria.

**leptospirosis** n. a disease caused by infection with *Leptospira* bacteria often transmitted through contact with contaminated urine or bodies of water. Affected individuals can develop fever, renal and liver failure, anemia, discolored urine, abortions, ocular abnormalities and may die. Treatment includes antibiotics, fluid therapy and supportive care. Preventative vaccines are available. Humans can become infected with *Leptospira* organisms.

**lesion** n. a visibly abnormal section of tissue.

**letdown** n. the movement of milk from glandular tissue into the ducts leading to an animal's teats.

**lethal white syndrome** n. *See* ileocolonic agangliosis.

**lethargy** n. an abnormal decrease in activity and responsiveness - **lethargic** adj.

**leukemia** n. a cancer of cells that produce a type of white blood cell. The leukemia is usually named for the white blood cell that is developing abnormally (e.g., lymphoblastic) and whether the disease came on rapidly (i.e., acute) or slowly (i.e., chronic). Affected animals can have abnormal white blood cell counts, anemia, fever, weakness, recurrent infections and enlargement of lymph nodes, liver and spleen. Treatment includes chemotherapy, antibiotics and supportive care. Response to treatment varies with the type of leukemia.

**leukemoid response** n. a greatly increased white blood cell count that is usually seen in response to infections but can be difficult to differentiate from leukemia.

**leukocyte** n. a type of cell that identifies and removes potentially harmful organisms or other substances (e.g., cancerous or damaged cells) from the body. *Also called* white blood cell.

**leukocyte adhesion deficiency** n. a genetic disease that prevents normal function of white blood cells and leads to poor wound healing and recurrent bacterial infections that do not respond well to antibiotics. Treatment is difficult. *Also called* granulocytopathy syndrome.

**leukocytosis** n. a white blood cell count that is higher than normal, which can be associated with infection, inflammation, stress, corticosteroid use or leukemia. *Compare* leukopenia.

**leukoderma** n. a loss of pigment from some areas of skin.

**leukodystrophy** n. a congenital disease of the white matter of the spinal cord and brain that can cause progressive weakness, difficulty walking and other neurologic disorders. There is no effective treatment.

**leukoencephalomalacia** n. degeneration of the white matter of the brain. *See also* fusariotoxicosis.

**leukoencephalomyelopathy** n. a disease of the white matter of the brain and spinal cord that is most frequently seen in adult Rottweilers and causes progressive weakness and difficulty walking. There is no effective treatment.

**leukogram** n. *See* hemogram.

**leukopenia** n. a white blood cell count that is lower than normal, which can be associated with severe infection or inflammation or bone marrow diseases. *Compare* leukocytosis.

**leukosis** n. *See* bovine leukosis.

**leukotrichia** n. the abnormal presence of white hairs.

**libido** n. the drive to breed.

**lice** n. *See* louse.

**licensed veterinary technician (LVT)** n. a person who has received training and certification in veterinary procedures, laboratory skills and the nursing care of animals.

**lichenification** n. an abnormal thickening and hardening of the skin.

**lick granuloma** n. *See* acral lick dermatitis.

**ligament** n. 1. a band of fibrous connective tissue that connects bones and supports joints. 2. a band of tissue that connects organs within the abdominal cavity.

**ligate** v. to tie off a blood vessel or other structure - **ligature** n.

**lily toxicosis** n. a disease caused by ingestion of parts of a lily plant.

Affected individuals can develop vomiting, loss of appetite, lethargy, abnormal heart rhythms and renal failure. Treatment may include medications and procedures to limit absorption of the toxin, fluid therapy, antiarrhythmic drugs and supportive care.

**limb** n. a leg or arm.

**limberneck** n. a disease of birds caused by a toxin produced by *Clostridium botulinum* bacteria. The toxin can be absorbed when animals eat decaying material or the maggots feeding on it or from bacteria present in the intestinal tract of infected birds. Affected animals exhibit progressive weakness and paralysis. Treatment can include antitoxin administration, supportive care and antibiotics. Some animals may recover without treatment if not too severely affected. *Also called* botulism.

**limbus** n. the outer edge of a body part.

**limping syndrome** n. shifting leg lameness and joint pain that can develop in kittens infected with feline calicivirus. Vaccines do not protect against this form of the disease.

**linear foreign body** n. a long, thin piece of material (e.g., a string) that when ingested can cause vomiting, loss of appetite and damage to the intestinal tract. Surgery to remove the linear foreign body and repair any intestinal damage is usually necessary.

**lingual** adj. pertaining to or oriented towards the tongue. *Compare* buccal.

**lipase** n. a substance measured in the blood the levels of which can rise with pancreatitis, other forms of pancreatic disease or with kidney disease.

**lipemia** n. increased amounts of fat in the blood, which can be associated with a recent meal, diabetes mellitus, hypothyroidism and other diseases - **lipemic** adj. *Also called* hyperlipidemia.

**lipid** n. any of a number of compounds that contain fat.

**lipid keratopathy** n. *See* stromal lipid keratopathy.

**lipidosis** n. *See* hepatic lipidosis.

**lipoma** n. a tumor of fat cells that is benign but can cause problems depending on its size and location. Surgical removal is curative, but subsequent lipomas at other locations are likely to develop.

**lipomatosis** n. a disease primarily affecting cattle in which masses of necrotic fat develop within the abdomen where they can be mistaken for a fetus or disrupt the gastrointestinal and urinary tracts. Some cases may be associated with ingestion of fescue grass infected with a fungus.

**lipophilic** adj. attracting or easily dissolved in fat. *Compare* hydrophilic.

**lipoprotein** n. a large compound that transports lipids through the circulatory system.

**liposarcoma** n. a malignant tumor of fat cells that can be invasive at its location or spread to other areas of the body. Treatment can include surgical removal and chemotherapy.

**lissencephaly** n. a congenital lack of ridges and grooves on the surface of the brain, which can lead to neurological disorders including behavioral abnormalities and seizures. There is no treatment.

**listeriosis** n. a disease caused by infection with the bacteria *Listeria monocytogenes* often contracted by eating spoiled or contaminated feed. Affected animals can develop loss of appetite, depression, lethargy, bizarre behavior, circling, abnormal facial expressions, drooling, inability to rise, paddling, abortion, diarrhea and may die. Treatment includes antibiotics and supportive care. *Also called* circling disease and silage disease.

**lithotripsy** n. the breaking apart of a stone, usually using shock waves, so that it can be more easily flushed from the bladder, gallbladder or other hollow organ.

**little white dog shaker syndrome** n. *See* generalized tremor syndrome.

**liver** n. a large, blood filtering abdominal organ with many functions, including detoxifying potentially harmful substances, producing bile, metabolizing and storing nutrients absorbed from the intestinal tract and producing proteins (e.g., clotting factors and albumin).

**liver enzymes** n. alanine aminotransferase, alkaline phosphatase and other substances that are produced within the liver, the levels of which are measured in the blood and can change with liver disease. *Also called* hepatic enzymes.

**liver failure** n. loss of the liver's ability to perform its normal functions, which may be caused by many different diseases. Animals with liver failure can develop behavioral changes, seizures, weakness, loss of appetite, abnormal fluid accumulations, bleeding, jaundice and may die. Therapy can include treatment of any underlying diseases, diet changes and supportive and symptomatic care. *See also* hepatic encephalopathy.

**liver fluke** n. a large and flat parasitic organism that infests and damages the liver. Affected individuals can develop vomiting, loss of appetite and weight, weakness, diarrhea, jaundice and may die. Treatment includes medications to kill the parasite. *See also* fascioliasis.

**liver function test** n. *See* bile acid test.

**liver profile** n. laboratory tests measuring the levels of different substances in the blood that are associated with liver health.

**loading dose** n. a first dose of a medication that is larger than subsequent doses and given to hasten an animal's clinical response.

**lobe** n. a part of an organ (e.g., liver or lung) that is partially separated from other similar portions by fissures or different tissues - **lobar** adj.

**lobectomy** n. the surgical removal of one or more lobes of an organ.

**lobule** n. a small lobe - **lobular** adj.

**local anesthesia** n. a lack of sensation that is induced in only a small area of the body without producing a loss of consciousness. Local anesthesia can be used for minor procedures such as suturing a small, superficial wound but may not be a good choice if an animal is unlikely to remain still. *Compare* general anesthesia.

**localized** adj. affecting only a limited area. *Compare* generalized.

**lochia** n. vaginal discharge seen after an animal gives birth. Normal lochia can initially be very bloody and copious but becomes less evident over the days to weeks following birth.

**lockjaw** n. *See* tetanus.

**locomotion** n. movement from one place to another.

**locus** n. a specific site - **loci** pl.

**longitudinal** adj. pertaining to the long axis of a structure. *Compare* transverse.

**lordosis** n. an abnormal downward curvature to the back when the animal is viewed from the side. *Compare* kyphosis.

**louse** n. a parasitic insect that can infest the skin and coat of animals - **lice** pl. *See* pediculosis.

**low dose dexamethasone suppression test (LDSS)** n. a laboratory test measuring the body's response to administration of a relatively low dose of dexamethasone, which is often used to help diagnose whether or not an animal has Cushing's disease.

**lower airway** n. the passages for air contained within the lungs. *Compare* upper airway. *Also called* lower respiratory tract.

**lumbar** adj. pertaining to the part of the back located between the rib cage and pelvis.

**lumbosacral** adj. pertaining to the area around the connection between the spine in the lower back and the pelvis.

**lumbosacral stenosis** n. anatomic abnormalities that lead to a narrowing of the spinal canal in the lumbosacral region. Affected individuals can develop hind end weakness, lameness and difficulty walking, lower back pain and incontinence. Treatment may include rest, anti-inflammatories and surgery to relieve pressure on nerves.

**lumen** n. a hollow channel or space within a body part or other object.

**lumps** n. *See* cervical lymphadenitis.

**lumpy jaw** n. *See* actinomycosis.

**lumpy wool** n. a disease of sheep caused by infection of the skin with the bacteria *Dermatophilus congolensis*. Infection is promoted by any factor that disrupts the normal, protective characteristics of skin (e.g., prolonged dampness). Lesions often consist of a raised, pyramid-shaped scab or crust matted to the wool. Treatment can include improving environmental conditions, antibiotics and medicated shampoos or dips. *Also called* streptothricosis and dermatophilosis.

**lung** n. one of two organs in the chest cavity responsible for transferring oxygen, carbon dioxide and other gasses to and from the bloodstream.

**lung fluke** n. *See* paragonimiasis.

**lungworm** n. any of many different types of parasitic worms that can invade the lungs and airways causing coughing, difficulty breathing, weight loss and sometimes death. Treatment includes medications that kill the parasites and supportive care. *Also called* verminous bronchitis and pneumonia. *See also* capillariasis.

**lupus** n. *See* discoid lupus erythematosus and systemic lupus erythematosus.

**luteal** adj. pertaining to the corpus luteum.

**luteal cyst** n. a persistent fluid-filled structure on the ovary that prevents affected individuals from coming into heat. Treatment includes hormone therapy.

**luteinizing hormone (LH)** n. a hormone produced by the pituitary gland or used as a drug that stimulates ovulation and the development of the corpus luteum.

**luteolysis** n. the destruction of the corpus luteum.

**luxating patella** n. *See* patellar luxation.

**luxation** n. the movement of a body part into an abnormal location. *See also* lens luxation, patellar luxation and dislocation.

**Lyme disease** n. a disease caused by infection with *Borrelia burgdorferi* bacteria that are transmitted by the bite of *Ixodes* ticks. Affected individuals can exhibit many different symptoms depending on where the infection localizes, but enlarged lymph nodes and painful, swollen joints are most commonly noted. Antibiotics can help control the disease but may not completely eliminate the infection. A preventative vaccine exists for dogs. *Also called* borreliosis.

**lymph** n. the fluid that carries lymphocytes, chyle and other substances as it circulates through special ducts and in the bloodstream, surrounds tissues, is filtered by lymph nodes.

**lymph node** n. accumulations of tissue that are located at various sites throughout the body, filter lymph and produce lymphocytes.

**lymphadenitis** n. inflammation of the lymph nodes, which often causes their enlargement. *See also* cervical and caseous lymphadenitis.

**lymphadenopathy** n. any disease affecting and often enlarging the lymph nodes.

**lymphangiectasia** n. a disease in which the ducts carrying lymph leak protein and other substances into the intestinal tract. Affected individuals can develop diarrhea, abnormal fluid accumulations and lose weight. Treatment may include dietary changes and corticosteroids.

**lymphangiosarcoma** n. an aggressive cancer of lymph vessels, which is most often located in or just under the skin and can vary in appearance. Surgical excision may be curative but reoccurrence at the site of surgery or spread to other organs is likely.

**lymphangitis** n. inflammation of the lymphatic channels. *See also* ulcerative lymphangitis.

**lymphatic system** n. the network of ducts, tissues and organs that produce, carry and filter lymph.

**lymphedema** n. swelling that occurs because of an accumulation of lymph within tissues. Lymphedema can develop because of obstruction of lymph channels by inflammation, trauma or tumors.

**lymphoblast** n. an immature lymphocyte. *See also* lymphosarcoma.

**lymphocyte** n. a type of white blood cell that produces antibodies or otherwise aids in the normal functioning of the immune system - **lymphocytic** adj. *See also* B and T cells.

**lymphocytic-plasmacytic enteritis** n. *See* inflammatory bowel disease.

**lymphocytic-plasmacytic stomatitis** n. a disease usually seen in cats that is thought to be caused by an abnormal immune reaction to oral bacteria, tartar and plaque or to the teeth and their supportive tissues. Affected individuals may develop oral inflammation and pain, reluctance to eat, bad breath, drooling and weight loss. Treatment can include antibiotics for secondary infections, medications to reduce the immune response and extraction of most or all of the teeth. *Also called* feline gingivitis-stomatitis syndrome and plasma cell stomatitis.

**lymphocytopenia** n. *See* lymphopenia.

**lymphocytosis** n. an increased number of lymphocytes in the bloodstream, which can be seen with infections and immune mediated diseases.

**lymphoma** n. *See* lymphosarcoma.

**lymphopenia** n. a decreased number of lymphocytes in the bloodstream, which can be seen with stress, loss of lymph (e.g., lymphangiectasia) and some infections.

**lymphosarcoma (LSA)** n. a cancerous proliferation of immature lymphocytes (i.e., lymphoblasts) that may cause enlargement of the lymph nodes, liver and spleen, skin lesions and abnormal function of any invaded organ (e.g., the intestinal tract or kidneys). Treatment can include surgical removal of affected tissues if the disease is localized and chemotherapy. Remissions can be lengthy, but the disease is eventually fatal. *Also called* lymphoma. *See also* epitheliotropic lymphoma.

**lysis** n. rupture or destruction of cells or tissues - **lytic** adj.

**lysosomal storage disease** n. any of a number of genetic diseases in which an animal does not produce an enzyme necessary for normal metabolism. As a result, substances build up within the brain causing progressive neurologic dysfunction in young animals. No effective, long-term treatment exists.

# M

**macaw wasting disease** n. *See* proventricular dilatation disease.

**maceration** n. a softening and weakening of tissues or other objects that can occur with prolonged wetness.

**macropalpebral fissure** n. a larger than normal opening between the eyelids that predisposes an animal to irritation and recurrent eye infections. Treatment can include antibiotic and anti-inflammatory ointments or surgery. *Also called* euryblepharon.

**macrophage** n. a type of cell that is located within tissues and removes microorganisms, abnormal cells and debris. *Also called* histiocyte.

**macrophthalmia** n. *See* buphthalmos.

**macroscopic** adj. visible to the naked eye. *Compare* microscopic.

**macule** n. an area of skin that is discolored but not raised - **macular** adj. *Also called* **macula**.

**mad cow disease** n. *See* bovine spongiform encephalopathy.

**mad itch** n. *See* pseudorabies.

**maedi-visna** n. *See* ovine progressive pneumonia.

**maggot** n. the larva of a fly that lays its eggs in wounds, on skin soiled with urine or feces or on carcasses. *See also* myiasis.

**magnesium** n. an element that is an important part of the diet and necessary for normal body function. *See also* hypomagnesemic tetany.

**magnesium ammonium phosphate urolith** n. *See* struvite urolith.

**magnetic resonance imaging (MRI)** n. a method of imaging the body that uses a magnetic field and a computer to create detailed pictures.

**malabsorption** n. an inability to absorb some nutrients from the intestinal tract into the bloodstream, which causes diarrhea and weight loss. Treatment usually includes diet changes and addressing any underlying diseases - **malabsorptive** adj. *See also* small intestinal bacterial overgrowth and inflammatory bowel disease.

**malacia** n. an abnormal softening of a tissue.

**malady** n. any illness or disease.

**malaligned** adj. not correctly positioned with regards to other parts or similar structures - **malalignment** n.

**Malassezia** n. a type of yeast that is normally present on the skin and in the ears of some animals (e.g., dogs and cats). When the normal protective properties of the skin are disrupted, Malassezia organisms can cause infections, foul odors and itchiness. Treatment includes medications that decrease itching and inflammation and kill the yeast as well as addressing any underlying conditions (e.g., allergies).

**malassimilation** n. an inability to digest and/or absorb nutrients from the intestinal tract into the bloodstream, which causes diarrhea and weight loss. Inflammation, autoimmune diseases, cancer, parasites, bacteria and viruses that disrupt the function of the digestive tract can lead to malassimilation.

**maldigestion** n. an inability to break down some nutrients in the intestinal tract, which causes diarrhea and weight loss - **maldigestive** adj. *See also* exocrine pancreatic insufficiency.

**malformation** n. abnormal anatomy that is caused by a disorder of development.

**malignant** adj. describes a disease, often cancer, that has the tendency to spread or otherwise worsen. *Compare* benign.

**malignant catarrhal fever (MCF)** n. a contagious, viral disease most commonly affecting cattle. Affected individuals can develop fever, ulcers of and discharge from mucous membranes, eye abnormalities, swollen lymph nodes, neurologic abnormalities and bloody diarrhea and urine. The disease is usually fatal despite any treatment.

**malignant edema** n. a disease caused by infection of wounds with *Clostridium septicum* and some other types of bacteria. Affected individuals develop a fever, loss of appetite, soft swellings that rapidly enlarge around the infected wound and may die quickly. Early treatment with antibiotics can be successful. Preventative vaccines are available.

**malignant fibrous histiocytoma** n. a type of cancer that is most commonly located in and under the skin. It does not tend to spread to distant tissues but can be very invasive at its location. Some cases in cats have been associated with injectable vaccines. Treatment can include wide surgical excision, which can be difficult to achieve, chemotherapy and radiation treatment. *Also called* giant cell tumor, hemangiopericytomas and dermatofibrosarcoma.

**malignant hyperthermia** n. a suspected genetic disorder that is initiated by a stressful event or general anesthesia and causes muscle stiffness, rapid breathing, abnormal heart rhythms, very high body temperatures and sometimes death. Treatment can include stopping the administration of anesthetic gasses, cooling the body, oxygen therapy and medications to relax muscles, normalize arrhythmias and correct acid-base disturbances.

**malnutrition** n. ingestion of only poor quality or insufficient amounts of food.

**malocclusion** n. a disorder in which the teeth in the upper and lower jaws are improperly aligned and do not contact each other in a normal manner. Cases that cause pain or hinder normal chewing can be treated with tooth extractions or orthodontic techniques.

**malpresentation** n. the passage of a fetus into the birth canal in an abnormal position. *See also* dystocia.

**malunion** n. a broken bone that has fused incorrectly. Treatment includes surgery to break the bone and affix the pieces in better alignment to allow proper healing.

**mammary gland** n. the tissues that can produce and secrete milk in female animals or their nonfunctional counterparts in males.

**mammary gland hyperplasia** n. a disease of cats that is caused by excessive production or administration of progesterone or similar hormones. Affected animals develop very large mammary glands that may be associated with inflamed or damaged skin. Treatment can include ovariohysterectomy or mastectomy. *Also called* mammary gland hypertrophy or fibroadenoma complex.

**mandible** n. the lower jaw - **mandibular** adj.

**mandibulectomy** n. the surgical removal of a part or all of the mandible.

**mange** n. infestation of the skin and/or ears with mites that can cause hair loss, itching, secondary bacterial infections and other lesions. See entries for specific diseases (e.g., demodicosis, sarcoptic mange, psoroptic mange) for detailed information.

**mania** n. an abnormal mental state characterized by excessive activity and bizarre behavior.

**mare** n. a female horse four years of age or older.

**mare reproductive loss syndrome (MRLS)** n. a disease of horses that is thought to be related to the ingestion of tent caterpillars and causes abortions or the birth of very sickly foals. There is no treatment but feeding hay to pregnant mares on pasture or otherwise limiting access to tent caterpillars can prevent abortions.

**Marek's disease** n. a contagious, viral disease most commonly affecting chickens. Some infected individuals develop tumors throughout the body, which can lead to depression, weight loss and death. Others may stand abnormally and have difficulty walking but soon recover. Effective preventative vaccines exist.

**marking behavior** n. the production of urine and/or feces or rubbing parts of the body (e.g., scent glands) against surfaces for the purpose of communication with other individuals.

**masculinization** n. *See* virilization.

**mass** n. an abnormal lump of tissue, which after diagnostic testing (e.g., cytology or histopathology) may be more specifically diagnosed as a cyst, abscess, granuloma or tumor.

**mast cell** n. a type of cell that is part of the immune system and plays a role in allergies.

**mast cell tumor** n. a tumor that is composed primarily of mast cells and most commonly located in the skin. Surgery to remove isolated mast cell tumors can be curative, but wide margins are necessary or they are likely to recur. Disease that has or is likely to spread can be treated with chemotherapy. *Also called* mastocytoma.

**mastectomy** n. the surgical removal of a mammary gland.

**mastication** n. the act of chewing.

**masticatory muscle myositis** n. an autoimmune disease in which the body inappropriately attacks the muscles responsible for moving the jaw. Early in the disease, animals develop swollen muscles on top of the head or behind the jaw, and attempts to open the mouth fully are painful. Treatment with corticosteroids will usually control the immune reaction. Some animals can be slowly weaned off the drugs while others may require life-long treatment. If the disease progresses, the affected muscles are replaced with scar tissue, and the individual may no longer be able to open its mouth wide enough to eat and drink.

**mastitis** n. inflammation of the mammary glands, which is usually caused by infection. Affected animals produce less milk than normal and/or milk that is unsuitable for consumption. Individuals may develop fevers, be in pain, have abscesses that rupture and, if the infection spreads to the bloodstream, they can die. Treatment with antibiotics is often successful but permanent damage to the mammary gland can result.

**mastocytoma** n. *See* mast cell tumor.

**maternal** adj. pertaining to a female parent. *Compare* paternal.

**maternal aggression** n. inappropriate attacks or related behaviors (e.g., growling, hissing or snapping) initiated by the dam against her offspring or against people or animals that are perceived to be a threat to her offspring. Maternal aggression can be related to a genetic predisposition or stress. Treatment includes avoiding situations that initiate aggressive behavior, weaning the offspring and preventing future pregnancies.

**maternal immunity** n. transfer of antibodies from the dam to her offspring through the placenta or the suckling of colostrum. Maternal immunity protects the newborn until its own immune system matures.

**matted** adj. describes hair or fur that is tangled and clumped together. A matted coat does not provide the protection against the elements that a healthy coat does and can be painful and lead to skin lesions.

**mature** adj. fully developed. *Compare* immature.

**maxilla** n. the upper jaw - **maxillary** adj.

**maxillectomy** n. the surgical removal of some or all of the upper jaw.

**meal feeding** n. a method of feeding animals in which a specific amount of food is offered at specific times during the day. *Compare* free choice feeding.

**meconium** n. the feces that are formed by the fetus while still within the uterus. Meconium is usually soft and should be passed within the first few hours of life.

**meconium impaction** n. meconium that becomes stuck in the colon causing straining to defecate and abdominal pain in a newborn. Treatment with laxatives and enemas is usually successful.

**medial** adj. situated towards the center of the body. *Compare* lateral.

**mediastinum** n. the central portion of the chest that is surrounded by the lungs and contains the heart, trachea, esophagus, thymus, lymph nodes, large blood vessels and other structures - **mediastinal** adj.

**medical** adj. pertaining to the prescription of drugs and the diagnosis, treatment and prevention of disease, excluding surgical methods.

**medulla** n. the inner portion of an organ or tissue - **medullary** adj. *Compare* cortex.

**medullary cavity** n. the inner chamber of a bone, which contains marrow.

**medulloblastoma** n. an aggressive type of brain tumor most commonly seen in young dogs. Treatment is difficult.

**megacolon** n. a distended and poorly functioning colon. Some cases are initiated by prolonged constipation while others have no known underlying cause. Affected individuals are constipated and may strain to defecate, vomit, become dehydrated and lose weight. Treatment includes addressing any underlying conditions, removing feces from the colon, diet changes, supportive care and medications to soften feces and improve colonic contractions.

**megaesophagus** n. a distended and poorly functioning esophagus. Some cases are associated with congenital defects, myasthenia gravis or other diseases, but most have no known underlying cause. Affected individuals regurgitate, drool, frequently swallow and can develop aspiration pneumonia. Treatment includes addressing any underlying disorders, changes in the consistency of foods and methods of feeding and medications that may stimulate esophageal function.

**megakaryocyte** n. a type of large cell that is normally located in the bone marrow and produces platelets.

**meibomian gland adenoma** n. a small, benign growth arising from a gland on the edge of the eyelid. The mass can rub on and damage the surface of the eye. Treatment includes the surgical removal of the tumor. *Also called* meibomian gland cyst or chalazion.

**melanin** n. a brown to black pigment that can give a dark color to the skin, hair and irises.

**melanocyte** n. a cell that produces melanin.

**melanocytoma** n. a benign, usually dark tumor of cells that produce melanin within the skin. Surgical removal is curative. *Compare* melanoma.

**melanoma** n. a tumor of cells that produce melanin. In small animals, the term refers specifically to malignant cancers that are usually located in the mouth and skin. These melanomas may or may not be pigmented. In large animals, melanomas are usually dark, can be benign or malignant and are most commonly seen in gray or white horses. Treatment includes surgery to remove the tumor or affected body part (e.g., toe or part of the jaw). Horses that cannot be treated surgically may benefit from medications that can modulate the immune system. *Compare* melanocytoma.

**melena** n. digested blood in the stool, which makes the feces appear very dark or tarry. *Compare* hematochezia.

**melting ulcer** n. an infected corneal ulcer that rapidly becomes bigger and deeper and can lead to rupture of the eyeball. Treatment often includes antibacterial and/or antifungal medications, pain relief and surgery to support the eye as it heals.

**menace response** n. the normal, involuntary reaction to blink when an object is rapidly moved towards an eye. Air currents and touching the eye must be avoided when testing for the menace response. A lack of the normal reaction can indicate blindness or disorders affecting the nerves running to the eyelids.

**meninges** n. the membranes that cover and surround the brain and spinal cord - **meningeal** adj.

**meningioma** n. a benign tumor of the meninges that can produce neurologic abnormalities by pressing on or invading the tissues of the brain or spinal cord. Treatment can include surgical removal of the tumor, radiation therapy and chemotherapy.

**meningitis** n. inflammation of the meninges that can be caused by infection, toxins, cancer or immune mediated disease. Affected animals often

develop pain, fever and stiffness. Treatment can include addressing any underlying disease and anti-inflammatories. *See also* steroid responsive meningitis.

**meningoencephalitis** n. inflammation of the meninges and brain. *See also* meningitis and encephalitis.

**meningoencephalomyelitis** n. inflammation of the meninges, brain and spinal cord. *See also* meningitis and encephalomyelitis.

**meniscus** n. a cartilaginous structure within the stifle joint that is often torn with a cranial cruciate ligament rupture. Removal of the damaged portion of the meniscus is commonly included in the surgical treatment of the injury.

**mentation** n. an animal's mental status (e.g., bright, alert and responsive).

**mesentery** n. the membranous structure within the abdomen that connects many abdominal organs to the body wall - **mesenteric** adj.

**mesial** adj. situated towards the center of the body or mouth.

**mesothelioma** n. a malignant tumor of the cells that line body cavities (e.g., the abdomen, chest and pericardium), which often causes an abnormal buildup of fluid. Symptoms depend on the location of the cancer within the body. Treatment is difficult but can include repeated removal of fluid accumulations.

**metabolic bone diseases** n. any disease of bone that is caused by a disorder of metabolism. Metabolic bone disease is frequently seen in reptiles fed a diet that is imbalanced in calcium, phosphorous and/or vitamin D. Affected individuals develop bones that are painful and bend or break easily. Treatment can include correcting the diet and nutritional supplements. *See also* nutritional and renal secondary hyperparathyroidism, hypervitaminosis A and mucopolysaccharidosis.

**metabolic disease** n. any of a number of diseases in which an aspect of metabolism does not function correctly, leading to an accumulation or deficiency of a substance that further disrupts the body.

**metabolic encephalopathy** n. neurologic dysfunction arising from diseases that disrupt metabolism. *See also* hepatic encephalopathy.

**metabolic epidermal necrosis** n. *See* hepatocutaneous syndrome.

**metabolism** n. the body processes that combine to digest and absorb nutrients, eliminate waste and produce energy for growth and maintenance of tissues - **metabolic** adj., **metabolize** v.

**metacarpal** adj. pertaining to the bones or region of the forelimb located between the carpus and digits.

**metaldehyde toxicity** n. disease caused by ingestion of a type of poison commonly used against slugs and snails. Affected individuals can develop fever, tremors, difficulty walking and breathing, abnormal eye movement, seizures, other neurologic disorders, vomiting, diarrhea, drooling and may die. Treatment may include procedures that limit absorption of the poison, sedatives, fluid therapy and symptomatic and supportive care.

**metaphysis** n. the portion of a long bone that is located between its shaft and end and is responsible for bone growth in young animals.

**metastasis** n. the spread of a disease (e.g., cancer) from one part of the body to another - **metastatic** adj., **metastasize** v.

**metatarsal** adj. pertaining to the bones or region of the hindlimb located between the tarsus and digits.

**methemoglobinemia** n. the abnormal presence in the bloodstream of large amounts of a type of hemoglobin that does not carry oxygen well. Ingestion of some types of toxic substances is the most common cause of methemoglobinemia. Affected individuals often develop a brown discoloration to their mucous membranes and urine and can have difficulty breathing. *See also* acetaminophen and nitrate toxicity.

**metritis** n. inflammation of the uterus, which is often associated with infection. *See also* endometritis and contagious equine metritis.

**microalbuminuria** n. the presence of small but still abnormal amounts of the protein albumin in a urine sample. In the absence of infection or inflammation, microalbuminuria can be an early indicator of kidney disease.

**microbe** n. *See* microorganism.

**microchip** n. a small object that can be injected under the skin and scanned to help identify an animal.

**microfilaremia** n. the presence of microfilariae in the bloodstream.

**microfilariae** n. the larval forms of some parasites (e.g., heartworms).

**microfilaricide** n. a drug that kills microfilariae.

**microhematocrit** n. a laboratory test that can quickly estimate an animal's red blood cell count (i.e., packed cell volume).

**microorganism** n. a microscopic organism (e.g., bacteria, virus and some types of parasites).

**microphthalmia** n. the condition of having smaller than normal eyes.

**microscopic** adj. pertaining to an instrument used to magnify objects - **microscope** n. 2. visible only under the microscope.

**microvascular dysplasia** n. *See* hepatoportal microvascular dysplasia.

**microvasculature** n. all of the small blood vessels in the body (e.g., capillaries).

**micturition** n. the process of urinating.

**midbrain** n. the part of the brain that connects other areas within the brain and is involved with visual and auditory reflexes.

**middle ear** n. the portion of the ear containing three small bones that transmit vibrations from the eardrum to the nerves of the inner ear. *See also* inner and outer ear.

**midge** n. a type of very small flying insect. *See also Culicoides* hypersensitivity.

**midline** n. the center of an animal's body running from the head to the tail.

**miliary dermatitis** n. a disease seen in cats that is usually caused by an allergic reaction to external parasites, foods, inhaled allergens or other substances. Affected individuals develop small bumps on the skin, scabs and are usually itchy. Treatment can include corticosteroids, antibiotics for secondary bacterial infections and addressing any underlying allergies.

**milk fever** n. *See* parturient paresis.

**milk replacer** n. manufactured liquids or powders that can be mixed with water used to feed young animals without access to natural milk. Improper formulation of milk replacers can cause diarrhea.

**milk teeth** n. *See* deciduous teeth.

**milk tetany** n. *See* hypomagnesemic tetany.

**miller's disease** n. a disease of horses that may be seen with a diet rich in grain and deficient in grass or hay because of imbalances in the amounts of phosphorous, calcium and vitamin D. Affected animals have abnormal bones (especially of the head) that are painful and easily injured. Correcting the diet is usually curative unless too much bone damage has occurred. *Also called* osteomalacia, nutritional secondary hyperparathyroidism, rickets, bran disease and big head.

**mineral** n. an inorganic substance (e.g., calcium) that is required in the diet for normal body function.

**mineral oil** n. a slippery liquid often used to promote passage of materials through the digestive tract or as an aid in the identification of external parasites under the microscope.

**mineralization** n. the deposition of minerals within a tissue or other object, which makes it harder and more visible on a radiograph.

**mineralocorticoids** n. one of several substances that affect the body's fluid and electrolyte balance and are made by the adrenal glands or manufactured as a drug. Aldosterone is a common mineralocorticoid. *See also* Addison's disease.

**minimum database (MDB)** n. initial laboratory tests that are often required to diagnose an illness or injury. A minimum database often consists of a biochemical profile, complete blood cell count and urinalysis but can vary depending on the suspected cause of disease.

**minimum inhibitory concentration (MIC)** n. a laboratory test that measures the effectiveness of antibiotics against bacteria that have usually been collected from a patient and cultured in the lab.

**miosis** n. contraction of an iris, which makes the pupil appear small - **miotic** adj. *Compare* mydriasis.

**mismating shot** n. a high dose of estrogen given to terminate a pregnancy in a recently bred dog. Mismating shots have a high incidence of serious side effects and are generally no longer used.

**mite** n. a type of very small insect that can infest the skin or other parts of the body. *See also* mange and the specific type of mite (e.g., ear mite or chigger) for details.

**mitosis** n. a process through which cells can divide and reproduce - **mitotic** adj.

**mitral valve** n. the heart valve separating the left atrium and left ventricle. *Also called* bicuspid valve.

**mitral valve dysplasia** n. a birth defect in which the heart's mitral valve did not form normally. Affected individuals can have a murmur, arrhythmias, difficulty breathing, abnormal fluid accumulations and may die. No specific treatment for the underlying condition exists, but medications and other treatments that improve heart function and control fluid accumulations can be helpful.

**modified live vaccine (MLV)** n. a type of vaccine containing live viruses or bacteria that have been modified so that they cannot cause disease but are still capable of stimulating immunity. *Also called* attenuated vaccine.

**moist dermatitis** n. a skin condition that is initiated by something (e.g., a flea bite or allergies) that causes an animal to bite or scratch at a particular area. The individual quickly can traumatize the patch of skin leading to hair loss, infection, inflammation, oozing and even more itchiness. Treatment may include clipping and cleansing the area, antibiotics, corticosteroids and addressing any underlying conditions. *Also called* hot spot. *See also* wet dewlap.

**molar teeth** n. the teeth at the back of the mouth that are used to grind food.

**mold** n. a type of fungus that often grows under damp conditions or on decaying organic material.

**moldy corn poisoning** n. *See* fusari-otoxicosis.

**molt** v. to shed skin, hair or feathers, often in response to environmental changes.

**Monday morning disease** n. *See* exertional rhabdomyolysis.

**moniliasis** n. *See* candidiasis.

**monkey mouth** n. the condition of having an upper jaw that is shorter than the lower jaw.

**monoclonal gammopathy** n. an abnormally large amount of a single type of antibody in the blood, which can be associated with certain types of cancer (e.g., myeloma). *Compare* polyclonal gammopathy.

**monocyte** n. a type of white blood cell that plays an important role in chronic infections or inflammation.

**monocytopenia** n. a decreased number of monocytes in the bloodstream.

**monocytosis** n. an increased number of monocytes in the bloodstream.

**monogastric** adj. describes an animal with a stomach consisting of a single chamber. *Compare* ruminant.

**monorchid** adj. describes a male animal that was born with one testicle. *Compare* cryptorchid.

**moon blindness** n. *See* recurrent uveitis.

**morbidity rate** n. the number of animals within a group that become sick with a particular disease. *Compare* mortality rate.

**moribund** adj. on the verge of death.

**mortality rate** n. the number of animals within a group that die from a particular disease. *Compare* morbidity rate.

**motility** n. 1. the ability of a cell to move itself. 2. movement within an organ (e.g., the gastrointestinal tract).

**motion sickness** n. nausea and vomiting that is instigated by movement (e.g., car rides). Medications can help alleviate motion sickness.

**motor neurons** n. nerves that carry signals from the brain and spinal cord to muscles. *Compare* sensory neurons.

**mouth breathing** n. the passage of air in and out of the lungs through the mouth rather than the nose. Mouth breathing can be a sign of serious respiratory disfunction in animals that normally breathe through their noses (e.g., cats).

**mouth gag** n. a piece of equipment that prevents an animal from fully closing its mouth, which can be used to protect hands or equipment from being bitten or allow full examination and treatment of the mouth.

**mouth rot** n. *See* infectious stomatitis.

**mucocele** n. an abnormal, hollow structure filled with a mucus-like liquid. *See also* salivary mucocele.

**mucociliary elevator** n. the action of small, hair-like projections that line the inner surface of parts of the respiratory tract and clear mucus and particles from within the lungs up through the trachea and out into the mouth.

**mucocutaneous junction** n. a part of the body where skin and mucous membranes are joined (e.g., around the lips).

**mucoid** adj. pertaining to, or similar to, mucus.

**mucoid enteropathy** n. a disease of rabbits with an unknown cause. Affected animals often develop mucus covered or gelatinous stools, loss of appetite and an enlarged abdomen. Treatment can include fluid therapy, antibiotics, pain relief and enemas, but most animals die even with aggressive therapy.

**mucolytic** adj. having properties that break down mucus.

**mucometra** n. a uterus that is filled with mucus. Treatment can include surgical removal of the uterus or hormones that stimulate expulsion of the fluid.

**mucopolysaccharidosis** n. a genetic disease that can cause abnormal formation and growth of bones throughout the body (especially the face), cloudy corneas and weakness. The disease stops progressing after maturity.

**mucopurulent** adj. having characteristics of both mucus and pus.

**mucosa** n. *See* mucous membrane.

**mucosal disease** n. an especially severe form of bovine viral diarrhea seen in some individuals with persistent infections of the virus. Affected animals develop diarrhea, ulcers of the skin, nose and gastrointestinal tract and usually die.

**mucous membrane** n. the moist, inner lining of many body parts (e.g., the mouth and eyelids).

**mucus** n. a sticky liquid or film that is produced by some glands and tissues - **mucous** adj.

**mule** n. the offspring of a mating between a female horse and a male donkey. *Compare* hinny.

**multicentric** adj. describes the presence of similar lesions affecting multiple locations throughout the body.

**multipara** n. a female that has had two or more successful pregnancies - **multiparous** adj. *Compare* nullipara and primipara.

**multiple cartilaginous exostoses** n. a suspected genetic condition in which many benign growths of cartilage and bone develop along the ribs and other bones. Treatment can include surgical removal of any masses that cause pain.

**multivalent vaccine** n. a single dose of a vaccine that contains several antigens to provide protection against multiple diseases or forms of the same disease. *Compare* univalent vaccine.

**mummified fetus** n. a fetus that died within the womb and subsequently dried out and shrunk.

**murmur** n. an abnormal sound that is heard when listening to the heart with a stethoscope and indicates the presence of turbulent blood flow. Different types of murmurs can be heard with specific diseases, but a murmur does not always adversely affect the animal. *See also* innocent murmur.

**muscle** n. a tissue that can contract and cause movement of or within a structure. *See also* striated and smooth muscle.

**muscle relaxant** n. a drug that decreases the ability of muscles to contract, which can be used to treat muscle spasms.

**muscle wasting** n. a loss of muscle mass that can be seen with neurologic or musculoskeletal diseases, cancer or poor nutrition.

**muscular dystrophy** n. any of a number of genetic or nutritional diseases that cause progressive degeneration of muscles. *See also* white muscle disease.

**musculoskeletal** adj. pertaining to the muscles, bones, cartilage, ligaments and tendons of an animal.

**mushy chick disease** n. infection of the yolk sac of a recently hatched bird that can cause lesions around the navel, depression and death. Improved environmental conditions can prevent the disease. Treatment includes antibiotics and supportive care but is difficult. *Also called* omphalitis and navel ill.

**mutation** n. an alteration in one or more of an animal's genes that can cause disease (e.g., cancer).

**muzzle** n. 1. the portion of the face that consists of the nose and mouth. 2. a device that is placed around an animal's mouth to prevent biting or other unwanted behaviors.

**myalgia** n. muscle pain.

**myasthenia gravis** n. a disorder in which the immune system attacks receptors for the neurotransmitter acetylcholine within muscles. Some cases in young animals are related to a congenital defect, not abnormal immune function. Affected animals can develop weakness, stiffness and tremors that may worsen with exercise and megaesophagus, which leads to regurgitation. Treatment can include medications that increase levels of acetylcholine and immunosuppressants.

**mycetoma** n. a draining mass that is caused by a fungal or bacterial infection.

**mycobacteriosis** n. disease caused by infection with mycobacteria. *See also* tuberculosis, leprosy and paratuberculosis.

**mycoplasmosis** n. disease caused by infection with *Mycoplasma*, a type of very small bacteria. Clinical signs vary with the part of the body affected. *See also* contagious agalactia.

**mycosis** n. a disease caused by a fungus - **mycotic** adj.

**mycosis fungoides** n. *See* epitheliotropic lymphosarcoma.

**mycotoxicosis** n. disease caused by ingestion of toxins produced by fungal organisms. See the specific mycotoxicosis (e.g., ergotism or fescue toxicosis) for details.

**mydriasis** n. widening of an iris, which makes the pupil appear large - **mydriatic** adj. *Compare* miosis.

**myectomy** n. the surgical removal of some or all of a muscle.

**myelin** n. a fatty substance that surrounds and insulates some types of nerve fibers promoting rapid and accurate transmission of signals.

**myelitis** n. inflammation of the spinal cord. *See also* encephalomyelitis.

**myelodysplasia** n. abnormal development of the spinal cord.

**myeloencephalitis** n. inflammation of the brain and spinal cord. *See also* encephalomyelitis, equine herpes myeloencephalitis and equine protozoal myeloencephalitis.

**myelogram** n. a radiograph that is taken after injection of a contrast agent into the space surrounding the spinal cord. A myelogram can be used to help diagnose lesions in and around the spinal cord.

**myeloid** adj. pertaining to the bone marrow or spinal cord.

**myeloma** n. a cancer of plasma cells within the bone marrow. Affected individuals may develop bone pain, fractures, anemia, bleeding, bruising and an increased susceptibility to infection. Chemotherapy can significantly prolong and improve the quality of life.

**myelomalacia** n. softening and degeneration of tissues within the spinal cord, which can be caused by trauma, decreased blood flow and inflammation.

**myelopathy** n. any disease affecting the spinal cord. *See also* wobbler syndrome and degenerative myelopathy.

**myeloproliferative disorder** n. one of a number of diseases in which a type of cell proliferates in the bone marrow. *See also* leukemia, myeloma and polycythemia vera.

**myelosuppression** n. decreased activity of the bone marrow, which results in low blood cell counts.

**myiasis** n. infestation of damaged or soiled skin and fur with maggots hatching from eggs laid by flies. Animals can become extremely depressed, weak and die. Treatment includes removal of the maggots, medications or pesticides that kill them, antibiotics and supportive care. *Also called* fly strike.

**myocardial infarction** n. blockage of the blood supply to a portion of the heart muscle causing tissue damage and sometimes heart failure or sudden death. The condition is most frequently seen in horses. *Also called* heart attack.

**myocarditis** n. inflammation of the myocardium, which can be caused by infection or toxins and lead to heart failure.

**myocardium** n. the muscles that compose the walls of the heart and heart chambers - **myocardial** adj.

**myoclonus** n. abnormal, repeated contractions of a group of muscles. Myoclonus can be seen in some types of infections (e.g., canine distemper) or genetic diseases - **myoclonic** adj.

**myoglobin** n. a protein that carries oxygen within muscles.

**myoglobinuria** n. the abnormal presence of myoglobin in the urine, which can be associated with muscle damage. *See also* exertional rhabdomyolysis.

**myopathy** n. any disease affecting muscles. See the specific myopathy (e.g., cardiomyopathy, hypokalemic polymyopathy and capture myopathy) for details.

**myositis** n. inflammation of muscle tissues. *See also* masticatory muscle myositis.

**myositis ossificans** n. abnormal mineralization of muscle tissue, which can follow injury or inflammation.

**myotonia congenita** n. a genetic disease that causes stiff muscles and difficulty walking. Medications can improve but not cure the condition.

**myringitis** n. inflammation of the eardrum.

**myringotomy** n. a surgical incision through the eardrum.

**myxedema** n. a swelling of tissues that can be seen with hypothyroidism. Myxedema of the skin can produce skin folds around the face while myxedema of the brain can lead to dullness and coma.

**myxoma** n. a benign tumor of connective tissue. Surgical removal can be curative.

**myxomatosis** n. a fatal, viral disease of rabbits that is transmitted through the bites of insects. Affected individuals can develop red eyes, fever, skin swelling and/or nodules (especially around the head), nasal and ocular drainage and difficulty breathing. There is no effective treatment.

# N

**nanophthalmos** n. a condition in which one or both eyes are abnormally small but otherwise normal.

**narcolepsy** n. a disorder of the brain that causes animals to intermittently fall asleep and lose muscle tone at inappropriate times. Attacks may be initiated by excitement. Medications can lessen the severity of the disease.

**narcotic drug** n. a type of medication that is often used to relieve pain. The prescribing of narcotics is strictly regulated by the federal government because of the possibility of abuse. Morphine is a commonly used narcotic.

**nares** n. nostrils.

**nasal** adj. pertaining to the nose.

**nasal bots** n. the larvae of the fly *Oestrus ovis*, which can invade the nasal passages and sinuses of sheep and goats. Affected individuals develop nasal discharge, sneezing and difficulty breathing. Treatment includes medications that kill the larvae.

**nasal catarrh** n. *See* snuffles.

**nasal conchae** n. *See* nasal turbinates.

**nasal meatus** n. one of the passageways that lies in between the nasal turbinates through each nasal cavity.

**nasal mite** n. a very small insect that can infest the nasal cavities of dogs causing sneezing, reverse sneezing and nasal discharge. Treatment includes medications to kill the mites.

**nasal septum** n. the structure that separates the two sides of the nose and is composed of bone, cartilage and mucous membrane.

**nasal solar dermatitis** n. lesions on the skin of the nose and sometimes other areas on the face that develop in response to sunlight exposure. The disorder is most commonly seen in breeds of dogs with white hair in this region and different underlying disorders (e.g., lupus and pemphigus) may be involved. Treatment can include protection from the sun, medications to reduce the immune response and vitamin E. *Also called* collie nose.

**nasal turbinates** n. scrolls of thin bone that lie within the nasal cavities. *Also called* nasal conchae.

**nasogastric tube (NG tube)** n. a flexible tube inserted through the nose and into the stomach, which can be used to provide nutrition, give medications or remove liquid and gas.

**nasolacrimal duct** n. a channel that allows passage of tears from each eye into the nasal cavity.

**nasopharyngeal polyp** n. an abnormal mass of connective tissue that can develop within the outer and middle ear, eustachian tube and nasopharynx of cats and cause difficulty breathing, sneezing and nasal discharge. Treatment includes the surgical removal of the entire polyp.

**nasopharynx** n. the area within the throat that lies behind the nasal cavities and above the soft palate - **nasopharyngeal** adj.

**natural cover** n. mating that occurs via insertion of the penis into the vagina. *Compare* artificial insemination.

**nausea** n. the feeling that vomiting is about to occur. Nauseous animals often drool and lick their lips - **nauseous** adj.

**navel** n. *See* umbilicus.

**navel ill** n. *See* omphalitis.

**navicular bone** n. the boat-shaped bone that lies towards the back of a horse's foot.

**navicular disease** n. degeneration, inflammation and pain affecting a horse's navicular bone and its surrounding structures. Causes include poor conformation, genetics, overwork on hard ground, activities that stretch the tendons running over the navicular bone and heavy body weight. Individuals may point an affected leg forward and develop a lameness that usually worsens with exercise. Treatment can include rest, therapeutic hoof trimming and shoeing, anti-inflammatories, medications that improve blood flow to the damaged tissues and surgeries that lessen pain and stress around the navicular bone.

**near side** n. the left side of a horse's body, described as such because a person usually leads and mounts a horse from the left side. *Compare* far side.

**nebulization** n. a type of treatment that involves inhaling a fine mist of medication and/or water into the lungs.

**neck lesion** n. *See* feline odontoclastic resorptive lesion.

**necrobacillosis** n. disease caused by infection with the bacteria *Fusobacterium necrophorum*. *See also* necrotic laryngitis and footrot.

**necrolytic migratory erythema** n. *See* hepatocutaneous syndrome.

**necropsy** n. the examination of a dead animal, usually to determine the cause of death.

**necrosis** n. death and degeneration of cells within a tissue, which can have many causes including trauma and a deficient blood supply - **necrotic** adj.

**necrotic dermatitis** n. *See* scale rot.

**necrotic laryngitis** n. a disease of young cattle caused by infection of the throat with the bacteria *Fusobacterium necrophorum*. Affected animals often have a cough, difficulty breathing and swallowing, nasal discharge, a fever and drool. Treatment includes antibiotics, anti-inflammatories and sometimes surgery to remove diseased tissue or to perform a tracheostomy. *Also called* calf diphtheria and necrobacillosis.

**necrotizing** adj. causing necrosis.

**necrotizing ulcerative gingivostomatitis** n. a disease of dogs in which bacteria that are normally found in the mouth produce a severe infection, sometimes as a result of an underlying disorder (e.g., stress). Affected animals develop very red and swollen oral mucous membranes, tissue loss, bad breath and reluctance to eat. Treatment can include antibiotics, antiseptics, dental prophylaxes, the surgical removal of diseased tissue and addressing any underlying conditions. *Also called* trench mouth.

**needle holder** n. a surgical instrument used to grasp a needle and suture material while placing stitches.

**negative reinforcement** n. a method of behavioral training in which unwanted behavior quickly results in an unpleasant consequence (e.g., being scolded or ignored). *Compare* positive reinforcement.

**neonatal isoerythrolysis** n. an immune mediated disease in which antibodies ingested through the colostrum destroy a newborn's red blood cells. Affected individuals become very weak and jaundiced within days of being born. Treatment includes preventing access to colostrum, blood transfusions and supportive care. *Also called* alloimmune hemolytic anemia.

**neonatal maladjustment syndrome** n. a disorder of newborn foals that is thought to be associated with inadequate oxygen delivery to the brain during the birthing process. Affected individuals may initially appear normal but then develop one or more of the following signs: an inability to stand or to nurse adequately, excitability or depression, wandering or other abnormal behaviors, infections and seizures. Treatment can include fluid and antibiotic therapy, feedings through a nasogastric tube, plasma transfusions, medications to control seizures and supportive care. *Also called* peripartum asphyxia, dummy foal, and hypoxic ischemic encephalopathy.

**neonatal ophthalmia** n. a disorder in which very young puppies and kittens develop an eye infection before the eyelids open. Treatment can include separating the eyelids, cleaning the eyes and applying topical antibiotics.

**neonate** n. a newborn animal - **neonatal** adj.

**neoplasia** n. *See* cancer - **neoplastic** adj.

**neosporosis** n. a disease caused by infection with *Neospora* protozoal parasites, which are transmitted through ingestion of contaminated tissues and dog feces. A fetus can be infected while still in utero. Neosporosis can cause paralysis that often progresses up the legs, abortion and other disorders. Treatment includes medications to kill the parasite and supportive care.

**neovascularization** n. the development of new blood vessels.

**nephrectomy** n. the surgical removal of a kidney.

**nephritis** n. inflammation of the kidneys. *See also* glomerulonephritis and pyelonephritis.

**nephroblastoma** n. a type of cancer usually affecting the kidneys of young animals. The tumor can become extremely large and spread to other parts of the body. Treatment includes the surgical removal of the kidney and chemotherapy.

**nephrolith** n. *See* kidney stone.

**nephrolithiasis** n. a condition associated with the presence of a kidney stone.

**nephron** n. the kidney's structural and functional unit that filters blood, conserves water and excretes waste products in the form of urine. Each kidney contains numerous nephrons.

**nephropathy** n. any disease of the kidneys. *See also* protein losing nephropathy.

**nephrosplenic entrapment** n. *See* left dorsal displacement of the colon.

**nephrotic syndrome** n. a kidney disorder in which albumin leaks from the blood into the urine often causing fluid to accumulate throughout the body. Glomerulonephritis or other disorders can lead to nephrotic syndrome.

**nephrotoxic** adj. capable of damaging the kidneys.

**nerve** n. cells that transmit electrochemical impulses throughout the body - **neural** adj. *See also* motor and sensory nerve. *Also called* neuron.

**nerve block** n. an injection of a local anesthetic around a nerve, which prevents the sensation of pain from being transmitted to the brain.

**nerve sheath tumor** n. *See* neurofibroma.

**nerving** n. *See* neurectomy.

**nervous system** n. the brain, spinal cord and all of the nerves in the body. *See also* central, peripheral and autonomic nervous system.

**nesting box** n. an enclosed area within a birdcage where the animals can lay and hatch eggs and rear young.

**neuralgia** n. pain that emanates from along a nerve's path.

**neuraxonal dystrophy** n. a genetic disease that causes progressive weakness, difficulty walking and head tremors in young animals. There is no effective treatment.

**neurectomy** n. the surgical removal of a portion of a nerve, which can be performed to relieve pain from chronic degenerative diseases (e.g., navicular disease). *Also called* nerving.

**neurilemmoma** n. *See* neurofibroma.

**neuritis** n. inflammation of a nerve, which can lead to pain and loss of function.

**neurodermatitis** n. skin lesions that develop as a result of compulsive self-trauma. *See also* acral lick dermatitis and twitchy cat disease.

**neuroendocrine system** n. the tissues of the nervous and endocrine systems that often interact to control many body functions.

**neurofibroma** n. a tumor of the cells that produce myelin around nerves. The tumor does not tend to spread from its initial site but can cause significant pain and loss of function (e.g., muscle atrophy and lameness). Treatment can include the surgical removal of the tumor and radiation therapy. *Also called* neurofibrosarcoma, perineuroma, neurilemmoma, nerve sheath tumor and schwannoma.

**neurogenic shock** n. inadequate delivery of oxygen to tissues caused by an injury to the brain or spinal cord that leads to a sudden drop in blood pressure and often organ failure and death. Treatment can include fluid and oxygen therapy, corticosteroids and medications to increase blood pressure.

**neuroleptanalgesia** n. a combination of medications that together provide both pain relief and sedation.

**neurologic** adj. pertaining to the nervous system. *Also called* neurological.

**neuroma** n. a tumor of nerve tissue that can form after injury to or excision of a portion of a nerve and cause pain. Surgical removal is curative.

**neuromuscular blocker** n. drugs that inhibit the transmission of signals through the neuromuscular junction and cause muscle relaxation or paralysis.

**neuromuscular junction** n. the connection between a nerve fiber and a muscle through which signals to contract are transmitted.

**neuron** n. *See* nerve.

**neuropathy** n. any disorder that adversely affects the functions of nerves. *See also* diabetic neuropathy and polyneuropathy.

**neuropraxia** n. a temporary loss of function of a nerve, usually due to trauma.

**neurotoxin** n. a poison that adversely affects the nervous system.

**neurotransmitter** n. a chemical that transmits signals between nerves or between nerves and other body parts (e.g., muscles).

**neuter** v. to surgically remove or otherwise disable the testicles. The term can also refer to the removal of the ovaries. *Also called* castrate.

**neutropenia** n. a lower than normal number of neutrophils in the bloodstream.

**neutrophil** n. a type of white blood cell that plays an important role in fighting infections and in inflammation. *Also called* polymorphonuclear leukocyte.

**neutrophilia** n. a higher than normal number of neutrophils in the bloodstream.

**nevus** n. a benign area of abnormal tissue, often describing a spot of dark pigmentation - **nevi** pl.

**Newcastle disease** n. a contagious, viral disease in birds. Affected individuals can develop difficulty breathing, neurologic abnormalities, diarrhea and tissue swelling. Treatment is limited to supportive care. Preventative vaccines are available. *Also called* pneumoencephalitis. *See also* viscerotropic velogenic Newcastle disease.

**niacin** n. a type of vitamin B that is important for maintaining the health of the gastrointestinal tract and skin.

**nictitating membrane** n. *See* third eyelid.

**nidus** n. a localized point of origin for a disease within the body.

**night feces** n. *See* cecotrope.

**nitrate poisoning** n. a disease most often seen in cattle that ingest forage, fertilizers or other chemicals containing high levels of nitrate, which makes red blood cells less able to carry oxygen. Affected individuals can develop tremors, weakness, difficulty walking and breathing, dark discoloration of tissues and urine and may die. Treatment includes medications that improve the oxygen carrying capacity of blood and supportive care. *Also called* nitrite poisoning.

**nit** n. an egg that is laid by a louse and is attached to the hair of an infested individual.

**nocardiosis** n. a disease caused by infection with *Nocardia* bacteria that usually enter the body through wounds or by inhaling organisms present in the environment. Individuals can develop draining nodules, fever and loss of energy, appetite and weight. The infection may persist despite treatment with appropriate antibiotics.

**nociception** n. the ability to sense pain.

**nocturnal** adj. pertaining to or active during the nighttime. *Compare* diurnal.

**nodular episcleritis** n. *See* canine fibrous histiocytoma.

**nodular fasciitis** n. *See* canine fibrous histiocytoma.

**nodular hyperplasia** n. a benign proliferation of tissue most commonly affecting the livers of older dogs, which can cause mild to moderate increases in liver enzymes but requires no treatment.

**nodular necrobiosis** n. a disease of horses with a suspected allergy to insect bites that causes them to develop firm nodules in the skin. Treatment can include corticosteroids and surgery. *Also called* equine collagenolytic granuloma.

**nodule** n. a small, rounded mass of tissue - **nodular** adj.

**nondiagnostic** adj. said of a laboratory test or other procedure that was hoped to help in the diagnosis of an animal's condition but did not provide useful information.

**nonfunctional tumor** n. a glandular tumor that does not secrete large amounts of a hormone or other substances that adversely affect the body.

**non-protein nitrogen poisoning** n. a disease usually seen in cattle caused by eating too much or a new type of urea or non-protein nitrogen in their feed. Affected individuals often drool, tremble, grind their teeth and have abdominal pain, difficulty breathing and bizarre behavior. Treatment includes procedures that limit the absorption of ammonia from the gastrointestinal tract and supportive care, but death can occur rapidly. *Also called* ammonia toxicosis, bovine bonkers, urea poisoning and ammoniated forage poisoning.

**nonregenerative anemia** n. a lower than normal red blood cell count that is not associated with the bone marrow responding to produce more red blood cells. Nonregenerative anemias can be seen with nutritional deficiencies (e.g., iron), disorders affecting the bone marrow or kidneys and many chronic diseases. *Compare* regenerative anemia.

**nonresponsive** adj. not responding to external stimuli.

**nonsteroidal anti-inflammatory drug (NSAID)** n. a type of medication that decreases inflammation and pain. Phenylbutazone and Rimadyl® are commonly used NSAIDs. *See also* NSAID toxicity.

**nonsuppurative polyarthritis of lambs** n. a disease of young sheep and sometimes other species caused by infection of wounds with *Erysipelothrix rhusiopathiae* bacteria. Affected individuals can develop painful, warm and sometimes enlarged joints. Treatment with antibiotics can be successful in early infections.

**nonunion** n. a broken bone that has not fused despite the passage of adequate time since the injury.

**nose bot** n. *See* nasal bot.

**nosocomial** adj. pertaining to the hospital. For example, a nosocomial infection is an infection that was contracted while in the hospital.

**notoedric mange** n. an intensely itchy, contagious skin disease of cats caused by the *Notoedres cati* mite. Individuals often develop skin lesions around the head and neck. Other animals, including people, can become infected. Treatment includes medications to kill the mite.

**NSAID toxicity** n. disease caused by an abnormal sensitivity to or overdosage with nonsteroidal anti-inflammatory drugs. Affected individuals can develop bleeding ulcers in the gastrointestinal tract, vomiting, diarrhea, kidney and liver dysfunction and other disorders. Treatment may include procedures to limit absorption of the drug from the digestive tract, medications that prevent or treat ulcers, fluid therapy and supportive care.

**nuchal ligament** n. a band of fibrous connective tissue that runs through the neck and supports the head.

**nuclear sclerosis** n. *See* lenticular sclerosis.

**nucleated red blood cell (NRBC)** n. an immature red blood cell that can be seen under the microscope when an animal's bone marrow is responding to an anemia or is affected by toxins or disease.

**nucleic acid** n. *See* deoxyribonucleic acid and ribonucleic acid.

**nucleus** n. 1. a structure within cells that contains chromosomes and controls the activities of the cell. 2. a group of cells in the brain that together perform a specific function - **nuclei** pl.

**nullipara** n. a female that has never had a successful pregnancy - **nulliparous** adj. *Compare* primipara and multipara.

**nurse** v. 1. to provide nutrition to a young animal through lactation. 2. to generally care for and provide comfort to a sick animal.

**nutraceutical** n. a substance that is normally found in food and can be used to treat or prevent disease.

**nutrient** n. a substance required in the diet to maintain normal body function. Vitamins, minerals, carbohydrates, fats, proteins and water are all important nutrients.

**nutrition** n. the ingestion, digestion, absorption and utilization of dietary substances that are necessary to maintain normal body function.

**nutritional myopathy** n. any disease of muscle that is caused by poor nutrition. *See also* white muscle disease.

**nutritional secondary hyperparathyroidism** n. a disease caused by imbalances in the amounts of phosphorous, calcium and vitamin D in the diet. Affected animals have bones that

easily bend or break and are painful. Correcting the diet is usually curative unless too much bone damage has occurred. *Also called* rickets, osteomalacia or in horses, bran disease, miller's disease and big head.

**nyctalopia** n. an inability to see under conditions of very low light.

**nymphomania** n. prolonged or exaggerated estrus behavior that is often caused by ovarian abnormalities (e.g., granulosa-theca cell tumors and follicular cysts).

**nystagmus** n. a rhythmic and involuntary movement of the eyes, which can be an indication of damage to the vestibular system or cerebellum.

# O

**oak bud poisoning** n. *See* acorn poisoning.

**obese** adj. having significantly more body fat than is healthy - **obesity** n.

**oblique** adj. at an angle.

**obsessive-compulsive disorder** n. normal behavior that is done with such frequency or intensity as to become a problem. For example, animals may chew on themselves to the point of developing skin lesions. Treatment can include behavior modifying protocols and drugs. *Also called* stereotypy.

**obstetrics (OB)** n. the care of animals during pregnancy and labor.

**obstipation** n. a blockage of the large intestine with feces, which may be due to dehydration, intestinal disorders or ingestion of undigestible materials. Affected animals may develop abdominal pain, reluctance to eat and straining and an inability to defecate. Treatment can include fluid therapy, stool softeners, enemas and manual or surgical removal of the feces.

**obstruction** n. an object or lesion that prevents normal movement of materials past a particular point - **obstructive** adj.

**obtunded** adj. describes a dull mental state or deadened pain.

**obturator nerve paralysis** n. *See* calving paralysis.

**occipitoatlantoaxial malformation** n. a disorder, often genetic, in which the bones that connect the back of the head to the top of the spine are not formed correctly. Affected individuals can develop weakness, difficulty walking and other neurologic abnormalities. Surgery to relieve pressure on the spinal cord is sometimes successful.

**occlusion** n. 1. the manner in which two opposing teeth meet when the mouth is closed. 2. the blockage of a structure through which material normally flows - **occlusive**, **occlusal** adj.

**occult** adj. not easily observed.

**ocular** adj. pertaining to the eye.

**oculocardiac reflex** n. a slowing of the heart rate that is seen with manipulation of, or application of, pressure to the eye.

**oculocephalic reflex** n. an eye motion that is seen in a comatose patient when the head is moved. The eyes should appear as if they are fixed on a stationary object as the head is rotated. If this does not occur, there is damage to the brainstem or inner ear. *Also called* doll's eye reflex.

**odontoma** n. a benign mass composed of the substances normally found in teeth (e.g., enamel). Surgical removal is curative.

**odynophagia** n. pain during swallowing.

**off-label drug use** n. *See* extra-label drug use.

**offset cannon** n. *See* bench knee.

**old dog encephalitis** n. a condition seen in some older dogs chronically infected with the canine distemper virus. Affected individuals can have difficulty walking, bizarre behavior and other neurologic abnormalities. Frequently, these animals never showed the more typical signs of canine distemper infection. Corticosteroids can help control the disorder.

**olecranon** n. the bony point of the elbow located at the top of the ulna.

**olfactory** adj. pertaining to the sense of smell.

**oligodontia** n. a birth defect in which fewer teeth are present in the mouth than is normal.

**oligogalactia** n. the production of less milk than is normal.

**oligospermia** n. the presence of fewer sperm in the ejaculate than is normal.

**oliguria** n. the formation of less urine than is normal.

**omasum** n. one of the four chambers of the ruminant stomach - **omasal** adj.

**omentalization** n. a surgical procedure in which the omentum is used to promote healing (e.g., as a patch over a potentially weak area of intestinal wall).

**omentum** n. a membrane within the abdomen that contains blood vessels and fat and surrounds and attaches to the stomach, liver and other organs.

**omnivore** n. an animal that eats both plants and other animals.

**omphalitis** n. infection of the umbilical stump, which can spread into the bloodstream of a newborn animal. *Also called* navel ill.

**onchocerciasis** n. disease caused by *Onchocerca* parasites. Adult worms can form nodules in the nuchal ligament and their larvae congregate in the skin and may cause itching and lesions, especially along the bottom of the abdomen. Medications can kill the larvae, but no treatment is available for the adult worms.

**oncology** n. the study and treatment of cancer.

**oncotic pressure** n. the ability of an animal's blood to hold fluid within the circulatory system. Oncotic pressure is primarily maintained by the presence of proteins (e.g., albumin) within the bloodstream. *Also called* colloid osmotic pressure.

**onion toxicosis** n. ingestion of sufficient quantities of onion to cause anemia, weakness, discolored urine and sometimes diarrhea, collapse and death. Treatment includes removing the source of onion and supportive care.

**onychectomy** n. the surgical removal of the nails and all of the tissues that could allow them to regrow. *Also called* declawing.

**onychomycosis** n. a fungal infection of the nails.

**oophorectomy** n. *See* ovariectomy.

**opaque** adj. not allowing light or other radiation to pass through - **opacity, opacification** n.

**open** adj. 1. exposed to the environment. 2. not pregnant.

**open fracture** n. *See* compound fracture.

**open herd** n. a number of animals that are managed together and into which individuals from outside of the group are occasionally added. An open herd has a higher risk for outbreaks of infectious disease than does a closed herd.

**ophthalmic** adj. pertaining to the eyes.

**ophthalmoscope** n. an instrument that magnifies and allows the veterinarian to thoroughly examine the eye.

**opioid** n. a type of medication that is often used to relieve pain or as a cough suppressant. The prescribing of opioids is strictly regulated by the federal government because of the possibility of abuse. Morphine and butorphanol are commonly used opioids. *Also called* opiate.

**opisthotonos** n. an abnormal body position that is characterized by backwards extension of the head and an arched back, which can be seen with brain lesions or other diseases (e.g., tetanus).

**opportunistic infection** n. an infection with microorganisms that are typically present in the environment or within an animal but do not generally cause disease. Opportunistic infections often develop because of a breakdown in an animal's immune defenses.

**optic** adj. pertaining to the eyes.

**optic disk cupping** n. an abnormal appearance to the part of the eye into which the optic nerve runs. Optic disk cupping can be seen with glaucoma.

**optic nerve** n. the nerve that transmits visual signals from the eye to the brain.

**optic neuritis** n. inflammation of the optic nerve, which can be associated with systemic infections, trauma or granulomatous meningoencephalitis. Affected individuals may become blind. Treatment can include corticosteroids and addressing the underlying disease.

**oral** adj. pertaining to the mouth.

**oral hypoglycemia agent** n. a type of medication that can be taken by mouth and will reduce blood sugar levels in some diabetic animals.

**orbit** n. the socket for the eye within the skull - **orbital** adj.

**orchiectomy** n. the surgical removal of one or both testicles. *Also called* **orchidectomy**.

**orchiepididymitis** n. inflammation of one or both testicles and the attached epididymides.

**orchitis** n. inflammation of one or both testicles, which is usually associated with infection.

**orf** n. a contagious, viral disease of sheep and goats. Affected individuals often develop lesions around the lips, within the mouth and sometimes around the feet or on the udder. Infected animals may transmit the virus to people. Antibiotics can help treat or prevent secondary bacterial infections as the viral lesions heal. Preventative vaccination is effective. *Also called* contagious ecthyma, contagious pustular dermatitis and sore mouth.

**organomegaly** n. enlargement of an organ, usually referring to those located in the abdomen.

**organophosphate toxicity** n. poisoning by exposure to organophosphate chemicals, which are commonly used as insecticides. Affected animals can exhibit drooling, ocular discharge, urination, diarrhea, muscle tremors, weakness, depression, difficulty breathing and may die. Treatment can include washing the animal if the exposure was topical, treatments to limit absorption from the gastrointestinal tract if the poison was ingested, medications to block or reverse the effects of the poison and supportive care.

**orifice** n. an opening into or out of a cavity.

**ornithosis** n. *See* psittacosis.

**orogastric intubation** n. the insertion of a flexible tube through the mouth and into the stomach, which can be used to temporarily provide nutrition, give medications or remove liquid and gas.

**oronasal** adj. pertaining to the mouth and nose.

**oropharynx** n. the area within the throat that lies behind the tongue and soft palate and moves food towards the esophagus - **oropharyngeal** adj.

**orthodontics** n. treatments that realign improperly oriented teeth.

**orthopedic** adj. pertaining to bones and their associated structures (e.g., ligaments and cartilage).

**Orthopedic Foundation for Animals (OFA)** n. an organization concerned with lowering the incidence of orthopedic and genetic diseases of dogs.

**orthopnea** n. difficulty breathing that is partially relieved by a particular body position. For example, dogs with congestive heart failure will often stand or sit with their elbows pushed away from their chest and are reluctant to lie down.

**Ortolani sign** n. an abnormal movement that can be felt when the rear leg of a dog with hip dysplasia is pressed up and moved away from the midline of the animal.

**osselets** n. inflammation and subsequent bony growth affecting the surface of the bones around a horse's fetlock joint, which causes pain, swelling and lameness. Overtraining a young horse on hard ground is often to blame. Treatment includes rest and procedures and medications that reduce inflammation and pain. *Also called* periostitis.

**osseous** adj. pertaining to bones or bony substances.

**ossicle** n. a small bone. For example, the three bones in the middle ear that transmit vibrations from the ear drum to the nerves of the inner ear are called auditory ossicles.

**ossification** n. the process of becoming bone or a bone-like substance - **ossifying** adj.

**ossifying myopathy** n. *See* fibrotic and ossifying myopathy.

**osteoarthritis** n. progressive deterioration of the cartilage that covers the surfaces of many bones involved in joints. Affected individuals can develop pain, joint swelling, muscle atrophy, stiffness and bony proliferation around the joint. Many factors may lead to the development of osteoarthritis including trauma, abnormal joint development, genetics, infections, immune disorders and poor conformation. Treat-ment can include anti-inflammatories, chondroprotective agents, pain relief, acupuncture and surgery. *Also called* degenerative joint disease.

**osteochondritis dissecans (OCD)** n. a disease most commonly seen in young, rapidly growing animals in which a portion of cartilage within a joint develops abnormally. Individuals may have swollen joints and become stiff and lame. Treatment can include rest, reduced feeding, anti-inflammatories, chondroprotective agents and surgery to remove affected areas of cartilage and underlying bone. *Also called* osteochondrosis.

**osteochondroma** n. *See* exostosis.

**osteochondromatosis** n. *See* multiple cartilaginous exostoses.

**osteodystrophy** n. any disease that causes abnormal bone development or changes in bony tissue because of nutritional or metabolic disorders. *See also* fibrous and hypertrophic osteodystrophy.

**osteogenesis imperfecta** n. a genetic disease that causes the development of loose joints and easily broken bones. No effective treatment is available.

**osteohemochromatosis** n. *See* erythropoietic porphyria.

**osteolysis** n. the destruction of bone - **osteolytic** adj.

**osteoma** n. a benign tumor of bone. Treatment can include surgical removal of the mass.

**osteomalacia** n. *See* nutritional secondary hyperparathyroidism.

**osteomyelitis** n. infection and inflammation of bone.

**osteopathy** n. any disorder affecting bones. *See also* craniomandibular and hypertrophic osteopathy.

**osteophyte** n. an abnormal growth of bone around a joint that can cause pain if it is traumatized or impinges on other tissues. *Also called* bone spur or exostosis.

**osteoporosis** n. a condition producing bones that are weak and easily fractured. Osteoporosis is often caused by calcium being removed from bone because of increased demand by the body (e.g., milk/egg production).

**osteosarcoma (OSA)** n. a malignant cancer of bone that causes pain, hard swellings and lameness when a leg is affected. Treatment can include amputation of a limb or removal of the diseased portion of bone. Chemotherapy in addition to surgery can help prolong survival times.

**osteosclerosis** n. abnormally hard or dense bones.

**osteotomy** n. the surgical cutting of a bone.

**ostertagiasis** n. infestation of the abomasum of cattle or other ruminants with *Ostertagia* worms. Heavily infested individuals can develop diarrhea and weight loss. Many dewormers are effective. *Also called* brown stomach worm.

**otitis** n. inflammation of the ear, which is often associated with infection. *See also* otitis externa, media and interna.

**otitis externa** n. inflammation of the outer ear, which is often associated with infection. Affected individuals can be itchy or in pain, shake their head and have discharge from the ear. Some infections develop because of underlying problems such as abnormal anatomy or allergies. Treatment can include repeated cleaning of the ear, medications to kill yeast, bacteria or mites, corticosteroids and addressing any underlying disorders.

**otitis interna** n. infection and inflammation of the inner ear. Otitis interna usually occurs because of extension of an outer ear infection through the ear drum and middle ear. Affected animals can develop a head tilt, circling, abnormal eye movements and difficulty walking. Treatment includes the long term use of systemic antibiotics.

**otitis media** n. infection and inflammation of the middle ear. Otitis media usually occurs because of extension of an outer ear infection through the ear drum. Symptoms are similar to otitis externa, but may also include Horner's syndrome and facial nerve paralysis. Treatment can include surgical procedures to facilitate removal of infected material from the middle ear in addition to therapy as is described for otitis externa.

**otodectic mange** n. infestation of the ears with *Otodectes cynotis* mites. *See also* ear mite.

**otoplasty** n. the surgical reconstruction of the ear.

**otoscope** n. an instrument used to look in the ear canal.

**ototoxic** adj. capable of damaging the sense of hearing or balance.

**outbreeding** n. the mating of individuals that are not closely related to one-another, which can decrease the chances of producing offspring with genetic abnormalities. *Compare* inbreeding.

**outer ear** n. the external portion of the ear that collects sound waves and funnels them towards the eardrum. *See also* inner and middle ear.

**ovarian remnant syndrome** n. a condition that is seen when an animal is spayed but both ovaries are not completely removed. Affected individuals will continue to appear to come into heat. Treatment includes the surgical removal of any remaining ovarian tissue.

**ovariectomy** n. the surgical removal of one or both ovaries. *Also called* oophorectomy.

**ovariohysterectomy (OHE)** n. the surgical removal of the ovaries and uterus. *See also* spay.

**ovary** n. one of the two organs that are located in the abdomen of females, release eggs and produce hormones related to reproduction.

**over at the knee** n. a conformation flaw usually described in horses in which the middle of the front leg appears to bow forward when viewed from the side. *Also called* buck knee. *Compare* back at the knee.

**overbite** n. the condition of having upper front teeth that protrude further forward than is normal. *Compare* underbite.

**overeating disease** n. a disease most commonly seen in sheep and goats that is caused by infection with *Clostridium perfringens* type D bacteria. Infections usually occur in newborns drinking excessive quantities of milk or animals rapidly switched to a high carbohydrate diet. Affected individuals can develop difficulty walking, bizarre behavior, seizures, diarrhea and may die rapidly. Treatment is difficult but can include antibiotics, antitoxin injections, antiserum and supportive care. Modifying the diet and vaccination can help prevent the disease. *Also called* pulpy kidney disease.

**overhydration** n. a higher than normal amount of water within the body, which may be caused by overuse of intravenous fluids or kidney disfunction. Overhydration can cause abnormal fluid accumulations and difficulty breathing.

**Overo lethal white disorder** n. *See* ileocolonic agangliosis.

**overreaching** n. moving the rear feet too far forward when in motion and striking the front legs. *Also called* forging.

**overriding dorsal spinous processes** n. *See* kissing spines syndrome.

**overshot jaw** n. *See* brachygnathism.

**over-the-counter (OTC)** adj. pertaining to a medication that is available without a prescription.

**oviduct** n. the passageway through which an egg released by the ovary travels to the uterus (mammals) or to the outside of the body (birds and reptiles).

**ovine** adj. pertaining to sheep.

**ovine progressive pneumonia (OPP)** n. a contagious, viral disease of sheep that causes difficulty breathing, weight loss and sometimes neurologic abnormalities, including difficulty walking, weakness and paralysis. No effective treatment or vaccine exists. *Also called* maedi-visna.

**ovulate** v. to release an egg from an ovary after which it can be fertilized by sperm - **ovulation** n.

**ovum** n. the female reproductive cell capable of forming an embryo after fertilization (i.e., an egg) - **ova** pl.

**oxygen (O₂)** n. an element that is essential for normal respiration and metabolism.

**oxygen cage** n. an enclosed cage into which oxygen can be pumped in order to provide oxygen therapy.

**oxygen saturation** n. the amount of oxygen carried within the bloodstream. *Also called* oxygenation.

**oxygen therapy** n. supplementing a higher concentration of oxygen into the air that an animal breathes. Oxygen therapy is often used in the treatment of diseases affecting the lungs and circulatory system.

**oxyuriasis** n. infestation of the large intestine with pinworms. Affected individuals can have pinworm eggs crusted around their anus and be very itchy. Many dewormers can eliminate the parasites.

## P

**p wave** n. a peak recorded on an electrocardiogram, which can change shape, size and frequency with different types of diseases affecting the heart, especially those of the atria.

**pacemaker** n. anything that controls the rate at which something occurs, often specifically referring to a device that can be implanted in the body to stimulate rhythmic contractions of the heart.

**Pacheco's disease** n. a contagious, viral disease of some types of birds (e.g., parrots) that can cause lethargy, loss of appetite, nasal discharge, diarrhea and sudden death. Some individuals remain carriers capable of spreading the virus after recovering from their illness. Treatment can include supportive care and antiviral medications. A preventative vaccine is available.

**pachydermatitis** n. abnormally thickened skin.

**packed cell volume (PCV)** n. a measure of an animal's red blood cell count.

**paintbrush lesion** n. a tuft of hair with an attached crust that is easily pulled from the skin. Paint brush lesions can be seen with dermatophilosis and other skin diseases.

**palate** n. the roof of the mouth - **palatal** adj. *See also* hard and soft palate.

**palliate** v. to make an animal more comfortable without otherwise altering the course of disease - **palliation** n., **palliative** adj.

**pallor** n. a pale tone to the skin or mucous membranes.

**palmar** adj. pertaining to the back of a front limb below the carpus. *Compare* plantar.

**palpate** v. to use the hands to feel parts of an animal's body - **palpation** n.

**palpebra** n. an eyelid - **palpebral** adj.

**palpebral nerve block** n. *See* auriculopalpebral nerve block.

**palpebral reflex** n. the normal, involuntary reaction to close the eyelids when they are touched.

**pancreas** n. an abdominal organ, parts of which produce insulin while other areas secrete digestive enzymes - **pancreatic** adj.

**pancreatic acinar cell atrophy** n. *See* exocrine pancreatic insufficiency.

**pancreatic lipase immunoreactivity (PLI)** n. a laboratory test that can be used to help diagnose pancreatitis.

**pancreatitis** n. inflammation of the pancreas, which can cause loss of appetite, lethargy, vomiting, abdominal pain and diarrhea. Pancreatitis may be initiated by eating a high fat or an otherwise abnormal meal, but many cases do not have an identifiable origin. Treatment can include fluid therapy, withholding food and water, plasma transfusions and medications to relieve nausea and pain.

**pancytopenia** n. lower than normal numbers of red and white blood cells and platelets in circulation. Pancytopenia can be seen with diseases affecting the bone marrow. *See also* aplastic anemia.

**pandemic** n. an outbreak of disease that is occurring in many locations and spreading more rapidly than is normally seen.

**panhypopituitarism** n. a disease caused by a genetic failure of pituitary gland development or a tumor or other lesion that disrupts its function. Affected newborns initially appear normal but grow slowly, retain their juvenile coat and have other developmental abnormalities and a shortened life span. Hormone supplements can improve quality and duration of life. *Also called* pituitary dwarfism. Adult animals that develop tumors or other lesions affecting the pituitary gland often are uncoordinated, depressed, blind, urinate excessively, lose weight and behave abnormally. Treatment is difficult.

**panleukopenia** n. *See* feline panleukopenia.

**panniculitis** n. inflammation of the fat underneath the skin. *See also* yellow fat disease.

**panniculus reflex** n. the normal, involuntary reaction of twitching the skin along the sides of the chest and abdomen when the area is pinched or poked.

**pannus** n. an immune mediated disease that causes abnormal tissue to develop on the surface of the eye. The tissue begins to infiltrate the cornea at the corners of the eye but may progress to cover the entire surface, leading to blindness. Treatment can include medications to suppress the immune response on the surface of the eye, or surgery.

**panophthalmitis** n. inflammation that is usually associated with infection and affects all parts of the eye.

**panosteitis** n. a disease seen most frequently in young, large breed dogs that may be caused by genetics or the excessive use of dietary supplements. Affected individuals can develop lameness that seems to shift between legs, a fever, loss of appetite and pain when pressure is applied to the long bones of the legs. Treatment includes rest and medications to reduce pain and inflammation. Once the period of bone growth ends, the disease resolves.

**pansteatitis** n. *See* yellow fat disease.

**pant** v. to take rapid, shallow breaths in and out of the mouth. Panting is a mechanism for heat loss in some animals (e.g., dogs) but can also be seen during times of stress.

**papilla** n. a small projection off the surface of a tissue - **papillae** pl., **papillary** adj.

**papillary acanthoma** n. *See* aural plaque.

**papillary stomatitis** n. *See* papillomatosis.

**papilloma** n. a warty growth that can be caused by a virus, particularly when young animals are affected. *See also* papillomatosis, sebaceous adenoma and sebaceous epithelioma - **papillomatous** adj.

**papillomatosis** n. a disease characterized by the presence of multiple papillomas. In young animals, papillomatosis is often caused by a contagious virus producing warts around the lips and within the mouth or on the genitalia and udder. The disease will usually resolve without intervention, but vaccines made from the warts themselves or surgery can hasten healing.

**papule** n. a small, solid, raised mass in the skin - **papular** adj.

**paracentesis** n. the insertion of a hollow needle into a cavity, usually to withdraw fluid.

**paragonimiasis** n. a disease that is caused by infestation of the lungs with *Paragonimus* flukes contracted through the ingestion of raw crabs and crayfish. Affected individuals can develop weakness and a cough. Treatment includes medications that kill the flukes.

**parainfluenza** n. a group of related viruses that often cause respiratory disease. *See also* kennel cough and bovine respiratory disease complex.

**parakeratosis** n. a disorder in which affected animals develop skin with thick, horny scales and cracks. Some cases are genetic while others are related to oversupplementation with calcium or a dietary zinc deficiency. Treatment can include changing the diet and zinc supplements.

**paralumbar** adj. pertaining to the area around the part of the back located between the rib cage and pelvis.

**paralysis** n. a loss of the ability to move or to feel sensations in a part of the body. See the particular type of paralysis (e.g., calving or facial nerve paralysis) for details. *Compare* paresis.

**paranasal sinus** n. one of several hollow cavities in the bones of the skull that connect with the nasal passageways.

**paraneoplastic** adj. occurring as a result of cancer.

**paraparesis** n. weakness or incomplete paralysis of the hind end of the body.

**paraphimosis** n. an inability to retract the penis because of penile engorgement or the presence of something that constricts the passageway into the sheath (e.g., a fur ring). *Compare* phimosis.

**paraplegia** n. paralysis affecting the hind end of the body.

**parasite** n. an organism that draws its nourishment from and adversely affects the animal in or on which it lives - **parasitic** adj.

**parasitemia** n. the presence of para-sitic organisms within the bloodstream.

**parasiticide** n. a medication that kills parasites.

**parasitology** n. the science and study of parasites and the diseases that they cause.

**parasympathetic nervous system** n. part of the autonomic nervous system that acts to slow the heart rate, increase some digestive functions and constrict the pupils. *Compare* sympathetic nervous system.

**parasympatholytic** adj. *See* anticholinergic.

**parasympathomimetic** adj. *See* cholinergic.

**parathyroid gland** n. several, small glands that lie adjacent to the thyroid gland in the neck and secrete parathyroid hormone.

**parathyroid hormone (PTH)** n. a substance produced by the parathyroid gland that helps regulate blood calcium levels. *Also called* parathormone. *See also* hyperparathyroidism and hypoparathyroidism.

**parathyroidectomy** n. the surgical removal of the parathyroid gland.

**paratuberculosis** n. a contagious disease that is seen most frequently in cattle and caused by infection with *Mycobacterium paratuberculosis* bacteria. Affected individuals develop chronic diarrhea, weight loss and eventually die. No effective treatment exists. Many countries have eradication programs in place, and suspected cases must be reported to appropriate regulatory agencies. *Also called* Johne's disease.

**paratyphoid** n. *See* salmonellosis.

**parenteral** adj. not given through the intestinal tract (e.g., injected under the skin or infused into a vein).

**parenteral nutrition** n. water, carbohydrates, proteins and other nourishing substances given by an intravenous infusion to an animal that cannot absorb nutrients through its intestinal tract. *Compare* enteral nutrition.

**paresis** n. incomplete paralysis that is often exhibited as weakness and an inability to rise or walk without assistance. *Compare* paralysis.

**paresthesia** n. an abnormal sensation (e.g., tingling) that can be associated with nerve damage.

**parietal** adj. pertaining to the walls of a body cavity.

**parotid duct transposition** n. a surgery used to treat keratoconjunctivitis sicca in which a duct that normally carries saliva to the mouth is moved so that it lubricates the surface of the eye.

**paroxysmal** adj. occurring intermittently, suddenly and intensely.

**parrot fever** n. *See* psittacosis.

**parrot mouth** n. *See* brachygnathism.

**partial seizure** n. a type of seizure during which an animal remains conscious but can display unusual behaviors or movement, such as biting at the air. Partial seizures result from abnormal electrical activity originating from only a small portion of the brain. *See also* seizure. *Also called* focal seizure. *Compare* generalized seizure.

**partial thromboplastin time (PTT)** n. a test that measures the clotting ability of blood. A prolonged PTT indicates abnormalities affecting particular coagulation factors. *Also called* activated partial thromboplastin time.

**partial-thickness** adj. not involving the entire depth of skin or another tissue. *Compare* full-thickness.

**parturient paresis** n. a disease of cows, sheep and goats caused by an increased demand for calcium by a fetus or milk production, which lowers blood calcium levels in the dam around the time of birth. Affected females can develop weakness, difficulty walking, bizarre behavior, bloat and may collapse and die. Treatment includes calcium supplements, which should not be given before parturient paresis develops as it actually decrease the animal's ability to mobilize calcium from the body as demand increases. *Also called* milk fever and hypocalcemia.

**parturition** n. *See* labor.

**parvovirus** n. a group of related viruses that can affect different species often causing vomiting, diarrhea or abortions. *See also* canine and porcine parvovirus and feline panleukopenia.

**passive immunity** n. resistance to disease that is transferred from one animal to another through colostrum, while within the womb or through administration of serum containing antibodies. *Compare* active immunity.

**pastern** n. the part of the lower leg located between the fetlock and the hoof.

**pasteurellosis** n. a disease caused by *Pasteurella* bacteria, which often infect the respiratory tract causing fever, difficulty breathing, nasal discharge, a cough and sometimes death. Treatment can include antibiotics, anti-inflammatories and supportive and symptomatic care. Preventative vaccines are available for some animal species. *See also* snuffles (rabbits).

**pasture** n. a field of grass and/or other plants from which grazing animals can gain the majority of their nutrition.

**pasture bloat** n. *See* frothy bloat.

**patella** n. the bone that lies over the front of the stifle joint (i.e., the kneecap) - **patellar** adj.

**patellar luxation** n. an abnormal movement of the patella to the side of its normal groove over the stifle joint, which can be caused by trauma or anatomic abnormalities. Affected individuals will intermittently skip on a hind leg, during which time they may be in pain. Treatment can include surgeries that prevent the patella from slipping to the side of the knee. *See also* upward fixation of the patella (horses and cattle).

**patellar reflex** n. the normal, involuntary response of kicking the lower leg forward when one of the ligaments attached to the patella is struck.

**patent** adj. open (e.g., describing a tube through which fluid can flow) or readily evident.

**patent ductus arteriosus (PDA)** n. a disease caused by the failure of a vessel that shunts blood past the lungs in a fetus to close after birth. Affected individuals can develop congestive heart failure and arrhythmias. In most cases, treatment involves surgery to close off the abnormal vessel.

**patent urachus** n. an abnormal opening that allows urine to flow from the umbilical stump of a newborn animal. Treatment can include surgical repair and antibiotics to treat infections of the bladder or skin damaged by dribbling urine.

**paternal** adj. pertaining to a male parent. *Compare* maternal.

**pathogen** n. a microorganism or substance that can cause disease - **pathogenic** adj.

**pathologic** adj. pertaining to or occurring because of disease. For example, a pathologic fracture is a broken bone that occurs because an underlying disease (e.g., cancer) has weakened the bone.

**pathology** n. the study of the cause and effects of disease, especially as it relates to tissues within the body.

**pathophysiology** n. the study of the mechanisms by which diseases arise and the body functions that are disturbed by them.

**pectoral** adj. pertaining to the chest.

**pectus excavatum** n. a birth defect in which the bottom of the chest is pushed inwards. Surgical repair is possible for animals adversely affected by the condition.

**pedal osteitis** n. inflammation, degeneration and pain involving the large bone encased within a horse's hoof, which is often caused by overwork on hard surfaces. Treatment can include rest, corrective shoeing and anti-inflammatories.

**pediatric** adj. pertaining to young animals.

**pediculosis** n. a disease caused by lice that infest the skin and coat of animals. Affected individuals can become very itchy and may develop anemia if heavily infested with certain types of lice. Lice that infest one species of animal generally cannot cause disease in an unrelated species. Treatment includes medications that kill the parasites.

**pedigree** n. a chart or other representation of an animal's ancestry.

**pedunculated** adj. attached by a stalk. *Compare* sessile.

**PEG tube** n. a feeding tube that is placed into the stomach through the abdominal wall using an endoscope. A PEG tube allows food, water and medications to be placed directly into the stomach. PEG stands for percutaneous endoscopic gastrostomy.

**pelvic limb** n. a hind leg.

**pelvis** n. the bony, box-like structure attached to the spinal column, hind legs and tail - **pelvic** adj.

**pemphigus foliaceus** n. a disease caused by an abnormal autoimmune reaction against some parts of an animal's skin. Individuals can develop lesions affecting the skin and mucocutaneous junctions. Treatment with

medicines that suppress the immune system can be effective.

**pemphigus vulgaris** n. an autoimmune disease causing animals to develop lesions primarily around mucocutaneous junctions and within the mouth. Treatment is difficult but can include medicines that suppress the immune system.

**pendulous** adj. hanging down further than is normal.

**penis** n. the external organ used for urination and reproduction in male animals - **penile** adj.

**PennHIP** n. a service run by the University of Pennsylvania's veterinary school that involves analysis of a specific type of hip radiograph to determine the likelihood of a dog developing osteoarthritis from hip dysplasia.

**Penrose drain** n. a piece of soft tubing sutured into a wound or other cavity to prevent the buildup of pus, blood or other unwanted fluids.

**pentastomiasis** n. a disease caused by a type of parasite that affects reptiles and causes a variety of clinical signs depending on where the infestation localizes. Treatment is difficult, and the parasite can be transmitted to people.

**per os (PO)** adj. by mouth.

**peracute** adj. describes a condition in which symptoms develop very rapidly, usually over the course of a few hours. *Compare* acute.

**percussion** n. striking parts of an animal's body with the tips of the fingers to investigate underlying structures through the sounds that result.

**percutaneous** adj. through the skin.

**perforation** n. a hole through the wall of an organ allowing leakage of its contents, which can be caused by injury or disease that weakens the tissues (e.g., an ulcer) - **perforate** v., **perforated** adj.

**perfusion** n. delivery of oxygen and nutrients carried by blood that flows into tissues.

**perianal** adj. around the anus.

**perianal fistula** n. a disease with an unknown cause that is most frequently seen in dogs, especially German Shepherds. Affected individuals can develop draining lesions around the anus, discomfort and difficulty defecating. Treatment may include medications that suppress the immune system, antibiotics, antiseptics and surgery.

**perianal gland tumor** n. tumors of the small glands in the skin most commonly found around the anus. Unneutered male dogs are at highest risk for perianal gland tumors, most of which are benign but can still be locally problematical. Treatment includes castration and the surgical removal of the mass. *Also called* hepatoid gland and circumanal gland tumors.

**periapical** adj. pertaining to the area around the end of a tooth root.

**pericardial effusion** n. an abnormal fluid accumulation between the heart and the membranes that surround it, which can be caused by infection or cancer. In some cases, no underlying disorder can be found. The fluid puts

pressure on the heart preventing its normal function and often causing lethargy, rapid breathing and an accumulation of fluid within the abdomen or chest. Treatment can include removal of the fluid from around the heart and elsewhere in the body, the surgical removal of a portion of the pericardium and addressing any underlying disorders.

**pericardiectomy** n. the surgical removal of a portion of the pericardium.

**pericardiocentesis** n. insertion of a hollow needle or catheter between the heart and its surrounding membranes to remove fluid.

**pericarditis** n. inflammation of the pericardium, which is often associated with infection.

**pericardium** n. the membranes that surround the heart - **pericardial** adj.

**perinatal** adj. around the time of birth.

**perineal hernia** n. a protrusion of tissues between muscles on one or both sides of the anus, which is most commonly seen in middle-aged, intact, male dogs. Prostatic disease and constipation can increase the likelihood of an animal developing this type of hernia. Affected individuals have a soft swelling beside the anus and can have difficulty defecating or urinating. Treatment includes surgical repair and castration.

**perineal laceration** n. an injury that occurs when the feet or another part of the fetus catches on a fold of tissue at the end of the female's reproductive tract during birth. The wounds are ranked as first, second or third degree in increasing order of severity. Third degree perineal lacerations create an opening that allows fecal material to enter the reproductive tract. Treatment includes surgical repair and antibiotics.

**perineal urethrostomy (PU)** n. a surgery usually performed in male cats that are not able to urinate because of a persistent or recurring urethral blockage. A permanent hole is formed in the upper part of the urethra through which urine can flow. *See also* blocked cat.

**perineum** n. the tissues between the anus and genitalia - **perineal** adj.

**perineuroma** n. *See* neurofibroma.

**periocular** adj. around the eye.

**periodic ophthalmia** n. *See* recurrent uveitis.

**periodontal disease** n. inflammation and destruction of the tissues surrounding teeth. Periodontal disease can be caused by an accumulation of food particles, plaque and tartar on and around teeth, which often leads to infection. Affected animals may have red, swollen gums that bleed easily, bad breath and loose or missing teeth. Treatment can include routine dental cleanings, tooth extractions, antibiotics and procedures that reduce the depth of gingival pockets around teeth.

**perioperative** adj. around the time of surgery.

**periorbital** adj. around the eye's socket.

**periosteal stripping** n. a surgery that can be performed to remove a portion of periosteum in order to encourage bone growth in young animals affected by some types of angular limb deformities.

**periosteum** n. the fibrous membrane that covers the surface of bones - **periosteal** adj.

**periostitis** n. inflammation of the periosteum. *See also* osselets.

**peripartum** adj. around the time of birth.

**peripartum asphyxia** n. *See* neonatal maladjustment syndrome.

**peripheral** adj. pertaining to the outer aspect of the body or other structure. *Compare* central.

**peripheral Cushing's disease** n. *See* equine metabolic syndrome.

**peripheral nervous system (PNS)** n. all of the nerves in the body excluding those of the brain and spinal cord. *Compare* central nervous system.

**perirenal pseudocysts** n. a disorder with an unknown cause that is seen in cats. Affected animals develop a large fluid filled structure on the outside of one or both kidneys, which can press on and damage the kidney. Treatment includes the removal of the fluid from within the cyst or of the cyst itself.

**peristalsis** n. rhythmic contractions of the gastrointestinal tract, which move ingesta from the esophagus towards the anus. Reverse peristalsis moves materials in the opposite direction and can cause vomiting.

**peritoneal cavity** n. the part of the body that is located between the diaphragm and the pelvis and contains the stomach, intestines, liver and other organs.

**peritoneal dialysis** n. a procedure used to remove unwanted substances from the body. Fluid is infused into the abdominal cavity where it collects toxins or waste products by diffusion. The fluid is then removed, and the process may be repeated.

**peritoneopericardial diaphragmatic hernia** n. a birth defect that allows abdominal contents to pass through a hole in the diaphragm and into the space between the heart and its surrounding membranes. If the individual's organ function is compromised by the situation, surgical repair is necessary.

**peritoneum** n. the membrane that lines the inner surface of the abdominal wall (i.e., parietal peritoneum) and the outer surface of abdominal organs (i.e., visceral peritoneum) - **peritoneal** adj.

**peritonitis** n. inflammation of the peritoneum, which is often associated with infection arising from perforation of the gastrointestinal tract or abdominal wall. Irritating substances (e.g., bile or urine) that leak into the abdomen also cause peritonitis. Affected individuals can develop abdominal pain, vomiting, reduced defecation and a fever. Treatment includes fluid therapy, antibiotics and surgery to flush the abdomen and repair any underlying abnormalities. *See also* hardware disease, egg peritonitis and feline infectious peritonitis.

**perivascular** adj. around a blood vessel.

**peroneal nerve paralysis** n. loss of function of a nerve running to the lower hind leg that can be caused by trauma or in large animals, a prolonged period of time spent lying down. Affected individuals often walk on the top surface of their foot and cannot flex their hock.

**persistent pupillary membrane (PPM)** n. the abnormal presence of membranous strands within the eye that arise from fetal vessels. Some cases are genetic in origin. Treatment may include surgical removal of the membranes if vision is adversely affected.

**persistent right aortic arch** n. the abnormal presence after birth of a structure associated with the fetal heart that in combination with other nearby body parts encircles the esophagus causing regurgitation and sometimes aspiration pneumonia. Treatment includes surgery to correct the defect and changes in feeding schedules and techniques. *Also called* vascular ring anomaly.

**pesticide** n. a chemical used to kill insects, rodents or other animals deemed to be a nuisance.

**petechia** n. a small area of purple discoloration resulting from blood pooling under the skin - **petechial** adj., **petechiae** pl.

**petit mal seizure** n. a type of seizure involving a brief loss of consciousness and few other clinical signs. *Compare* generalized seizure.

**petroleum toxicosis** n. poisoning with petroleum-based products (e.g., gasoline) through ingestion, inhalation or topical exposure. Affected animals may develop difficulty breathing, coughing, vomiting, diarrhea, bloat (ruminants), abnormal behavior, tremors and difficulty walking. Treatment can include bathing, antibiotics and medications to protect the gastrointestinal tract. Therapy for bloat may be necessary but can greatly increase the risk of complications (e.g., aspiration pneumonia).

**pH** n. a measure of the acidity or alkalinity of a material. A pH of seven is considered neutral. Lower values indicate the presence of an acid and higher numbers, the presence of a base.

**phacoemulsification** n. a surgical method of treating cataracts that uses ultrasonic vibrations to break apart the lens allowing it to be more easily removed from the eye.

**phalanx** n. any one of the major bones in the finger, toe, claw or hoof - **phalanges** pl., **phalangeal** adj.

**pharyngeal lymphoid hyperplasia** n. a condition most commonly seen in young horses in which nodules develop in the pharynx. Many cases do not adversely affect the individual and regress with age, but others may be associated with viral infections, reduced appetite and painful swallowing. Treatment can include rest and anti-inflammatories.

**pharyngeal paralysis** n. a loss of function of the nerves that are necessary for normal pharyngeal function, which can be caused by infections, trauma or tumors. Affected individuals have difficulty swallowing and breathing. Treatment can include

anti-inflammatories, antibiotics, supportive care and addressing any underlying disorders.

**pharyngitis** n. inflammation of the pharynx, which is often associated with infection.

**pharyngostomy** n. the surgical creation of an opening from the pharynx directly to the outside of the body. A pharyngostomy may be performed to allow insertion of a feeding tube or an endotracheal tube.

**pharynx** n. the area behind the nasal cavities and mouth that moves food towards the esophagus and air to and from the larynx - **pharyngeal** adj. *See also* nasopharynx and oropharynx.

**phenobarbital level** n. a laboratory test used to determine if an animal taking phenobarbital for the treatment of seizures is receiving the correct amount of the drug.

**pheochromocytoma** n. a tumor of particular cells within the adrenal gland that can cause high heart rates and blood pressure, difficulty breathing, abnormal behavior, fluid accumulations, tissue swelling and bleeding. Surgical removal is the best treatment but can be difficult if the tumor has invaded nearby large blood vessels. Medications to decrease blood pressure can be helpful.

**pheromone** n. a substance secreted by an individual that can be sensed by another animal and affect their behavior.

**philtrum** n. area where the two sides of the nose and the upper lip meet.

**phimosis** n. an abnormally small opening into the penile sheath that does not allow movement of the penis through the structure. *Compare* paraphimosis.

**phlebitis** n. inflammation of a vein, which can disrupt blood flow through the structure.

**phlebotomy** n. the puncture of or incision into a vein, often to remove a blood sample or inject a medicine. *Also called* venipuncture.

**phlegm** n. a thick, mucoid secretion arising from the respiratory tract. *Also called* sputum.

**phobia** n. an abnormally strong, fearful reaction to a stimulus (e.g., a loud noise). Treatment can include behavioral modification protocols and antianxiety medications.

**phosphorus** n. a mineral that is an important component of the diet and necessary for normal metabolism and the maintenance of healthy bones. *See also* hyperphosphatemia and hypophosphatemia.

**photophobia** n. avoidance of light, which can be seen when an animal has a disease (e.g., pinkeye) that becomes more uncomfortable with light exposure.

**photosensitization** n. a condition in which discomfort and skin lesions develop as a result of sunlight exposure. Photosensitization may be caused by ingestion of various plants or poisons and some types of liver disease. Treatment can include avoiding exposure to sunlight and the causative substance and symptomatic and supportive care. *See also* erythropoietic porphyria and facial eczema.

**phthisis bulbi** n. a process by which the eyeball degenerates and shrinks, which can be caused by severe disease (e.g., glaucoma) affecting the eye. Surgical removal of the eye can be considered if it is bothersome or painful.

**physeal dysplasia** n. *See* physitis.

**physeal fracture** n. a break in a bone that involves that portion responsible for bone growth in young animals. Surgery is often necessary to prevent uneven growth as the animal matures.

**physical exam (PE)** n. the inspection of an animal using various senses (e.g., sight, hearing, smell and touch) to aid in the diagnosis of disease or determination of health.

**physical therapy** n. exercises and procedures that can be used to promote function of the musculoskeletal or nervous systems and aid in recovery from injury or illness. *Also called* physiotherapy.

**physiology** n. the processes (e.g., metabolism and respiration) that combine to allow a body to function.

**physis** n. the portion of a bone in a young animal that is responsible for bone lengthening during growth - **physeal** adj. *Also called* growth plate.

**physitis** n. inflammation of a bone's growth plate. Specifically, a disease of young horses with several possible causes including rapid growth, a dietary imbalance of calcium and phosphorous, poor conformation and exercise on hard surfaces. Affected animals develop swelling of the growth plates around some of their leg joints and may be in pain and reluctant to move. Treatment can include rest, exercise restriction, weight loss and dietary changes *Also called* epiphysitis and physeal dysplasia.

**phytobezoar** n. a mass of plant material that accumulates in and disrupts the function of the gastrointestinal tract. Treatment can include medications that encourage the evacuation of the phytobezoar or surgery.

**pica** n. the tendency to eat abnormal and often indigestible materials. Pica can be associated with a nutritional imbalance, diseases that disrupt normal metabolism or behavioral disorders. *Also called* depraved appetite.

**pigeon breast** n. a disease of horses caused by infection with the bacteria *Corynebacterium pseudotuberculosis.* Affected individuals develop deep abscesses in their chest muscles. The infection may spread to other regions of the body. Treatment includes lancing, draining, flushing or the surgical removal of abscesses, antibiotics and supportive care. *Also called* pigeon fever, dryland distemper and false strangles.

**piloerection** n. an elevation of hair or fur that can help keep animals warm or is used as a method of communication.

**pilomatricomas** n. a tumor arising from cells within hair follicles. Most are benign but some rarer forms can be malignant. Treatment includes surgery to remove the tumor.

**pilonidal sinus** n. *See* dermoid sinus.

**pin** n. a thin, metal rod that can be surgically inserted through and stabilize broken bones.

**pin feather** n. a growing feather with a blood supply to its shaft that, if broken can bleed profusely. Bleeding may be stopped with pressure or substances applied to the broken shaft, or the entire feather can be removed. *Also called* blood feather.

**pin firing** n. the process of applying a very hot instrument to the legs of horses, which was thought to encourage healing of tendons or ligaments. The procedure is now considered inhumane and ineffective.

**ping** n. the high-pitched sound heard when the skin over an abdominal organ distended with gas is flicked with a fingertip.

**pinioning** n. a surgical procedure that is used to prevent flight in birds and usually involves amputating the end of one wing.

**pinkeye** n. *See* infectious keratoconjunctivitis.

**pinkie** n. a very young, hairless mouse that is often fed to some types of reptiles.

**pinky syndrome** n. *See* Arabian fading syndrome.

**pinna** n. the external flap of the ear. *Also called* auricle.

**pinworms** n. *See* oxyuriasis.

**piroplasmosis** n. *See* babesiosis.

**pithomycotoxicosis** n. *See* facial eczema.

**pitting edema** n. a condition in which pressure applied to a swollen tissue causes a depression to develop and remain visible for a period of time.

**pituitary dwarfism** n. *See* panhypopituitarism.

**pituitary gland** n. a gland within the brain that secretes many different hormones (e.g., antidiuretic hormone, adrenocorticotrophic hormone, follicle stimulating hormone, luteinizing hormone and growth hormone).

**PIVKA test** n. a laboratory test that can help diagnose animals poisoned with anticoagulant rodenticides.

**pizzle rot** n. a contagious disease that most frequently affects castrated male sheep and is caused by infection with *Corynebacterium renale* bacteria. Pizzle rot is often associated with a diet high in protein. Individuals develop inflammation, swelling, discharge and lesions affecting the prepuce and penis, which if severe enough can prevent urination and lead to death. Treatment includes cleaning the affected area, diet changes and antibiotics. *Also called* enzootic balanoposthitis, ulcerative posthitis and vulvitis and sheath rot.

**placebo** n. a substance without any therapeutic activity or harmful side effects that may be given to an animal as part of a drug study or to appease a caretaker who expects some type of medication to be given to the patient.

**placenta** n. the structure contained within the uterus during pregnancy that secretes hormones and allows transfer of substances between the blood supply of the mother and fetus. The placenta must be expelled or removed from the uterus after birth.

**placentitis** n. inflammation of the placenta, which is often associated with infection.

**plague** n. 1. a disease most commonly seen in cats that is caused by infection with *Yersinia pestis* bacteria often transmitted through the bites of infected fleas or ingestion of infected rodents. In the bubonic form, individuals develop swollen lymph nodes (i.e., buboes) that may drain pus. Vomiting, diarrhea, weakness, difficulty breathing and a cough can be seen in the septicemic and pneumonic forms of the disease. All types of plague can produce a high fever and may result in death. Treatment includes antibiotics and supportive and symptomatic care. Plague can be transmitted to people. 2. an outbreak of any disease that causes a large number of deaths.

**plantar** adj. pertaining to the back of a rear leg below the tarsus. *Compare* palmar.

**plantigrade** adj. bearing weight on all of the lower hind leg up to the tarsus. The condition is normal in some animals (e.g., bears) but can be seen with neurologic or musculoskeletal disorders in other species.

**plaque** n. 1. a film of bacteria, saliva and other substances that can stick to the surface of teeth promoting the formation of tartar, gingivitis and periodontal disease. 2. a flat, raised lesion visible on the surface of a tissue.

**plasma** n. the liquid part of blood that is present after the cells have been removed without allowing the blood to clot. *Compare* serum.

**plasma cell** n. a type of white blood cell that develops from a lymphocyte and secretes antibodies - **plasmacytic** adj. *Also called* plasmacyte. *See also* myeloma.

**plasma cell stomatitis** n. *See* lymphocytic-plasmacytic stomatitis.

**plasma protein (PP)** n. a measurement of the amount of all proteins (e.g., albumin and antibodies) present in plasma. *Also called* total protein.

**plasmacytic-lymphocytic enteritis** n. *See* inflammatory bowel disease.

**plasmacytic-lymphocytic stomatitis** n. *See* lymphocytic-plasmacytic stomatitis.

**plasmacytoma** n. *See* extra-medullary plasmacytoma.

**plastron** n. the external, protective and supportive structure that covers the bottom of turtles and tortoises.

**plate** n. 1. a thin, flat piece of metal that can be surgically implanted to support broken bones or other orthopedic injuries. 2. a flat structure within the body. 3. a flat container containing a substance that promotes the growth of bacteria or other microorganisms.

**platelet** n. a cell that helps blood to clot. *Also called* thrombocyte.

**play aggression** n. inappropriate attacks or related behaviors (e.g., growling, hissing or snapping) that are initiated by an animal during play. Treatment can include avoidance of any type of confrontational play and behavioral modification protocols.

**pleomorphic** adj. having many forms.

**pleura** n. the membrane that lines the inner surface of the chest cavity (i.e., parietal pleura) and the outer surface of lungs (i.e., visceral pleura) - **pleural** adj.

**pleural effusion** n. an abnormal accumulation of fluid within the chest cavity, which can be caused by heart disease, infections, low blood protein levels, bleeding and cancer. Treatment includes removing the fluid from around the lungs and addressing any underlying disorders. *See also* chylothorax and pyothorax.

**pleuritis** n. inflammation of the membranes surrounding the lungs, which may be associated with infections, tumors or trauma. Affected individuals can be in pain and reluctant to take deep breaths. *Also called* pleurisy. *See also* pleuropneumonia.

**pleuropneumonia** n. inflammation of lung tissue and surrounding membranes that is often associated with viral and/or bacterial infections, although other causes and organisms can be involved. Affected individuals may cough, be in pain and have difficulty breathing, nasal discharge and lethargy. Treatment can include antibiotics, anti-inflammatories, oxygen therapy, surgical drainage of fluid from around the lungs and supportive care.

**plexus** n. an interwoven network of vessels or nerves. *See also* brachial plexus.

**plication** n. a folding of a tissue upon itself, which may occur secondary to disease (e.g., a linear foreign body) or be performed surgically to limit movement of a body part - **plicate** v.

**pneumocystography** n. the taking of radiographs after injection of air into the urinary bladder to allow for better visualization of the organ.

**pneumoencephalitis** n. *See* Newcastle disease.

**pneumomediastinum** n. the abnormal presence of air around the organs contained within the mediastinum, which is often caused by injury to the trachea, esophagus or lungs. The air will usually be absorbed with treatment of the underlying disorder.

**pneumonia** n. inflammation of lung tissue, which is often associated with viral and/or bacterial infections, although other causes (e.g., inhalation of foreign material) and organisms can be involved. Affected individuals may cough and have difficulty breathing, nasal discharge and lethargy. Treatment can include antibiotics, bronchodilators, antiinflammatories, oxygen therapy, supportive care and procedures and drugs to loosen mucus within the airways.

**pneumonic** adj. pertaining to pneumonia or to the lungs.

**pneumonitis** n. inflammation of lung tissue, which is usually associated with infections or allergies. *See also* hypersensitivity pneumonitis, pneumonia and feline chlamydiosis.

**pneumothorax** n. the abnormal presence of air surrounding the lungs in the chest cavity, which leads to rapid and shallow breathing. Causes include a penetrating wound through the chest wall or disorders causing rupture of parts of the respiratory tract. Treatment involves procedures to remove the air from around the lungs and addressing any underlying conditions.

**pneumovagina** n. an accumulation of air with the vagina, which is often caused by anatomical abnormalities and can limit the animal's ability to maintain a pregnancy. *Also called* windsucking.

**pocket pet** n. any of a number of very small animals (e.g., hamsters and guinea pigs) that make suitable human companions.

**pododermatitis** n. inflammation of the foot, which is usually associated with an infection. *See also* bumblefoot.

**point of maximal intensity (PMI)** n. the region of the heart around which a murmur is the loudest when listening with a stethoscope.

**polioencephalomalacia** n. degeneration of the gray matter of the brain. *See also* cerebrocortical necrosis.

**polioencephalomyelitis** n. inflammation of the gray matter of the brain and spinal cord, which can be caused by a viral infection.

**poll** n. the top of the head.

**poll evil** n. a disease of horses in which a fluid-filled sac on top of the head swells and ruptures, draining to the surface of the skin. Trauma or infection (e.g., *Brucella* bacteria) are potential causes. Treatment can include surgical removal of affected tissues and antibiotics.

**pollakiuria** n. the frequent elimination of only small amounts of urine.

**polled** adj. describes an individual or breed that does not grow horns, unlike other closely related individuals.

**polyarteritis** n. inflammation of multiple arteries.

**polyarthritis** n. inflammation of multiple joints, which can be associated with infection or immune mediated disease. *See also* transmissible serositis and nonsuppurative polyarthritis of lambs.

**polyarthritis-serositis** n. *See* transmissible serositis.

**polyclonal gammopathy** n. abnormally high levels of several different types of antibodies in the blood, which can be associated with infection, inflammation or autoimmune disease. *Compare* monoclonal gammopathy.

**polycystic kidney disease** n. a disorder, often genetic, in which multiple cysts develop within the kidneys. Mild or early cases many not significantly affect kidney function, while more severely affected individuals can develop chronic renal failure. There is no specific treatment for polycystic kidney disease, but addressing chronic renal failure when it develops can prolong and improve the quality of life.

**polycythemia** n. an abnormally large number of red blood cells in circulation, which can be caused by dehydration, low blood oxygen levels or bone marrow disease. *Also called* erythrocytosis. *See also* polycythemia vera and relative polycythemia.

**polycythemia vera** n. a disorder in which increased production by the bone marrow releases abnormally large numbers of red blood cells into circulation. Affected animals may drink and urinate more than normal

and have red mucous membranes, changes in behavior, blindness and seizures. Treatment can include repeated procedures to remove blood from the circulatory system and medications that slow the production of red blood cells. *Also called* absolute polycythemia. *Compare* relative polycythemia.

**polydactyly** n. the presence of a greater number of digits than is normal.

**polydipsia (PD)** n. excessive thirst and water intake.

**polyestrus** adj. having multiple heat cycles during each breeding season.

**polymorphonuclear** **leukocyte (PMN)** n. *See* neutrophil.

**polymyositis** n. a disease of adult dogs that is thought to be immune mediated. Some cases may be seen in association with other diseases (e.g., myasthenia gravis). Affected individuals can develop weakness, depression, loss of weight and muscle mass, lameness and muscle pain. Treatment includes immunosuppressive drugs.

**polyneuritis equi** n. *See* cauda equina neuritis.

**polyneuropathy** n. any disease that adversely affects multiple nerves. *See also* chronic inflammatory demyelinating polyneuropathy and distal polyneuropathy.

**Polyomavirus** n. *See* budgerigar fledgling disease.

**polyp** n. a small, rounded mass of tissue that usually arises from the surface of a mucous membrane.

**polyphagia** n. a greatly increased appetite.

**polyradiculoneuritis** n. inflammation of peripheral nerves and the areas where they connect to the spinal cord. *See also* idiopathic polyradiculoneuritis, neosporosis and toxoplasmosis.

**polysaccharide storage myopathy (PSSM)** n. a disease of horses caused by an abnormal accumulation of a type of carbohydrate within muscles. Affected Quarter Horses can develop muscle tremors, stiffness, sweating, pain and reluctance to move. Draft horses tend to flex their hind legs and tail and have muscle tremors, weakness, difficulty backing up and a loss of muscle mass. Symptoms tend to get worse after exercise. Treatment can include reducing or eliminating grain from the diet, decreasing stress and muscle relaxants. *Also called* shivers in draft horses.

**polysynovitis** n. inflammation of multiple synovial membranes throughout the body. *See also* synovitis.

**polytetrafluoroethylene (PTFE) poisoning** n. a disease of birds caused by fumes released during the overheating of nonstick cookware or some other devices (e.g., heat lamps). Affected individuals develop difficulty breathing and may die rapidly. Treatment can include fresh air, oxygen therapy and supportive care. *Also called* Teflon® toxicosis.

**polyuria (PU)** n. the production of larger than normal amounts of urine.

**popliteal** adj. pertaining to the area behind the knee.

**popped knee** n. *See* carpitis.

**porcine** adj. pertaining to pigs.

**porcine parvovirus** n. a contagious virus of pigs that usually causes abortions only during a sow's first pregnancy. Preventative vaccines are available.

**porphyria** n. *See* erythropoietic porphyria.

**porphyrin** n. any of a number of pigmented compounds (e.g., hemoglobin). A porphyrin pigment is responsible for the reddish-brown discoloration caused by dried tears or saliva.

**porphyrinuria** n. *See* erythropoietic porphyria.

**portal system** n. *See* hepatic portal system.

**portal vein** n. the large vessel that is formed as the smaller veins of the portal system combine before entering the liver.

**portocaval shunt** n. *See* portosystemic shunt.

**portography** n. the taking of radiographs after a contrast agent is injected into the portal system to allow for better visualization of the vessels.

**portosystemic shunt** n. a disorder in which one or more abnormal blood vessels connect the portal system to other veins (e.g., the vena cava) thereby bypassing the liver. Cases in young animals are generally related to birth defects, while older animals can form shunts because of diseases that obstruct flow of blood through the liver. Affected individuals may develop behavioral abnormalities or seizures that get worse after eating, slow growth, vomiting, diarrhea and an accumulation of fluid within the abdomen. Treatment options include surgery to close the abnormal veins, diet changes, addressing any underlying diseases and medications that decrease the production and absorption of waste products from the intestinal tract.

**positive reinforcement** n. a method of behavioral training in which wanted behavior quickly results in a pleasant consequence (e.g., praise or a treat). *Compare* negative reinforcement.

**possessive aggression** n. inappropriate attacks or related behaviors (e.g., growling, hissing or snapping) that are initiated when an attempt is made to remove an object that is under an animal's control. Treatment can include avoidance of situations that incite the aggression and behavioral modification protocols.

**posterior** adj. in back of or pertaining to the hind end. *Compare* anterior.

**posterior presentation** n. *See* breech presentation.

**posthitis** n. inflammation of the prepuce, which is often associated with infection.

**postictal** adj. pertaining to the time just after seizures have ended. Animals will often appear disoriented and unsteady on their feet during the postictal phase. *Compare* ictal and preictal.

**post-legged** adj. a conformation flaw in which the joints of the back legs are straighter than normal when an animal is standing.

**postmortem** adj. occurring after death.

**postoperative** adj. after surgery.

**postpartum** adj. pertaining to the time after birth.

**postparturient hemoglobinuria** n. a disease of lactating cattle that can be caused by dietary deficiencies (e.g., phosphorus, copper and selenium) or plant toxins. Affected individuals develop red blood cells that rupture easily, weakness, red-brown urine, low milk production, rapid breathing, yellow or pale mucous membranes and may die. Treatment can include correcting the diet, blood transfusions, fluid therapy and medications that slow the breakdown of red blood cells.

**postprandial** adj. after eating.

**postrenal** adj. pertaining to the structures within the urinary tract that drain urine from the kidneys (i.e., ureters, urinary bladder and urethra).

**postural reactions** n. *See* conscious proprioception.

**postvaccinal hepatitis** n. *See* Theiler's disease.

**potassium (K)** n. an important electrolyte, the correct levels of which are essential for maintaining normal body function. *See also* hyperkalemia and hypokalemia.

**pot-bellied** adj. having an abdomen that is prominent and enlarged in comparison to the rest of the body.

**potentiation** n. the combined actions of two substances (e.g., medicines) that is greater than the sum of their effects - **potentiated** adj.

**Potomac horse fever (PHF)** n. a disease of horses caused by ingestion of the bacteria *Neorickettsia risticii* (previously called *Ehrlichia risticii*) carried by freshwater snails. Affected animals may develop diarrhea, fever, colic, laminitis and abort their fetuses. Treatment can include antibiotics and supportive care. Vaccines exist that may provide protection in some cases. *Also called* ditch fever, equine monocytic ehrlichiosis, Shasta River crud and equine ehrlichial colitis.

**poultice** n. a moist, warm material applied to a part of the body to increase circulation and speed healing.

**poultry mite** n. *See* red mite.

**pox** n. a group of contagious, viral diseases affecting many different species in which animals develop skin lesions that often progress from a reddened area to a fluid-filled structure that ruptures producing a scab. In North America, poxvirus infections are generally mild and limited to cattle and pigs.

**preanesthetic** adj. occurring before anesthesia.

**precocious** adj. describes development that occurs at an earlier age than is normally seen. *Also called* precocial.

**precordial** adj. pertaining to the area of the chest through which heart beats can be felt or heard.

**predatory aggression** n. inappropriate attacks or related behaviors (e.g., stalking and chasing) that are initiated by an animal against other animals, people (especially young children) or moving objects. In many cases, it is best to simply avoid this problem by keeping the animal confined or restrained.

**preen** v. to clean the surface of the body (e.g., feathers or fur) with the beak or tongue.

**pregnancy** n. the time between the fertilization of the egg and birth, during which the female body nourishes and protects the developing embryo and fetus. *Also called* gestation.

**pregnancy toxemia** n. a disease seen in pregnant females that is caused by inadequate energy intake during late gestation. Affected animals can develop loss of appetite, depression, weakness, difficulty walking, seizures, other neurologic abnormalities and may die. Treatment may include feeding high-energy foods, delivery of the fetus, supportive care and medications that normalize the animal's acid-base balance and blood sugar and electrolyte levels. *Also called* ketosis and twin lamb disease.

**preictal** adj. pertaining to the time just before seizures develop. Animals will sometimes begin to act abnormally during the preictal phase. *Compare* ictal and postictal.

**premature** adj. occurring early or before full development has occurred.

**premature ventricular contraction (PVC)** n. an abnormal contraction of the heart that can be recorded on an electrocardiogram. Occasional PVCs may not be significant, but more frequent occurrences can be seen with serious underlying diseases and adversely affect heart function. *Also called* ventricular premature contraction.

**premedication** n. a drug that is given prior to anesthesia to decrease anxiety and lower the doses of or improve the response to anesthetics.

**premolar teeth** n. the teeth located behind the canines and in front of the molars.

**prenatal** adj. pertaining to the time before birth. *Also called* antenatal.

**preoperative** adj. before surgery.

**prepatent period** n. the time after an animal has become infected with an organism but before the disease can be detected.

**prepubertal** adj. occurring before puberty.

**prepuce** n. the skin and other tissues that surround the non-erect penis - **preputial** adj. *Also called* sheath.

**prepurchase exam** n. an examination of an animal by a veterinarian for a potential buyer with the goal of identifying problems that could adversely affect the animal's future usefulness.

**prerenal** adj. pertaining to something that occurs before the kidney, in a physiological sense. For example, prerenal azotemia refers to a higher than normal blood level of creatinine and/or blood urea nitrogen that results from inadequate blood flow to the kidney.

**presbycusis** n. hearing loss that commonly affects some animals (e.g., dogs) as they get older.

**presbyopia** n. a loss of visual sharpness that can affect some older animals because of a decreased ability of the eye's lens to change shape and focus an image on the retina.

**prescription** n. a written or verbal order for a particular drug, therapy or medical device given by a veterinarian to be acted upon by another person (e.g., pharmacist).

**presentation** n. 1. the orientation of a fetus within the birth canal. *See also* anterior and breech presentation. 2. the initial clinical signs displayed by an animal upon being brought to a veterinarian for diagnosis and treatment.

**pressure sore** n. *See* decubital ulcer.

**prevalence** n. the number of animals affected by a disease within a particular population at a given time.

**preventive medicine** n. veterinary care aimed at preventing rather than treating disease. Vaccinations, dental cleanings, physical exams, consultations and some medications (e.g., flea control) can all play a part in preventative medicine.

**priapism** n. a painful and persistent erection of the penis.

**primary** adj. initial, most important or not occurring as a result of another, underlying disorder. *Compare* secondary.

**primary hyperparathyroidism (PHP)** n. a disease caused by a tumor of the parathyroid gland that produces excess parathyroid hormone. Affected individuals may have bones that bend or break easily, drooling, loose teeth and be unable to fully close their mouths. Treatment can include surgical removal of the tumor and post-operative calcium supplements.

**primary teeth** n. *See* deciduous teeth.

**primipara** n. a female that has had only one successful pregnancy - **primiparous** adj. *Compare* nullipara and multipara.

**prion** n. an abnormally folded protein that can infect animals and cause their cells to reproduce the protein leading to disease. *See also* bovine spongiform encephalopathy, chronic wasting disease and scrapie.

**probiotic** n. a dietary supplement containing bacteria and/or yeast that may promote a beneficial balance of microorganisms within the gastrointestinal tract.

**proctitis** n. inflammation of the rectum.

**prodromal** adj. pertaining to the earliest signs of the development of a disease or other problem (e.g., seizures).

**productive cough** n. a cough that expels phlegm from the respiratory tract into the mouth.

**proestrus** n. the period of time during which ovarian follicles develop prior to ovulation and estrus.

**progesterone** n. a hormone that is produced primarily by the corpus luteum and placenta and helps maintain pregnancies. Progesterone may also be used as a drug.

**prognathism** n. a longer than normal jaw, usually referring to the lower jaw. *Also called* undershot jaw

and sow mouth. *Compare* brachygnathism.

**prognosis** n. a prediction of the likely outcome of a disease and course of treatment in a particular animal.

**progressive** adj. becoming increasingly worse.

**progressive retinal atrophy (PRA)** n. a genetic disease seen most frequently in dogs that initially causes decreased vision at night but eventually leads to complete blindness. No effective treatment is available.

**prokinetic drug** n. a medicine that promotes the movement of ingesta through the gastrointestinal tract.

**prolactin** n. a hormone made by the pituitary gland that encourages mammary gland development and milk production.

**prolapse** n. the slipping of an organ or other body part out of its normal position. See the particular type of prolapse (e.g., rectal or uterine) for details.

**proliferative** adj. characterized by an increased amount of tissue.

**proliferative enteritis** n. a disease caused by infection of the gastrointestinal tract with *Lawsonia intracellularis* bacteria. Affected animals have diarrhea that varies in its severity. Treatment can include antibiotics and fluid therapy. A preventative vaccine is available for pigs. *Also called* proliferative enteropathy, proliferative bowel disease, proliferative hemorrhagic enteropathy and wet tail.

**proliferative keratoconjunctivitis** n. *See* canine fibrous histiocytoma.

**prophylaxis** n. a procedure or treatment aimed at preventing a disease or other condition - **prophylactic** adj.

**proprioception** n. *See* conscious proprioception.

**proptosis** n. the abnormal movement of an eye towards the front or out of its socket.

**prostaglandin** n. any of a number of different substances produced within the body that can play a role in uterine contractions, inflammation, blood clotting, gastric acid secretion and many other body functions. Prostaglandins may be used as a drug, primarily for inducing estrus, pregnancy termination and stimulating uterine contractions.

**prostate** n. a gland that secretes important fluid components of semen into the urethra of male animals - **prostatic** adj.

**prostatitis** n. inflammation of the prostate, which is usually associated with infection. Affected individuals may have difficulty defecating, a fever, blood in their urine and recurrent urinary tract infections. Treatment can include antibiotics, surgery to drain any abscesses, castration and supportive care.

**prostatomegaly** n. enlargement of the prostate.

**prosthesis** n. an artificial object used to replace a body part.

**protein** n. molecules containing chains of amino acids that are an important part of the diet and have many functions within the body.

**protein losing enteropathy** n. any intestinal disease that results in a leakage of protein into the intestinal tract (e.g., lymphangiectasia, paratuberculosis and inflammatory bowel disease).

**protein losing nephropathy** n. any kidney disease that results in a leakage of protein into the urine (e.g., glomerulonephritis).

**protein:creatinine ratio** n. a laboratory test used to determine if an abnormally large amount of protein is being lost through the kidneys and into the urine.

**proteinuria** n. the presence of abnormally large amounts of protein in the urine, which can be associated with diseases of the kidneys and/or bladder.

**prothrombin time (PT)** n. a test that measures the clotting ability of blood. A prolonged prothrombin time indicates abnormalities affecting particular coagulation factors.

**proton pump inhibitor** n. a type of medication that can be used to reduce gastric acid secretion.

**protozoa** n. a single celled, animal-like organism, some types of which can cause disease - **protozoal** adj.

**proud cut** adj. describes a gelding displaying some behaviors more typically seen in stallions. In some cases, the behavior may be due to incomplete castration, but it may also be normal for the individual or a result of poor training.

**proud flesh** n. inappropriate over-production of granulation tissue most frequently seen with wounds to a horse's lower leg. Proud flesh can be prevented by quickly suturing any lacerations and limiting movement of the tissues with stall rest and bandaging. Once proud flesh has developed, treatment may include its surgical removal, skin grafts, bandaging, stall rest and topical medications that shrink the tissue or prevent its return.

**proventricular dilatation disease (PDD)** n. a disease of birds that is most commonly seen in macaws and is thought to be caused by a virus. Affected individuals lose weight, defecate undigested food, vomit and may develop neurological abnormalities. The disease is fatal, but diet changes, antibiotics and anti-inflammatories can prolong and improve the quality of life. *Also called* macaw wasting disease.

**proventriculus** n. a part of a bird's stomach.

**proximal** adj. situated away from the end of a structure (e.g., up the leg away from the foot). *Compare* distal.

**proximal enteritis-jejunitis** n. *See* anterior enteritis.

**pruritis** n. itching - **pruritic** adj.

**pseudocoprostasis** n. inability to defecate because of matted hair over and around the anus.

**pseudocowpox** n. a contagious, viral infection of cattle that causes red bumps, scabs and other skin lesions on the teats and udder. Humans can develop skin lesions through contact with infected cows. No treatment is usually necessary, and improved hygiene can slow or prevent the spread of disease within a herd.

**pseudocyesis** n. a condition most commonly seen in intact female dogs causing them to appear pregnant when they are not because of hormonal changes that occur after every heat cycle. Affected individuals can have enlarged mammary glands that may produce milk, exhibit nesting behavior and may even act as if they are undergoing labor. Symptoms disappear with time, and spaying prevents subsequent episodes. *Also called* false pregnancy and pseudopregnancy.

**pseudohermaphrodite** n. an animal that has genitalia with characteristics of both sexes and either ovarian or testicular tissue. *Compare* hermaphrodite.

**pseudorabies** n. a contagious disease caused by infection with a type of herpesvirus. Affected pigs can exhibit coughing, sneezing, difficulty breathing, abortion and nervous disorders. Affected cattle can have intense itching, convulsions and suddenly die. Preventative vaccines are available, and many regions have eradication programs in place. *Also called* mad itch or Aujeszky's disease.

**psittacine** n. a bird that belongs to the order that contains parrots and parakeets.

**psittacine beak and feather disease (PBFD)** n. a contagious, viral disease of some species of birds that can cause abnormal appearance to or loss of feathers, beak changes, depression, diarrhea, difficulty breathing and eventually is fatal. Treatment is limited to supportive care and antibiotics for secondary infections.

**psittacosis** n. a disease of birds caused by infection with the bacteria *Chlamydophila psittaci*. Affected individuals can develop discharge from the eyes and nose, fever, discolored and loose droppings, weight loss, weakness, difficulty breathing and may die. People can be infected through exposure to infected birds or their surroundings. Therapy includes supportive care and antibiotics, but birds may still be capable of infecting other birds or people despite treatment. *Also called* chlamydiosis, ornithosis and parrot fever.

**psoroptic mange** n. a disease caused by infestation with *Psoroptes* mites, which lead to itching and skin lesions. The disease in cattle is especially severe. Some forms of psoroptic mange (cattle and sheep) must be reported to appropriate regulatory agencies. Medications to kill the mite are generally effective. *See also* ear mange.

**psychogenic** adj. arising from a psychological or emotional disorder. For example, some cats will pull their hair out if they are anxious or bored, and the condition is called psychogenic alopecia.

**psychotropic drug** n. a type of medication that can affect the mental state of animals (e.g., relieve anxiety).

**ptosis** n. drooping of an upper eyelid, which can be caused by neurologic disorders.

**ptyalism** n. excessive salivation.

**puberty** n. the period of time during which a young animal begins to develop the traits necessary for reproduction.

**puerperal tetany** n. a disease most often seen in small breed dogs that are nursing large litters and is associated with low blood calcium levels. Affected individuals can pant, be restless and develop muscle tremors, difficulty walking, stiffness, behavioral changes, seizures and may die. Treatment includes calcium supplementation, supportive care and weaning of the litter, if possible. *Also called* eclampsia.

**pulmonary** adj. pertaining to the lungs.

**pulmonary adenomatosis** n. a contagious, viral disease of sheep and goats that causes tumors to develop in the lungs. Affected individuals lose weight and have nasal discharge and difficulty breathing. No effective treatment is available.

**pulmonary artery** n. a blood vessel that carries deoxygenated blood from the heart to the lungs.

**pulmonary edema** n. an abnormal accumulation of fluid in the lungs, which is most frequently caused by heart disease. Affected individuals can have rapid or difficult breathing. Treatment can include medications to remove the fluid, oxygen therapy and addressing any underlying disorders.

**pulmonary embolism** n. a blockage of an artery within the lungs by a blood clot or another substance that traveled through the circulatory system. Affected animals can develop difficulty breathing and coughing. Treatment can include oxygen therapy and medications that help blood clots dissolve and/or prevent new clots from forming.

**pulmonary emphysema** n. an abnormal accumulation of air within the lungs that can occur as a result of any disorder causing a prolonged increased effort to exhale (e.g., recurrent airway obstruction).

**pulmonary infiltrates with eosinophils (PIE)** n. a disease that is usually caused by allergies in which eosinophils accumulate within the lungs causing difficulty breathing. Treatment includes medications to suppress the immune system.

**pulmonary valve** n. the structure between the right ventricle of the heart and the pulmonary artery that prevents backward flow of blood into the heart. *Also called* pulmonic valve.

**pulmonary vein** n. a blood vessel that carries oxygenated blood from the lungs to the heart.

**pulmonic stenosis** n. a narrowing of or around the pulmonary valve that partially blocks blood flow from the heart into the lungs. Affected animals may tire easily and develop congestive heart failure. Treatment can include surgical procedures to relieve the blockage and medicines that ease the effects of the narrowing.

**pulp** n. 1. the central portion of teeth that contains blood vessels and nerves. 2. a spongy tissue.

**pulpotomy** n. the surgical removal of dental pulp from within a tooth.

**pulpy kidney disease** n. *See* overeating disease.

**pulse** n. the feel or sight of blood coursing through an artery that corresponds with a heart beat.

**pulse deficit** n. an inability to feel a pulse corresponding to every heart beat, which can be associated with some types of arrhythmias.

**pulse oximeter** n. a device that measures the concentration of oxygen carried within the bloodstream.

**pulse rate** n. the number of times a pulse can be felt per minute.

**pulsed electromagnetic field therapy (PEMF)** n. a form of treatment utilizing magnetic fields that may help with some forms of musculoskeletal or other diseases. *Also called* electromagnet therapy.

**pulsed therapy** n. treatment that occurs at regular intervals rather than continuously.

**punch biopsy** n. the removal of a small, circular piece of tissue by pressing and rotating a circular blade against the skin.

**punctum** n. a small spot or opening - **puncta** pl., **punctate** adj.

**puncture** n. a wound or incision that is caused by a sharp, pointed object and is often deeper than it is long.

**pupil** n. the circular opening in the middle of each eye's iris that allows light to pass through to the lens and retina.

**pupillary light reflexes (PLR)** n. the normal, involuntary widening of the pupil in response to light and narrowing of the pupil in response to darkness.

**puppy pyoderma** n. a superficial, bacterial infection most often seen on the abdominal skin of puppies. The infection often resolves on its own without antibiotics.

**puppy strangles** n. a disease of puppies with an unknown cause that is characterized by the development of pustules and abscesses around the head, ears and neck and often associated with fever, loss of appetite and swollen lymph nodes. Bacterial infections are not involved initially but can develop with time. Treatment may include corticosteroids and antibiotics. *Also called* juvenile cellulitis.

**puppy vaginitis** n. a disorder of female puppies in which they develop inflammation of and discharge from the vulva but are otherwise healthy. Treatment with antibiotics is often not needed. Anatomic and physiologic changes occur with the first heat cycle, which usually resolve the problem. Many affected individuals should not be spayed until going through a heat cycle.

**pure red cell aplasia (PRCA)** n. a disease in which the bone marrow fails to produce adequate numbers of red blood cells. PRCA may be caused by autoimmune diseases, infections, toxins and the use of some drugs. Treatment can include addressing any underlying disorders, corticosteroids and blood transfusions.

**purgative** n. a substance that stimulates the release of feces from the body, sometimes in the form of diarrhea.

**purpura** n. a disorder that causes spontaneous bleeding into tissues and abnormal bruising. Infections, toxins, immune mediated diseases and any disease that causes a low platelet count can result in purpura.

**purpura hemorrhagica** n. a disorder of horses, many of which are recovering from strangles. Affected individuals can develop swellings under the skin, bruises, skin lesions and may die. Treatment includes corticosteroids and supportive care.

**pus** n. a fluid produced by the body that can contain white blood cells, microorganisms and cellular debris and is often the result of an infection - **purulent** adj.

**pustule** n. a small area of pus contained within the skin - **pustular** adj.

**pyelogram** n. *See* intravenous pyelogram.

**pyelonephritis** n. infection of one or both kidneys, which can be caused by spread of infection through the bloodstream or from the bladder. Affected individuals often develop fever, pain, vomiting and increased thirst and urination. Some cases may progress to kidney failure. Treatment can include antibiotics, fluid therapy and the surgical removal of a severely damaged kidney.

**pyloric stenosis** n. a disease in which the pylorus becomes narrowed causing retention of food within the stomach and vomiting. Treatment can include diet changes, medications that encourage evacuation of the stomach and surgery.

**pylorus** n. the part of the stomach that lies closest to the opening for the small intestine - **pyloric** adj.

**pyoderma** n. a skin disease that is usually the result of a bacterial infection. In many cases, something (e.g., dampness, allergies or trauma) has disrupted the protective mechanisms of the skin allowing bacteria normally present on the surface to overgrow. Affected animals can develop itching, scaling, hair loss, and skin lesions that may drain pus. Treatment includes addressing any underlying disorders, antibiotics and medicated baths.

**pyogenic** adj. producing pus.

**pyogranulomatous** adj. characterized by discrete masses of inflammation and pus.

**pyometra** n. infection and accumulation of pus within the uterus. Affected individuals may develop a fever, vaginal discharge, vomiting and increased thirst and urination. Treatment can include the surgical removal of the uterus, flushing the uterus if the cervix is open and the administration of hormones to promote evacuation of uterine contents.

**pyothorax** n. an accumulation of pus within the chest cavity that often causes difficulty breathing and a fever. Treatment can include antibiotics and surgical procedures that allow drainage of the pus.

**pyramidal disease** n. *See* buttress foot.

**pyrethrin** n. a natural chemical that can be used to kill and repel external parasites (e.g., flies, fleas, ticks and lice).

**pyrethroid** n. a synthetic chemical that can be used to kill and repel external parasites (e.g., flies, fleas, ticks and lice).

**pyrexia** n. an abnormally high body temperature, which can be associated with infections, inflammation or high environmental temperatures - **pyrexic** adj. *Also called* fever.

**pyrogen** n. a substance that causes an animal to develop a fever.

**pyrrolizidine alkaloidosis** n. poisoning by ingestion of several types of plants (e.g., ragwort and rattleweed) that cause liver damage. Affected individuals can develop loss of appetite and weight, constipation or diarrhea, abnormal fluid accumulations, jaundice, bizarre behavior and often die. Treatment is difficult but includes preventing access to the plants, diet changes and medications that help protect the liver and encourage its healing.

**pythiosis** n. disease caused by infection with *Pythium insidiosum* microorganisms, which are related to algae and usually contracted through contact with contaminated bodies of water. Affected individuals can develop draining skin nodules (i.e., kunkers) and vomiting and diarrhea if the gastrointestinal tract is involved. Treatment can be difficult but includes surgical removal of affected tissues and medications that can kill the microorganisms.

**pyuria** n. the abnormal presence of pus in the urine. *See also* urinary tract infection.

# Q

**Q fever** n. a disease caused by infection with *Coxiella burnetii* bacteria, which can be spread through tick bites and contact with contaminated birth fluids, placentas, milk, urine and feces.

Affected animals may lose their appetite, become lethargic and abort. Antibiotics can eliminate the infection and prevent its spread through a herd. Humans can become infected with Q fever.

**QRS complex** n. a wave pattern recorded on an electrocardiogram, which can change shape, size and frequency with different types of diseases affecting the heart.

**quadriparesis** n. weakness or incomplete paralysis affecting all four legs. *Also called* tetraparesis.

**quadriplegia** n. paralysis of all four legs. *Also called* tetraplegia.

**quarantine** n. isolation of an animal to prevent the spread of contagious diseases.

**quarter** n. 1. one of the four sections of an udder. 2. the side of a horse's hoof.

**quarter crack** n. a vertical fissure on the side of a horse's hoof. *See also* sand crack and grass crack.

**queen** n. 1. a mature, sexually intact female cat. 2. v. to give birth to kittens.

**Queensland itch** n. *See Culicoides* hypersensitivity.

**quick** n. the tissues that lie just under a hoof or nail that will cause pain and bleed if cut or injured.

**quidding** n. a disorder in which food is dropped from the mouth while it is being chewed, which can indicate oral or neurologic disorders.

**quinolones** n. a class of antibiotics that includes enrofloxacin, ciprofloxacin, orb-ifloxacin and marbofloxacin.

**quittor** n. infection of cartilage located on the side of a horse's foot within the hoof. Quittor can be caused by a wound to the bottom of the foot or to the tissues above the hoof. Affected individuals develop swelling of and drainage from the coronary band and lameness. Treatment includes the surgical removal of the diseased tissues and antibiotics.

## R

**rabbit calicivirus** n. a contagious virus that affects some types of rabbits and can cause fever and rapid death. Cases must be reported to appropriate regulatory agencies. *Also called* viral hemorrhagic disease.

**rabies** n. a viral disease transmitted through the bites of infected animals or contact between their saliva and open wounds. Humans can become infected. In the furious form of rabies, animals often become agitated, irritable and aggressive and can have difficulty walking and seizures. The dumb or paralytic form of rabies is characterized by drooling, inability to swallow, weakness and paralysis. Rabies is fatal once clinical signs of the disease have developed. Cases must be reported to appropriate regulatory agencies. Effective preventative vaccines are available.

**radial nerve paralysis** n. a loss of function of the radial nerve, which is located in the forelimb and often damaged by traumatic injury. Affected animals may place the top of the foot on the ground or be unable to bear weight on that leg. Treatment can include rest and anti-inflammatories.

**radiation therapy** n. a procedure in which electromagnetic radiation is used to destroy diseased, often cancerous tissues. The radiation may be directed towards the body from an outside source or originate from an implanted object or injected substance (e.g., iodine-131). *Also called* radiotherapy.

**radiculitis** n. inflammation of the areas where spinal nerves attach to the spinal cord.

**radioactive iodine** n. *See* iodine-131.

**radioallergosorbent test (RAST)** n. a laboratory test that can be performed on a blood sample to help diagnose allergies.

**radiodense** n. *See* radiopaque.

**radiograph** n. a picture formed by passing electromagnetic energy of certain wavelengths through a structure and capturing the image on a sensitive film. *Also called* x-ray.

**radiolucent** adj. appearing dark on a radiograph because of characteristics that allow the passage of x-rays through a body part or other material- **radiolucency** n. *Compare* radiopaque.

**radiopaque** adj. appearing white or light gray on a radiograph because of characteristics that block x-rays from passing through a body part or other material - **radiopacity** n. *Compare* radiolucent.

**radiotherapy** n. *See* radiation therapy.

**radius** n. one of the two long bones that lie between the elbow and carpus.

**radius curvus** n. a developmental abnormality caused by damage to a growth plate that stops the ulna from lengthening. Continued growth of the radius causes the lower front limb to curve.

**rain rot** n. *See* dermatophilosis.

**rain scald** n. superficial scaling of the skin and hair loss along the top side of a horse that is caused by prolonged dampness. Dry conditions will cure the disorder. *Compare* dermatophilosis.

**rale** n. an abnormal sound heard when listening to the lungs with a stethoscope.

**ram** n. an adult, male sheep that has not been castrated.

**ram effect** n. the willingness of ewes to breed that occurs more quickly after a period of anestrus when a ram is introduced to the flock.

**range of motion (ROM)** n. the extent to which a joint can be flexed, extended or rotated.

**ranula** n. an abnormal accumulation of saliva within a cyst under the tongue that is caused by a blocked salivary duct. Treatment can include surgery to remove the salivary gland or create a channel for saliva to drain from the cyst.

**rapid eye movement (REM)** n. a period of sleep characterized by dreaming and movement of the eyes.

**rasp** v. to file down the surface of a structure (e.g., tooth, hoof or bone).

**ration** n. the amount and type of food offered to an animal.

**reactive** adj. describes a lesion or other finding that is the result of a tissue's response to a disease process.

**recessive gene** n. one of two paired genes that will produce its version of a trait only if the other copy calls for the same thing. *Compare* dominant gene.

**recombinant vaccine** n. a type of vaccine that contains only a single protein associated with a disease-causing microorganism. The protein is manufactured by bacteria or yeast that have had a section of DNA coding for the protein inserted into their own genetic material.

**rectal exam** n. insertion of a finger or hand into the rectum to examine structures that can be palpated within the end of the gastrointestinal tract or through the rectal wall. *Also called* rectal palpation.

**rectal prolapse** n. eversion of the rectum through the anus, which can be caused by straining associated with the intestinal, urinary or reproductive tracts. Treatment includes surgery to replace the rectum and hold it in the normal position and addressing any underlying conditions.

**rectovaginal fistula** n. an abnormal hole that connects the rectum and vagina. Surgical repair is necessary to repair the fistula. *See also* perineal laceration.

**rectum** n. the end of the gastrointestinal tract located just in front of the anus - **rectal** adj.

**recumbent** adj. describes an animal that is lying down - **recumbency** n.

**recurrent airway obstruction (RAO)** n. a disease of horses that is caused by allergies and leads to coughing, difficulty breathing and nasal discharge. Treatment involves limiting exposure to the allergen (e.g., dust associated with hay and straw), bronchodilators and corticosteroids. *Also called* heaves, broken wind and chronic obstructive pulmonary disease.

**recurrent uveitis** n. a disease of horses in which intermittent bouts of inflammation within the eyes can lead to squinting, ocular drainage, red eyes, small pupils, corneal opacities and other eye lesions. The inflammation may be initiated by infection (e.g., leptospirosis) or other causes, but eventually the disease is primarily a result of immune system dysfunction. Treatment can include addressing any underlying disorders, anti-inflammatories and drugs that dilate the pupil.

**red blood cell (RBC)** n. the cell in blood that carries oxygen. *Also called* erythrocyte.

**red blood cell parameters** n. calculations that are based on laboratory tests and help determine the likely cause of abnormal red blood cell counts. *Also called* red blood cell indices and erythrocyte parameters.

**red bug** n. *See* chigger.

**red mite** n. a small insect that can infest birds and cause weight loss, anemia and death. Treatment of the birds and their environment with substances that kill the mite can be effective. *Also called* chicken mite, roost mite and poultry mite.

**red nose** n. *See* infectious bovine rhinotracheitis.

**red water disease** n. *See* bacillary hemoglobinuria.

**redirected aggression** n. attacks or related behaviors (e.g., growling, hissing or snapping) against an inappropriate target because the actual inciting cause cannot be reached. Instituting appropriate behavioral modification protocols can be helpful.

**red-leg disease** n. a disease of amphibians that can be caused by microorganisms, often *Aeromonas hydrophila*, entering the bloodstream because of wounds, unsanitary conditions or stress. Affected individuals have reddened skin that is often visible on the inside of the rear legs, lose their appetite, become lethargic and can die. Treatment includes antibiotics and supportive care.

**reduce** v. to put body structures (e.g., the ends of a broken bone) back into their proper position. A closed reduction occurs without surgery while an open reduction involves an incision through the skin and down to the body parts in question to allow for their adequate manipulation - **reduction** n.

**refer** v. to send a patient to another veterinarian who is better able to handle the diagnosis and treatment of a particular disorder - **referral** n.

**referred pain** n. discomfort that is felt in a part of the body that is a distance from where the causative lesion is located.

**reflex** n. an involuntary response to a stimulus. See the particular reflex (e.g., patellar or oculocephalic) for details.

**reflux** n. the movement of a liquid or other substance in a direction that is the reverse of what is normally seen.

**refractometer** n. a device that is used most frequently to measure urine specific gravity or the protein concentration within a sample of serum.

**refractory** adj. not responding to treatment.

**regenerative anemia** n. a lower than normal red blood cell count that is associated with the bone marrow responding to produce more red blood cells. Regenerative anemias are often seen with bleeding or diseases that lead to the destruction of red blood cells. *Compare* nonregenerative anemia.

**registered veterinary technician (RVT)** n. a person who has received training and certification in veterinary procedures, laboratory skills and the nursing care of animals.

**regurgitation** n. 1. the backward flow of food from within the esophagus out through the mouth. *Compare* vomit. 2. the backward flow of blood through a heart valve.

**reinforcement** n. *See* positive and negative reinforcement.

**rejection** n. 1. activity of the immune system that acts to destroy material that is foreign to the body (e.g., a transplant). 2. unwillingness of a female to nurse and otherwise care for her offspring.

**relapse** n. the return of a disease after an apparent recovery because the source within the animal was not completely eradicated.

**relative polycythemia** n. an abnormally high red blood cell count that is caused by any disorder that leads to a loss of fluid from the circulatory system (e.g., dehydration). *Compare* polycythemia vera.

**remission** n. the state in which a disease that was previously causing significant clinical signs is still present in the body but having little adverse effect.

**renal** adj. pertaining to the kidney(s).

**renal failure** n. loss of the kidneys' ability to perform their normal functions, including excreting waste and conserving water. *Also called* kidney failure. *See also* acute and chronic renal failure.

**renal medullary washout** n. a loss of the kidneys' ability to conserve water because a prolonged period of increased urine production has resulted in reduced levels of sodium and chloride within renal tissues. Treatment includes salt supplements and addressing any underlying disorders.

**renal pelvis** n. the central portion of a kidney into which urine drains.

**renal profile** n. laboratory tests measuring the levels of different substances in blood and urine that are associated with kidney health.

**renal secondary hyperparathyroidism** n. overproduction of parathyroid hormone that develops as a result of chronic renal failure. Affected individuals can have increased thirst and urination, vomiting, bones that bend or break easily, inability to close their mouth, drooling and loose teeth. Treatment includes therapy for chronic renal failure and medications that help lower blood phosphorous and raise blood calcium levels.

**renomegaly** n. an enlarged kidney.

**reperfusion injury** n. the inflammation and damage to tissues that occurs when blood supply is restored after a period of time without adequate circulation.

**repositol** n. a form of a drug that will release medication over a prolonged period of time after injection.

**reproduction** n. the process through which animals, plants and other living beings produce offspring.

**reproductive tract** n. the ovaries, uterus, testicles, penis and other body parts that are all associated with producing offspring.

**resect** v. to surgically remove a portion of an organ or other structure - **resection** n.

**resistance** n. the ability of an organism to withstand the effects a disease, drug or other phenomenon. For example, dogs are naturally resistant to tetanus and rarely develop the disease, and bacteria may develop resistance to certain antibiotics after which these drugs have little to no effect - **resistant** adj.

**resorb** v. to break down and absorb a structure within the body - **resorption** n.

**respiration** n. 1. the transfer of oxygen and carbon dioxide through the lungs and between cells within the body and the circulatory system. 2. the process through which cells break down nutrients (e.g., carbohydrates) to produce energy - **respiratory** adj.

**respiration rate (RR)** n. the number of times an animal breathes per minute.

**respiratory tract** n. the nasal passages, trachea, bronchi, lungs and other structures that all work to exchange oxygen, carbon dioxide and other gasses between the environment and the circulatory system.

**responsive** adj. responding to external stimuli.

**restrictive cardiomyopathy** n. a disease in which the muscles of the heart's ventricles cannot relax and allow blood to fill the chambers. Affected individuals may develop difficulty breathing and lethargy and lose use of their hind legs. Treatment can include medications that improve heart function, removal of excess fluid and decreasing the formation of blood clots.

**resuscitate** v. to perform procedures (e.g., CPR) and use medications in an attempt to restart the heart and/or breathing in an animal that is dying - **resuscitation** n.

**retained** adj. failing to have moved into another location or to be shed from

the body as should have occurred. For example, a retained testicle is located within the abdomen or inguinal canal when it should have moved into the scrotum.

**retching** n. attempts at vomiting that do not produce any material.

**reticulocyte** n. an immature red blood cell.

**reticulocytosis** n. higher than normal numbers of reticulocytes in circulation, which can be seen when an animal is making more red blood cells in response to anemia.

**reticulopericarditis** n. *See* hardware disease.

**reticuloperitonitis** n. *See* hardware disease.

**reticulum** n. one of the four chambers of the ruminant stomach.

**retina** n. the tissue that lines the back of the inside of the eye, receives light and converts it into neurologic impulses to be transmitted to the brain - **retinal** adj.

**retinopathy** n. any disease of the retina.

**retractor** n. a surgical instrument that holds tissues out of the way of the surgeon allowing easier access to the region of interest.

**retrobulbar** adj. behind the eyeball.

**retrograde** adj. moving backwards.

**retroperitoneal** adj. between the peritoneum and the abdominal wall. For example, the kidneys lie within the retroperitoneal space.

**retropharyngeal** adj. behind the pharynx.

**retropulse** v. to push in a backwards direction - **retropulsion** n.

**retrovirus** n. a group of related viruses including those that cause feline leukemia, ovine progressive pneumonia and equine infectious anemia.

**reverse sneeze** n. a condition affecting dogs characterized by a sudden and harsh intake of air through the nose and snorting noises. Reverse sneezing can be associated with irritation to the nasopharynx and may continue for several minutes but is not dangerous and usually requires no treatment. If the condition becomes more frequent or severe or is associated with other clinical signs (e.g., nasal discharge) a search for an underlying cause should be initiated.

**rhabdomyolysis** n. *See* exertional rhabdomyolysis.

**rheumatoid arthritis** n. an autoimmune disease that can cause fever, lethargy, enlarged lymph nodes and swollen and painful joints. Smaller joints (e.g., those in the toes) are most often affected. Treatment can include anti-inflammatories and immunosuppressive drugs.

**rhinitis** n. inflammation of the nasal passages, which can be associated with infections, allergies or irritants.

**rhinoscopy** n. the use of an instrument (e.g., an endoscope) to allow visualization of the nasal passages and sometimes the removal of foreign objects and tissue samples.

**rhinosinusitis** n. inflammation of the nasal passages and sinuses, which can be associated with infections, allergies or irritants.

**rhinotracheitis** n. inflammation of the nasal passages and trachea. *See also* infectious bovine rhinotracheitis and feline viral rhinotracheitis.

**rhodococcosis** n. a disease, most commonly of foals, caused by infection with *Rhodococcus equi* bacteria. Individuals usually come into contact with organisms present in the environment and may develop fever, lethargy, difficulty breathing, coughing, diarrhea and abdominal pain. Treatment can include antibiotics, oxygen and fluid therapy, anti-inflammatories and supportive care.

**riboflavin** n. a type of vitamin B that plays an important role in many enzymatic reactions within the body.

**ribonucleic acid (RNA)** n. the genetic material within cells that helps form proteins. RNA is also the blueprint for the development, maintenance and reproduction of some types of viruses.

**rickets** n. *See* nutritional secondary hyperparathyroidism.

**rickettsia** n. a group of related bacteria that are often transmitted through the bites of parasites or the ingestion of infected organisms. Rickettsia can cause a variety of diseases (e.g., ehrlichiosis and Potomac horse fever).

**ridgeling** n. *See* cryptorchid. *Also called* rig.

**right displaced abomasum (RDA)** n. *See* displaced abomasum.

**right dorsal colitis** n. a disorder most frequently seen in horses treated with nonsteroidal anti-inflammatory drugs. Affected individuals may develop abdominal pain, fever, diarrhea and loss of appetite and weight. Treatment can include stopping administration of any causative drugs, diet changes, medications that help the gastrointestinal tract heal and surgery to remove severely damaged tissues.

**right dorsal displacement of the colon** n. movement and sometimes twisting of part of a horse's large intestine so that it lies between the cecum and the body wall causing abdominal pain. Treatment can include fluid therapy, pain relief and surgery.

**rigor mortis** n. the temporary stiffening of a body that occurs soon after death.

**ring womb** n. a disorder primarily affecting ewes in which the cervix fails to dilate enough to allow birth of the fetus. A cesarian section is usually necessary.

**ringbone** n. inflammation and abnormal bony growths around the joints of a horse's lower leg, which often causes lameness. Low ringbone affects the joint at the top of the hoof and high ringbone involves the next joint up a horse's leg. Potential causes include poor conformation, repeated exercise on hard ground, improper hoof trimming or shoeing, injury or infection. Rest, anti-inflammatories and for high ringbone, surgical fusion of the affected joint can all decrease discomfort associated with the disease.

**ringtail** n. a disorder seen in mice and rats housed under inappropriate environmental conditions (e.g., low humidity). Affected animals develop lesions around the base of their tails, which may fall off. Treatment includes improving environmental conditions and supportive care while the tail stump heals.

**ringworm** n. a disease caused by infection of the skin, hair or nails with a dermatophyte fungus. Affected individuals can develop areas of hair loss, flaky skin, crusting, secondary infections and misshapen and brittle nails. The fungus can be transmitted to other animals and people. Treatment may include medicated baths, shaving the coat and topical and oral medications to kill the fungus. *Also called* dermatophytosis.

**roach back** n. a convex curve to the back, most frequently seen as a conformational defect in horses. *Compare* swayback.

**roaring** n. *See* laryngeal hemiplegia.

**Robert Jones bandage** n. a thickly padded and stiff bandage that is often used to prevent unwanted motion of a musculoskeletal injury.

**Rocky Mountain spotted fever** n. a disease that is caused by *Rickettsia rickettsii* bacteria transmitted through the bites of infected ticks. Affected individuals can develop fever, swollen lymph nodes, lameness, bleeding, vomiting, diarrhea, coughing and difficulty breathing. Treatment includes antibiotics and supportive care.

**rod** n. a type of bacteria that appears like an elongated oval under the microscope. Determining that bacteria are rods can help diagnose and appropriately treat an infection. *Compare* cocci.

**rodent ulcer** n. *See* eosinophilic ulcer.

**rodenticide** n. a chemical used to kill rodents (e.g., mice and rats). *See also* anticoagulant rodenticide toxicity.

**rolling skin disease** n. *See* twitchy cat disease.

**rongeur** n. an instrument that can be used to break off pieces of a hard substance (e.g., bone or dental tartar).

**roost mite** n. *See* red mite.

**root** n. the portion of a structure (e.g., a tooth) that is buried in and attached to other tissues.

**root canal** n. removal and subsequent filling of the central portion of a tooth that contains blood vessels and nerves. Root canals are usually performed because of damage (e.g., fracture) to the tooth.

**root planing** n. scraping plaque and tartar from the accessible surfaces of tooth roots. *Also called* root scaling.

**root signature** n. pain felt in a leg that originates from pressure upon a nerve as it leaves the spinal cord.

**rostral** adj. 1. towards the front of the face. 2. pertaining to or resembling a beak.

**rotavirus** n. a group of related, contagious viruses that can cause diarrhea in a number of species. Young animals are most frequently affected.

Treatment includes fluid therapy and supportive care - **rotaviral** adj.

**roughage** n. types of feed that are mostly indigestible (i.e., high in fiber) and can promote the function and health of the gastrointestinal tract.

**round cell tumor** n. any of a number of types of tumors that are primarily composed of cells that appear round under the microscope. Lymphomas, histiocytomas, extramedullary plasmacytomas and transmissible venereal tumors can all be considered round cell tumors.

**roundworm** n. a type of parasite that attaches to the walls of the gastrointestinal tract and can cause poor growth, weight loss, a pot-bellied appearance, vomiting and diarrhea, especially in young animals. Larval forms can migrate throughout the body. Animals are infected through the ingestion of eggs in the environment, while in the uterus or through suckling milk from an infected dam. Many types of dewormers can kill the parasites.

**rubber jaw** n. *See* hyperparathyroidism.

**rudimentary** adj. not fully or properly developed.

**rugae** n. folds, particularly those of the stomach's inner lining.

**rumen** n. the largest of the four compartments of a ruminant's stomach, which is responsible for fermenting food.

**rumen impaction** n. *See* grain overload.

**rumenitis** n. inflammation of the rumen.

**rumenotomy** n. a surgical incision into the rumen.

**ruminal acidosis** n. *See* subacute ruminal acidosis and grain overload.

**ruminal drinking** n. a disorder most often seen in young ruminants fed milk from a bucket in which the reflex that should allow liquids to bypass the rumen does not occur normally. Affected individuals can have a poor appetite and growth, a distended abdomen and pasty feces. Treatment includes flushing out the rumen and encouraging the animal to suckle rather than gulp milk.

**ruminal tympany** n. an accumulation of gas within the rumen to the point of distention and pain. Passage of a stomach tube or surgery to release the gas is often necessary to provide relief and prevent death. *Also called* bloat. *See also* frothy and free gas bloat.

**ruminant** n. animals including cattle, sheep and goats that have a four-chambered stomach and regurgitate and rechew their food.

**runt** n. a young animal that is smaller, and sometimes weaker and less healthy than normal. Many disorders affecting a pregnant female or newborn animal can cause runting.

**rupture** n. a tear that can disrupt the normal function of a tissue.

## S

**sacrocaudal dysgenesis** n. a birth defect, sometimes genetic in origin, in which the bones of the sacrum and tail do not form correctly. Animals often are tailless and can have neurologic problems affecting urination, defecation and their hind legs.

**sacroiliac** adj. pertaining to the connection between the sacrum and the front part of the pelvis.

**sacrum** n. the bony structure that lies between and connects the hip bones, last spinal vertebra and tail - **sacral** adj.

**saddle sore** n. injury to the skin and sometimes deeper tissues caused by the friction of a poorly fitting saddle or other piece of tack. Eliminating the cause of the injury is essential. Additional treatment may include antibiotics, anti-inflammatories and surgery. *Also called* gall.

**saddle thrombus** n. a disorder most often seen in cats with heart disease in which a blood clot blocks circulation to the hind legs. Affected cats are in pain, cannot walk and their hind feet are cool to the touch. Return of hindlimb function is possible in some cases but additional clots may develop. *Also called* aortic thromboembolism.

**sagittal** adj. situated along the midline of the long axis of the body.

**salicylate** n. a type of medication that can decrease inflammation, pain and the tendency of blood to clot. Aspirin is the most commonly used salicylate. *See also* nonsteroidal anti-inflammatory drug and NSAID toxicity.

**saline** adj. containing salt.

**saliva** n. the liquid that is produced by glands draining into the mouth. Saliva helps lubricate food and begin the digestive process - **salivary** adj.

**salivary mucocele** n. an abnormal accumulation of saliva within a cyst under the skin that is caused by a blocked salivary duct. Treatment can include periodic drainage of the cyst or surgery to remove the salivary gland.

**salivation** n. the production of saliva.

**salmon poisoning** n. a disease of dogs that is caused by ingestion of fish infested with a parasite carrying the bacteria *Neorickettsia helminthoeca*. Affected individuals may develop fever, depression, loss of appetite, vomiting, diarrhea, discharge from the eyes and nose, enlarged lymph nodes and very often die. Treatment can include antibiotics, supportive care and blood transfusions.

**salmonellosis** n. a disease caused by infection with *Salmonella* bacteria, which are often contracted through the ingestion of feces containing the organism. Affected individuals can develop diarrhea, a fever, abdominal pain and may die. The infection may spread into the bloodstream and throughout the body. Pregnant females often will abort. Treatment can include antibiotics, anti-inflammatories, fluid therapy and supportive care. The bacteria may persist in and be intermittently shed from an animal that has recovered from salmonellosis. People can become infected with *Salmonella*. *Also called* paratyphoid.

**salpingitis** n. inflammation of a uterine tube, which is often caused by infection.

**salt** n. a compound that contains an acid bound to a base, often specifically referring to sodium chloride.

**salt lick** n. salt that is often mixed with minerals and other substances and offered to a grazing animal to prevent dietary deficiencies.

**salt poisoning** n. a disease caused by continued salt intake when water ingestion is limited. Affected animals can develop increased thirst, vomiting, diarrhea or constipation, drooling, bizarre behavior and may die. Treatment includes removing the source of the salt and fluid therapy.

**Salter-Harris classification** n. a system of identifying various types of fractures affecting animals' growth plates.

**sand colic** n. a disease of horses caused by the ingestion of sand that accumulates within the large intestine. Affected animals can develop abdominal pain, diarrhea and weight loss. Oral psyllium treatment will bind to and help eliminate the sand from the gastrointestinal tract. *See also* colic.

**sand crack** n. a vertical fissure in a horse's hoof that starts at the top of the foot and travels downwards. Sand cracks can be caused by poor conformation, injury or overgrown hooves and may be painful if they are deep or involve the coronary band. Corrective trimming and shoeing can promote healing of the crack. *Compare* grass crack.

**sanguinous** adj. bloody. *Also called* sanguineous.

**sarcocystosis** n. a disease caused by infection with *Sarcocystis* protozoal parasites contracted through ingestion of the tissues or feces of an infected animal. Affected individuals may develop a fever, weakness, bizarre behavior, loss of appetite and weight, a sparsely haired tail and may die. Pregnant females can abort. Many infected animals will show no clinical signs of disease. Treatment includes medications to kill the parasite and supportive care. *Also called* sarcosporidiosis. *See also* equine protozoal myeloencephalitis.

**sarcoid** n. a tumor affecting the skin of horses, which may be caused by a virus. These tumors generally do not spread to other parts of the body but may be locally invasive and get very large. Treatment can include surgery, cryosurgery, radiation therapy and medications that stimulate the immune system.

**sarcoma** n. a type of cancer that arises from tissues such as bone, muscle or connective tissue. Sarcomas often develop and spread rapidly. See the specific type of sarcoma (e.g., lymphosarcoma and fibrosarcoma) for details.

**sarcoptic mange** n. a contagious disease caused by infestation of the skin with a *Sarcoptes* mite. Affected animals are extremely itchy and may not eat well and lose weight. Transmission to humans is possible. The disease is to be reported to appropriate regulatory officials in some species. *Also called* barn itch and scabies.

**satiate** v. to eat and drink to the point where hunger and thirst are no longer evident.

**saucer fracture** n. *See* bucked shin.

**saw horse stance** n. an abnormal body position in which an animal stands with its legs spread wider apart than is normal. Tetanus and some types of neurologic disorders are possible causes.

**scabies** n. *See* sarcoptic mange.

**scale** n. 1. a thin plate or flake of skin - **scaly** adj. 2. v. to scrape away tartar and plaque from teeth.

**scale rot** n. a skin infection of reptiles sometimes caused by humid and unsanitary conditions. Affected individuals often have areas of redness, blisters, ulcers and pus on their skin. Treatment involves antibiotic therapy and cleaning the animal's environment. *Also called* blister disease, ulcerative dermatitis and necrotic dermatitis.

**scaler** n. an instrument used to scrape away tartar and plaque from teeth.

**scalpel** n. a surgical blade.

**scaly leg and face** n. a disease of birds caused by mites that produce raised, crusty skin lesions affecting the legs and/or face and sometimes permanent beak deformities. Treatment includes medications and chemicals that kill the mites on the bird and in the environment.

**scapula** n. the shoulder blade.

**scapulohumeral joint** n. the connection between the shoulder blade and the humerus.

**Schiff-Sherrington syndrome** n. an abnormal body position that is caused by damage to a part of the spinal cord and produces rigid extension of the front limbs and hind end paralysis.

**Schirmer tear test** n. a test that measures the amount of tears produced by the glands associated with the eye.

**schistosomus reflexus** n. a fatal birth defect in which the spine is severely bent so that the head and tail may touch over the back and the organs of the chest and abdomen protrude from the body.

**schwannoma** n. *See* neurofibroma.

**sciatic nerve paralysis** n. *See* calving paralysis.

**scintigraphy** n. a test that involves the administration of a mildly radioactive substance to an animal and observing its distribution as it is taken up by the tissues. The procedure is often used to detect areas of inflammation. *Also called* nuclear scintigraphy and bone scan.

**scirrhous cord** n. a painful infection and thickening of the part of the spermatic cord that remains after castration. Treatment can include antibiotics, anti-inflammatories and surgery to remove the diseased tissues.

**sclera** n. the outside of the eye that connects to the cornea and is usually white - **scleral** adj.

**sclerosis** n. an abnormal hardening of a tissue - **sclerotic** adj.

**scooting** n. dropping and dragging the rear end along the ground, which is most commonly seen in dogs affected by irritating disorders of the anal region (e.g., anal sac distension).

**scours** n. diarrhea.

**scrapie** n. a disease of sheep and goats caused by an abnormal protein called a prion that can be ingested or transmitted by an infected female to her unborn young. Affected animals develop itching, difficulty walking, abnormal behavior, excessive thirst and eventually die. There is no treatment, and suspected cases must be reported to appropriate regulatory agencies.

**scratches** n. skin lesions on the back of a horse's lower legs often associated with standing in damp, dirty conditions. Affected individuals can develop swelling, oozing, crusting, hair loss, thickened skin and pain at the site. Treatment may involve repeated, thorough cleansing of the area, antibiotics and improved hygiene. *Also called* cracked heel and greasy heel.

**screwworm** n. the larva of a type of fly that can invade healthy skin through wounds and cause tissue destruction and sometimes death. Cases of screwworm must be reported to appropriate regulatory agencies.

**scrotal circumference** n. a measurement of testicular size that can be used to assess potential fertility in adult male ruminants.

**scrotal hernia** n. a protrusion of abdominal contents into the scrotum, which is usually associated with trauma or birth defects that enlarge a normal passageway between the two body cavities. Affected individuals can be in pain and have an enlarged scrotum. Some congenital hernias may close with time, but surgery is often necessary to repair the defect.

**scrotum** n. the exterior pouch that holds the testicles - **scrotal** adj.

**scrub** n. *See* surgical scrub.

**scruff** n. the loose skin on the back of the neck of some animals. Grasping the scruff is a humane way to hold and restrain some species (e.g., cats and ferrets).

**scurvy** n. a disease caused by a deficiency of vitamin C in the diet, which is seen in guinea pigs, primates and some other species. Affected animals can develop lameness, swollen joints, loss of appetite and weight, diarrhea, poor quality coats, a tendency to bleed, secondary infections and may die. Treatment includes vitamin C supplements and supportive care.

**scute** n. a hard, scale-like structure on the surface of some reptiles (e.g., tortoises). *Also called* **scutum.**

**sebaceous adenitis** n. a disease of dogs in which the immune system destroys the glands that produce sebum causing flaky skin and hair loss. Treatment can include topical or oral treatments that reduce skin flaking.

**sebaceous adenoma** n. a benign, wart-like tumor of the skin that most commonly affects older dogs. Surgical removal is curative.

**sebaceous cyst** n. *See* epidermal inclusion cyst.

**sebaceous epithelioma** n. a benign, wart-like tumor of the skin. Surgical removal is curative.

**sebaceous gland** n. the tissues that produce and secrete an oily substance (i.e., sebum) onto the surface of the skin.

**seborrhea** n. a condition characterized by the excessive production of skin flakes. Some cases are related to genetics, but many others are the result of an underlying disorder (e.g., hormonal diseases or allergies). Some animals with seborrhea develop secondary skin infections. If the skin is greasy and the flakes clump together, the disorder is referred to as seborrhea oleosa. Animals with seborrhea sicca have dry, flaky skin. Treatment can include medicated shampoos and conditioners, drugs to treat infections and reduce itching, nutritional supplements and addressing any underlying disorders.

**sebum** n. an oily substance that is secreted onto the surface of the skin by the sebaceous glands.

**second degree burn** n. a moderately severe burn that damages superficial and deep layers of skin. *Compare* first and third degree burns.

**secondary** adj. 1. occurring as a result of another, underlying disorder. 2. not the most important. *Compare* primary.

**sedate** v. to give medications that lead to a decrease in alertness, anxiety and reactions to stimuli - **sedation, sedative** n.

**sediment** n. the particulate matter that collects at the bottom of a liquid over a period of time or during centrifugation.

**seed tick** n. a small, immature tick.

**seedy toe** n. a condition in which a gap develops between layers within the front of the hoof wall, which can be caused by laminitis or overgrown or poorly balanced hooves. Foreign material collects in the cavity and often leads to infection. Treatment can include cleaning out the area, removing the overlying hoof wall, corrective shoeing and medications to treat or prevent infection. *Also called* hollow wall.

**seizure** n. an involuntary change in muscular activity and/or mental awareness arising from abnormal electrical activity within the brain. Seizures may be caused by physical abnormalities (e.g., a brain tumor or injury), metabolic abnormalities (e.g., low blood sugar) or because of idiopathic epilepsy. Treatment for mild seizures may not be necessary or can be directed at any underlying causes. If seizures are frequent or of long enough duration to become dangerous, anticonvulsant medications will usually reduce their occurrence and severity. *See also* partial seizure and generalized seizure.

**selenium** n. an element, the correct levels of which are important in the diet. *See also* selenium toxicosis, white muscle disease and postparturient hemoglobinuria.

**selenium toxicosis** n. a disease seen in animals that consume forage that has a high selenium concentration or ingest too much selenium from supplements and other sources. Affected individuals often are lethargic, thin and have poor quality hooves leading to lameness. Their hair breaks easily and some horses can have very short manes and tails. Infertility can also be seen. *Also called* alkali disease.

**self-limiting** adj. describes a condition that resolves without specific treatment.

**semen** n. the material released during ejaculation that consists of sperm and fluids produced by glands (e.g., prostate) associated with the male reproductive tract.

**semilunar valve** n. either of the valves that control blood flow from the heart into the aorta or the pulmonary arteries. *See also* aortic and pulmonary valves.

**seminoma** n. a testicular tumor most commonly seen in older dogs. Most cases are benign, and castration is curative. Cryptorchidism increases the risk of developing a seminoma, and these tumors are more likely to be malignant.

**seneciosis** n. *See* pyrrolizidine alkaloidosis.

**senile** adj. 1. pertaining to old age. 2. pertaining to a loss of mental abilities that can accompany old age - **senility** n.

**sensory neurons** n. nerves that carry signals from sense organs (e.g., the eyes or skin) to the spinal cord and brain. *Compare* motor neurons.

**separation anxiety** n. distress that occurs when an animal is not in the presence of certain people. Affected animals can be very destructive, cry, urinate and defecate when left alone or when they fear being left alone. Treatment may include behavioral modification protocols and medications that relieve anxiety.

**sepsis** n. the presence of disease-causing microorganisms or their toxins within the blood or body - **septic** adj. *See also* septicemia and endotoxemia.

**septal defect** n. *See* atrial and ventricular septal defects.

**septic arthritis** n. infection and inflammation of one or more joints that can lead to swelling, lameness, fever, lethargy and loss of appetite. Bacteria may enter through the bloodstream or through wounds that penetrate into the joint. Treatment can include antibiotics, anti-inflammatories and surgery or procedures to remove infectious organisms and damaged tissue from within the joint. *Also called* infectious arthritis and joint ill.

**septic shock** n. inadequate delivery of oxygen to tissues that is caused by a severe infection. Septic shock may drastically lower blood pressure and result in organ failure and death. Treatment can include fluid and oxygen therapy, antibiotics and medications to increase blood pressure.

**septicemia** n. the presence of bacteria or other microorganisms within the blood. Affected individuals can develop a fever, lethargy, low blood pressure and may die without prompt and aggressive treatment - **septicemic** adj. *Also called* blood poisoning or bacteremia.

**septicemic cutaneous ulcerative disease (SCUD)** n. a disease of turtles caused by infection with some types of bacteria that can be associated with a dirty environment. Affected individuals can lose their appetite, become lethargic and develop lesions and hemorrhages on the skin and shell. The infection may spread to the bloodstream and cause death. Treatment can include iodine soaks and antibiotics.

**septum** n. a structure that divides an organ or body part - **septal** adj.

**sequela** n. an unwanted condition that develops as a result of a procedure, treatment or another disorder.

**sequestrum** n. a piece of tissue that has died but is surrounded by normal tissues. A sequestrum can be a source for recurrent infections, and its surgical removal is usually necessary. *See also* corneal sequestrum.

**serology** n. a type of laboratory test that looks for the presence of antibodies against a particular disease. Serology can provide evidence of a current or past infection or protection provided by a vaccine.

**seroma** n. a pocket of watery fluid (i.e., serum) that can develop after tissue damage. If the seroma is problematical, it can be drained, but in most cases the fluid will be absorbed without any intervention.

**serosa** n. the membrane that covers the surface of organs and body cavities - serosal adj. *Also called* serous membrane.

**serositis** n. inflammation of the serosa.

**serous** adj. pertaining to or like serum.

**serovar** n. a subtype of a particular bacterial species that can have different characteristics than other closely related subtypes.

**Sertoli cell tumor** n. a testicular tumor most commonly seen in older dogs. The tumor can secrete estrogen and cause male animals to lose hair, have darkened skin and develop feminine characteristics. Cryptorchidism increases the risk of developing a

Sertoli cell tumor, and these tumors tend to be more malignant than those contained within the scrotum. Treatment can include castration, chemotherapy and radiation therapy.

**serum** n. the liquid part of blood that is present after clotting has occurred and the cells are removed. *Compare* plasma.

**serum glutamic-oxaloacetic transaminase (SGOT)** n. *See* aspartate aminotransferase.

**serum hepatitis** n. *See* Theiler's disease.

**service** v. to breed.

**sesamoid bone** n. a small bone that is contained within a tendon, ligament or the capsule surrounding a joint.

**sesamoiditis** n. inflammation of a sesamoid bone, which is often caused by injury to surrounding soft tissues (e.g., ligaments). Animals can be lame and experience pain and swelling over the affected area. Treatment includes anti-inflammatories and prolonged rest.

**sessile** adj. fully attached along the base. *Compare* pedunculated.

**setfast** n. *See* exertional rhabdomyolysis.

**sex hormone** n. one of several hormones (e.g., estrogen, progesterone and testosterone) that play a role in reproduction and the development of male or female characteristics.

**sexing** n. a determination of the sex of an individual animal, which can be difficult in some species or in very young animals.

**sex-linked** adj. describes a trait, the genes for which are carried on the X or Y chromosome.

**shaker foal syndrome** n. *See* toxicoinfectious botulism.

**Shasta River crud** n. *See* Potomac horse fever.

**shear mouth** n. a greater than normal angle to the chewing surface of a horse's molars, which can make chewing difficult. Floating the teeth can improve the condition but may need to be repeated regularly.

**sheared heals** n. a condition of horses in which uneven weight bearing causes the development of asymmetrical heels, abnormal hoof wear, lameness and other foot problems. Treatment includes corrective hoof trimming and shoeing.

**sheath** n. a tubular structure that covers and surrounds another object. *See also* prepuce.

**sheath rot** n. *See* pizzle rot.

**sheep ked** n. a wingless fly that lives on and ingests the blood of sheep and can cause itching, wool damage and discoloration, skin lesions, anemia, lethargy and loss of appetite and weight. Treatment includes shearing the wool and chemicals to kill the insects on the animals.

**shell rot** n. a disease of turtles caused by a bacterial or fungal infection that often develops because of damage to the shell or a dirty environment. Affected individuals develop holes in the shell that may penetrate into the underlying body cavity. Treatment can include iodine soaks and antibacterial or antifungal medications.

**shipping fever** n. a disease that is characterized by respiratory infections and initiated by a stressful event (e.g., transport). *See also* bovine respiratory disease complex.

**shivers** n. *See* polysaccharide storage myopathy.

**shock** n. a potential outcome of different disorders that all cause inadequate delivery of oxygen to tissues. Shock may lead to organ failure and death. See the specific type of shock (e.g., cardiogenic, hemorrhagic or septic) for details.

**Shope fibroma** n. a mass under the skin of rabbits that have been infected with a virus usually transmitted through the bites of insects. Affected individuals develop one or more masses, which can grow rapidly but eventually regress without treatment.

**short bowel syndrome** n. a possible side effect of the surgical removal or congenital lack of a large portion of small intestine. Affected animals develop diarrhea and weight loss. Treatment can include diet changes, nutritional supplements and anti-diarrheal medicines.

**shunt** n. a channel that allows the flow of materials between two structures that are not usually connected. *See also* portosystemic shunt.

**shying** n. a sudden movement away from something that frightens an animal.

**sialadenitis** n. inflammation of a salivary gland, which can be caused by trauma or infection.

**sialocele** n. *See* salivary mucocele.

**sialolith** n. an accumulation of minerals and other substances that form a stone within a salivary gland or its draining ducts.

**sick sinus syndrome** n. a disease in which electrical impulses are not transmitted normally throughout the heart. Affected individuals often have alternating periods of high and low heart rates and/or irregular heart rhythms. Drugs that increase the heart rate can be helpful, or a pacemaker can be implanted. *Also called* bradycardia-tachycardia syndrome.

**sickle hocked** n. a conformational flaw most commonly described in horses in which the hock joints are too sharply angled when viewed from the side causing the hind feet to be placed too far under the body. The disorder can predispose an animal to lameness.

**side effect** n. a consequence of a medicine or procedure that is not related to the desired outcome and is usually unwanted.

**sidebone** n. mineralization of the cartilages that lie on either side of the bone encased within a horse's hoof. Sidebones can be caused by overwork on hard surfaces or conformational flaws, and may or may not be associated with lameness. Treatment can include anti-inflammatories and corrective hoof trimming and shoeing.

**signalment** n. the age, sex and breed of an animal.

**silage** n. the feed that results from the process of bacterial, anaerobic fermentation acting on fresh, chopped forage. Silage can be stored for an extended period of time without loosing its nutritional value.

**silage disease** n. *See* listeriosis.

**silent heat** n. an absence of the signs or behavior normally seen around the time when a female is receptive to mating and is capable of becoming pregnant. *Also called* silent estrus.

**silica urolith** n. a type of stone that can form within and disrupt the function of the urinary tract. Diets rich in plants containing high levels of silica might be linked to some cases of these uroliths. The stones must be physically removed, but increasing water intake and diet changes may prevent their return.

**silver nitrate** n. a chemical that can be applied topically to treat infections or stop bleeding from small vessels.

**simple fracture** n. *See* closed fracture.

**sinoatrial node** n. an area containing muscle and nerve cells within the wall of the right atrium of the heart that normally controls the frequency and timing of heart contractions.

**sinoatrial node block** n. an abnormal heart rhythm that results from a lack of normal conduction of impulses out of the sinoatrial node of the heart. Affected animals may be lethargic or faint and have a slow heart rate. Treatment can include medications that increase the heart rate or implantation of a pacemaker.

**sinus** adj. 1. pertaining to the sinoatrial node of the heart. 2. n. a cavity. *See also* paranasal, frontal and dermoid sinus.

**sinus arrest** n. an abnormal heart rhythm that results from a lack of

electrical impulse generation in the sinoatrial node of the heart. Affected animals may be lethargic or faint and have a slow heart rate. Treatment can include medications that increase the heart rate or implantation of a pacemaker.

**sinus arrythmia** n. a normal increase in heart rate that accompanies inhalation, followed by a decrease in heart rate that accompanies exhalation.

**sinus rhythm** n. a normal, regular heart rate and rhythm.

**sinusitis** n. inflammation of one or more of the paranasal sinuses, which can be caused by infections, allergies or irritants.

**sire** n. a male parent.

**situs inversus** n. a birth defect in which organs are located on the opposite side of the body from which they are normally found.

**skeletal muscle** n. *See* striated muscle.

**skin scraping** n. a technique in which a scalpel is used to lightly abrade the surface of the skin to collect samples to be viewed under the microscope. Skin scrapings are useful in the diagnosis of demodicosis and some other types of mange.

**skin tag** n. a benign overgrowth of skin most commonly seen in older dogs. If the skin tag is problematical, it can be removed surgically.

**slaframine toxicosis** n. a disorder caused by ingestion of forage (e.g., clover) infected with a fungus that produces the chemical slaframine. Affected animals drool excessively but recover within a day or two after ingestion of the forage has been stopped. Treatment is generally not necessary but can include fluid therapy and medications to decrease drooling. *Also called* slobbers.

**sleeping sickness** n. any of a number of diseases that cause apparent drowsiness. *See also* pregnancy toxemia and Eastern, Western and Venezuelan encephalomyelitis.

**slipped disk** n. *See* herniated disk.

**slipped shoulder** n. *See* sweeny.

**slipper foot** n. a disorder of cattle in which a claw dramatically curls upward to a blunt end. Laminitis is a common cause, and treatment is difficult.

**slit lamp** n. a piece of equipment that provides magnification and shines a narrow band of bright light, which allows for close examination of the eye.

**slobbers** n. excess drooling that is often caused by overgrown teeth or other dental disorders in rabbits, chinchillas and other animals with teeth that grow continually. Treatment includes routinely filing the teeth. *See also* slaframine toxicosis.

**slough** v. to fall off, particularly referring to dead pieces of tissue that are shed from a body surface during the healing process.

**small intestinal bacterial overgrowth (SIBO)** n. a disorder most frequently seen in dogs that can occur secondary to diseases adversely affecting digestion (e.g., exocrine pancreatic insufficiency) or for unknown reasons. Animals usually develop diarrhea and lose weight. Treatment can include diet changes, antibiotics and addressing any underlying disorders.

**small intestine** n. the part of the gastrointestinal tract that is located between the stomach and the colon and plays a major role in the digestion and absorption of nutrients. The small intestine is divided into three sections: the duodenum, jejunum and ileum.

**small strongyle** n. a type of intestinal worm of horses that can cause diarrhea and weight loss. Many dewormers are effective against the adult worms, but larvae residing in the intestinal wall are more difficult to remove.

**smear** n. the microscopic examination of a thin layer of cells or another substance placed upon a glass slide. *See also* impression and blood smear.

**smegma** n. the dead cells and other debris that can accumulate within the penile sheath.

**smooth mouth** n. a condition in which the normal edges on the chewing surfaces of a horse's teeth are absent because of excessive wear or filing. Affected animals have difficulty chewing and digesting their food. Diet changes can be helpful.

**smooth muscle** n. a muscle the action of which cannot be consciously controlled (e.g., muscles in the intestines that control peristalsis). *Also called* involuntary muscle.

**sneeze** n. a sudden and involuntary expulsion of air out of the nose and mouth that is usually caused by irritation to the nasal passages.

**snuffles** n. a disease of rabbits caused by a bacterial infection of the respiratory tract. *Pasteurella* bacteria are often involved. Animals can develop nasal discharge, coughing and sneezing. Treatment includes antibiotics and supportive care but may not completely eliminate the infection. *Also called* rhinitis, pasteurellosis and nasal catarrh.

**socialization** n. the process through which an animal acquires the ability to relate with people and other animals and to deal with a variety of situations. Young animals often have a limited socialization period during which they are most able to develop these traits.

**sodium (Na)** n. an important electrolyte, the correct levels of which are essential for maintaining normal body function.

**sodium chloride (NaCl)** n. table salt. Solutions containing sodium chloride are often used to replenish fluid and electrolytes in the body.

**soft palate** n. the fleshy area located towards the back of the roof of the mouth. *Compare* hard palate.

**soft tissue** n. any part of the body excluding bone or cartilage.

**solar dermatitis** n. *See* actinic dermatitis.

**solar keratosis** n. *See* actinic keratosis.

**sole** n. the bottom of the foot. In horses, the sole is encircled by the hoof wall and surrounds the frog.

**soluble** adj. capable of being dissolved in a liquid. *Compare* insoluble.

**solute** n. a substance that is dissolved within a liquid.

**solution** n. a mixture of liquids and/or dissolved substances.

**solvent** n. a liquid that is capable of dissolving another substance.

**somatic cell count (SCC)** n. a measurement of the number of white blood cells contained within a sample of milk. High SCCs are often associated with mastitis and adversely affect milk quality.

**somatotropin** n. a hormone produced by the pituitary gland or used as a drug that promotes growth, muscle mass and milk production. *Also called* growth hormone.

**Somogyi effect** n. a higher than normal blood glucose level that occurs after an animal is overdosed with insulin and the body has responded to the resulting hypoglycemia.

**song bird fever** n. a disease of cats that is caused by *Salmonella* bacteria contracted through hunting and ingesting song birds. *See also* salmonellosis.

**sonography** n. *See* ultrasonography.

**sore hocks** n. *See* bumblefoot.

**sore mouth** n. *See* orf.

**sorehead** n. bloody skin lesions on the head of sheep, goats and some other species caused by the larvae of *Elaeophora schneideri* parasites. *See also* elaeophorosis.

**sorghum toxicity** n. a disease primarily seen in horses eating grasses containing certain types of natural chemicals. Affected individuals develop difficulty walking in the hind end, urinary tract infections and incontinence. Birth defects and abortion are also possible. Treatment is difficult but includes eliminating access to the causative grasses, antibiotics and supportive care.

**soring** n. the inhumane and illegal practice of applying substances or objects to a horse's feet or legs to cause pain and cause the animal to lift its feet higher and have a more animated gait.

**soundness** n. the ability to perform an activity for which the animal is intended, often referring to the ability to breed or a lack of lameness - **sound** adj.

**sour crop** n. a fungal or bacterial infection of a bird's crop, which may develop because of crop impaction, unsanitary conditions, inappropriate feeding or antibiotic use. Treatment can include addressing any underlying problems and antibiotic or antifungal medications.

**sow** n. a female pig that has given birth to piglets.

**sow mouth** n. *See* undershot jaw.

**spasm** n. a sudden and involuntary contraction of muscles or narrowing of a passageway - **spasmodic, spastic** adj.

**spasmolytic** adj. *See* antispasmodic.

**spastic paresis** n. a genetic disease of cattle that causes young animals to hold one or both hind legs in extension. Eventually the disease progresses so that the affected limb(s) are almost completely rigid. Surgery may improve the situation. *Also called* Elso heel.

**spavin** n. a condition affecting the hock joint. *See also* blood, bog and bone spavin.

**spay** v. to remove the ovaries surgically. In most cases, the uterus is removed as well. *See also* ovariohysterectomy.

**specific gravity** n. *See* urine specific gravity.

**spectacle** n. a protective, normally clear covering over the surface of the eye of some reptiles, which should fall off and be regenerated during each cycle of skin shedding.

**speculum** n. an instrument that can be used to keep a part of the body (e.g., the mouth) open allowing for a more thorough examination and access to perform procedures.

**sperm** n. the male reproductive cells capable of fertilizing an ovum and producing an embryo. *Also called* spermatozoa.

**spermatic cord** n. the structure that runs between the testicles and the abdomen containing blood vessels, nerves, muscles and the duct that carries sperm.

**spermatogenesis** n. the process through which sperm are produced.

**sphincter** n. an anatomical structure that intermittently constricts and relaxes to prevent or allow flow of materials through an opening within the body.

**spider lamb syndrome** n. *See* hereditary chondrodysplasia.

**spina bifida** n. a birth defect in which the two halves of the spinal column do not fuse correctly along a portion of its length. Affected individuals can have varying degrees of hind end weakness, difficulty walking and incontinence.

**spinal canal** n. the passageway through the spinal column that contains the spinal cord and cauda equina. *Also called* vertebral canal.

**spinal column** n. the structures (e.g., vertebrae and intervertebral disks) that surround and protect the spinal cord and cauda equina from the top of the neck to the hind end of the animal. *Also called* vertebral column.

**spinal cord** n. the structure that is surrounded by the spinal column and contains nerves that transmit impulses to and from the brain and the rest of the body.

**spinal dysraphism** n. a birth defect that is sometimes genetic in origin and causes abnormal development of the spinal cord and surrounding tissues. Affected animals often have hind end weakness and an unusual "bunny hopping" gait. No effective treatment exists.

**spinal nerve** n. one of the many paired nerves that arise off the spinal cord and pass between vertebrae into the rest of the body.

**spinal tap** n. insertion of a hollow needle into a cavity within the spinal column usually to withdraw a sample of fluid for analysis.

**spindle-cell sarcoma** n. *See* hemangiopericytoma.

**spindly leg syndrome** n. a disease of young frogs and toads that is thought to be caused by improper diet or environmental conditions. Affected individuals have underdeveloped front legs that can break easily. No effective treatment is available.

**spinose ear tick** n. a type of tick (*Otobius*) that infests the ear canals of many species and can lead to intense itching and irritation. Treatment includes manual removal of ticks and medications to kill them. *Also called* spinous ear tick.

**spirochetosis** n. a disease caused by infection with one of several types of spiral shaped bacteria (e.g., leptospirosis). Spirochetosis may specifically refer to a disease of birds caused by *Borrelia anserina*, which is transmitted through tick bites. Affected individuals can develop diarrhea, depression, shivering and increased thirst. Treatment with antibiotics is often successful when started early enough in the course of the disease. Preventative vaccines are available. *See also* leptospirosis and treponematosis (rabbit).

**splayleg** n. an abnormal condition in which one or more of an animal's legs cannot be brought underneath the body, making it difficult or impossible to stand and walk. Causes include genetics, trauma (often from sliding on slippery floors), infections, toxins and poor diet. Treatment can include surgery, bandages or splints to hold the affected legs in a more normal position. *Also called* spraddle leg.

**spleen** n. an organ within the abdomen that removes damaged or old red blood cells from circulation, stores blood and is a part of the immune system.

**splenectomy** n. the surgical removal of the spleen.

**splenomegaly** n. enlargement of the spleen.

**splint** n. 1. a device secured around an unstable injury (e.g., a fractured bone) that provides rigidity and prevents unwanted movement. 2. v. *See* guarding.

**splint bone** n. the small bones that lie to the sides of a horse's cannon bones just below the carpus or hock.

**splints** n. inflammation and subsequent bone growth of the area around a horse's splint bones, which can be caused by trauma (e.g., overtraining of young animals), poor conformation and overfeeding. Affected animals are often lame during the early stages of the disease, but the pain usually resolves with time. Treatment includes rest and anti-inflammatories.

**spondylitis** n. infection and inflammation of a vertebrae. *See also* diskospondylitis.

**spondylopathy** n. any disease affecting a vertebrae.

**spondylosis** n. an abnormal bony growth off the spinal column that can become large enough to fuse the joints between adjacent vertebrae. Spondylosis is often caused by aging or injury. Some cases may cause pain or neurologic problems if nearby

nerves are affected. Treatment can include anti-inflammatories and pain relievers.

**spongy bone** n. *See* cancellous bone.

**spontaneous** adj. occurring without a known cause.

**sporotrichosis** n. a disease caused by infection with the fungus *Sporothrix schenckii*, which is usually contracted through wounds or contact with animals shedding large numbers of the organism. Individuals develop ulcerated and draining nodules that often occur at the site of a wound and along the nearby lymphatic channels. The infection can sometimes spread to the rest of the body. Antifungal medications can eliminate the infection. Humans are susceptible to sporotrichosis.

**spraddle leg** n. *See* splayleg.

**sprain** n. an injury to a joint that causes ligaments to stretch or rupture and often damages nearby blood vessels, nerves, muscles and tendons. Treatment can include rest, anti-inflammatories and supportive bandages.

**spraying** n. a behavior seen in cats during which they will usually emit a brief stream of urine against a vertical surface while their tail is erect and twitching. Spraying can be a form of territorial marking or a result of anxiety. Treatment includes providing multiple, well-cleaned litter boxes, preventing stressful situations (e.g., separating antagonistic cats) and behavior modifying drugs.

**springhalt** n. *See* stringhalt.

**sputum** n. *See* phlegm.

**squamous cell carcinoma (SCC)** n. a type of cancer arising from tissues that line body surfaces or cavities (e.g., the inner lining of the mouth). Squamous cell carcinomas on the skin commonly affect light colored or sparsely haired areas and are often related to sun exposure. The tumors tend to be locally aggressive and may spread throughout the body. Treatment can include surgical removal, chemotherapy, immunotherapy and radiation therapy.

**stabilize** v. 1. to prevent unwanted movement of an injured body part (e.g., a broken bone). 2. to perform treatments aimed at quickly improving a critically ill or injured animal's condition - **stabilization** n., **stable** adj.

**staging** n. a determination of how widespread or advanced a disease is.

**stain** n. a colored dye used to improve visualization and identification of cells or structures under the microscope.

**stall rest** n. strict restriction of activity by housing an animal in a stall small enough to prevent unwanted movements. Stall rest is often used to prevent damage to a healing injury.

**stallion** n. an uncastrated, male horse four years of age or older.

**standard of care** n. the accepted protocol that should be used to diagnose and treat a disease or injury. Legally, the standard of care is the quality of medical or surgical treatment that is provided by an average, conscientious veterinarian in a particular location.

**staphylectomy** n. the surgical removal of the back of the soft palate.

**staphylococcosis** n. disease caused by infection with *Staphylococcus* bacteria. Some species of *Staphylococcus* are normal residents on the surface of the skin and mucous membranes but can cause disease if the tissue's normal protective barriers are disrupted. Clinical signs depend on where the infection localizes (e.g., skin, joints or mammary glands). Treatment includes antibiotics, but resistance can be a problem.

**star-gazing** n. an abnormal body position in which the neck is twisted so that the animal appears to be staring at the sky. Star-gazing can be a sign of neurologic disease.

**stat** adv. immediately.

**status epilepticus** n. seizure activity that continues for a prolonged period of time without being interrupted by periods of awareness. Status epilepticus can lead to brain damage. Treatment may include anticonvulsant medications, oxygen therapy and procedures to cool the body.

**stay apparatus** n. the combination of muscles, tendons and ligaments that allow horses to lock their legs and remain standing while asleep.

**steatitis** n. inflammation of fat. *See also* yellow fat disease.

**steatorrhea** n. the presence of large amounts of fat in the feces, which causes the stool to be greasy, voluminous and foul smelling. Diseases that adversely affect digestion (e.g., exocrine pancreatic insufficiency) can cause steatorrhea.

**stenosis** n. an abnormally narrowed opening or channel - **stenotic** adj.

**stent** n. a device that can be surgically implanted to keep a hollow structure within the body (e.g., an artery) open.

**step mouth** n. an abnormal condition affecting horses in which one or more teeth are significantly longer or shorter than adjacent teeth. Step mouth can cause difficulty eating and is commonly seen if a tooth has been lost and can no longer wear down the opposing tooth. Treatment can include routine dental floating and diet changes.

**stephanofilariasis** n. *See* filarial dermatitis.

**stereotypy** n. *See* obsessive-compulsive disorder. *Also called* stereotypic behavior.

**sterile** adj. 1. not involving infection or contamination with microorganisms. *Also called* aseptic. 2. unable to produce offspring - **sterilize** v.

**sternal bursitis** n. *See* breast blister.

**sternebra** n. one of the bones that combine to form the sternum - **sternebrae** pl.

**sternum** n. the breast bone - **sternal** adj.

**steroid** n. one of a group of hormones produced by the body or similar compounds manufactured as drugs. Glucocorticoids, mineralocorticoids and sex hormones are all considered steroids.

**steroid-responsive meningitis** n. a disease most often seen in young dogs.

Affected individuals exhibit neck pain and fever and can usually be successfully treated with immunosuppressive drugs. *Also called* aseptic meningitis.

**stertor** n. noisy breathing (e.g., snoring), which can be associated with disorders that partially block the upper respiratory tract - **stertorous** adj.

**stethoscope** n. a device that amplifies sounds produced within the body making them easier to hear and interpret.

**stiff lamb disease** n. *See* white muscle disease.

**stifle** n. the joint in the rear leg between the hip and the hock. *Also called* knee in small animals.

**stillbirth** n. delivery of a mature but dead fetus - **stillborn** adj.

**stocking up** n. swelling of a horse's legs that is usually caused by fluid accumulating in the tissues because of a lack of exercise.

**stoma** n. an opening.

**stomach** n. the sac-like organ that receives ingesta from the esophagus, empties into the small intestine and plays an important role in digestion.

**stomatitis** n. inflammation of the mouth. *See also* vesicular, infectious, ulcerative and lymphocytic-plasmacytic stomatitis.

**stone** n. an abnormal, mineralized object within the body. *Also called* calculus. *See also* bladder stone, kidney stone and cholelithiasis.

**stool** n. *See* feces.

**storage disease** n. any disorder of metabolism that leads to an abnormal accumulation of a substance within the body. *See also* hemochromatosis and glycogen and lysosomal storage disease.

**strabismus** n. a condition in which both eyes are not pointed in the same, correct position (e.g., cross-eyed). Strabismus can be caused by birth defects, trauma or neurologic disease.

**strain** v. 1. to mildly injure a muscle or tendon usually by overuse or overstretching. Treatment can include rest and anti-inflammatories. 2. to use a greater than normal amount of effort.

**strangles** n. a contagious disease of horses caused by infection with the bacteria *Streptococcus equi equi*. Affected individuals often develop a fever, nasal discharge, abscesses around the head and neck and may have difficulty breathing and swallowing. Treatment includes supportive care, cleansing of ruptured abscesses and sometimes antibiotics. Vaccines are effective. *See also* puppy, bastard and false strangles.

**strangulation** n. constriction of a body part (e.g., intestine) by a surrounding structure, which often leads to an impaired blood supply, tissue damage and sometimes death.

**stranguria** n. slow and painful urination.

**straw itch mite** n. *See* forage mite.

**strawberry footrot** n. a disease of sheep caused by infection of the skin of the lower leg with the bacteria *Dermatophilus congolensis*. Infection is promoted by any factor that disrupts the normal, protective characteristics of skin (e.g., standing in wet, muddy conditions for a prolonged period of time). Lesions often consist of a red, raised area of tissue covered in crusts or scabs. Treatment can include improving environmental conditions, antibiotics and medicated shampoos or dips. *Also called* streptothricosis and dermatophilosis.

**streptococcal lymphadenitis** n. *See* cervical lymphadenitis.

**streptococcosis** n. disease caused by infection with *Streptococcus* bacteria. Some species of *Streptococcus* are normal residents on the surface of the skin and mucous membranes but can cause disease if the tissue's normal protective barriers are disrupted or if the animal is stressed. Clinical signs depend on where the infection localizes (e.g., skin, heart or brain). Treatment includes antibiotics, but resistance can be a problem. *See also* strangles and cervical lymphadenitis.

**streptothricosis** n. *See* dermatophilosis.

**stress** n. external or internal influences (e.g., disease, poor nutrition or emotional distress) that change an animal's behavior, anatomy or physiology. Stress can be debilitating when it is prolonged and unrelieved.

**stress leukogram** n. a pattern of changes in the numbers of different types of white blood cells that is seen in animals being treated with corticosteroids, affected by Cushing's disease or that are stressed for any reason.

**striated muscle** n. a muscle the action of which can be consciously controlled (e.g., muscles that flex the leg). *Also called* skeletal or voluntary muscle.

**stricture** n. an abnormal narrowing of a channel, which prevents the normal flow of materials through it. Strictures can be caused by inflammation, scarring or tumors.

**stridor** n. abnormal, high-pitched breathing noises, which are usually heard when an animal breathes in and can be associated with disorders that partially block the upper respiratory tract.

**stringhalt** n. a disorder of horses that causes affected individuals to spasmodically flex one or both hind legs. Some severe and progressive cases may be associated with exposure to toxins present in some plants, but most have no known cause. Treatment can include eliminating access to the toxic plants, surgery and medications that reduce the unwanted muscular contractions. *Also called* springhalt.

**strip** v. 1. to apply pressure with the fingers along a channel and move or extract the fluid (e.g., milk) contained within the structure. 2. to pull dead hair out of an animal's coat, often by using a special comb. 3. to surgically peel unwanted tissues from body structures.

**stroke** n. impairment of blood flow through blood vessels in the brain leading to destruction of brain tissue. Some return of normal function can be seen with time and rehabilitation. *Also called* cerebrovascular accident.

**stromal lipid keratopathy** n. the abnormal deposition of fats within the cornea, which can be caused by abnormal fat metabolism or disorders of the cornea. Affected animals develop white areas within the cornea. Treatment can include addressing any underlying diseases and medications that help extract fat from the cornea or decrease the local immune response.

**strongyle** n. a type of intestinal parasite. *See also* large and small strongyle.

**struvite urolith** n. a type of stone that can form within and disrupt the function of the urinary tract. Struvite uroliths often develop in association with infection or because of alkaline urine. Treatment can include antibiotics, diets or medications that acidify the urine and surgery to remove the stones. Urinary acidifiers can help prevent the return of the stones. *Also called* magnesium ammonium phosphate and triple phosphate uroliths.

**strychnine poisoning** n. disease caused by ingestion of strychnine, which may be used as a pesticide. Affected animals can develop abnormal behavior, stiffness, rigid extension of the legs, seizures, high body temperatures and may die quickly. Treatment options include procedures to reduce absorption of strychnine from the gastrointestinal tract, anticonvulsant medications, muscle relaxants and fluid and oxygen therapy.

**stump pyometra** n. infection within a part of the uterus that was not removed during an ovariohysterectomy. The development of a stump pyometra usually also requires the presence of some ovarian tissue remaining in the abdomen. Treatment includes the surgical removal of the uterine stump and any remaining ovarian tissue.

**stupor** n. profound lethargy and decreased responsiveness that verges on unconsciousness - **stuporous** adj.

**styptic** adj. describes a material that chemically induces the formation of a blood clot.

**subacute** adj. describes a condition in which symptoms develop somewhat quickly, usually over the course of a week or so. *Compare* acute and chronic.

**subacute ruminal acidosis** n. a disease of ruminants chronically fed diets high in grain and low in fiber, which intermittently causes a low pH that damages the lining of the rumen. Individuals can develop loss of appetite, poor weight gain and milk production, diarrhea, laminitis, infections throughout the body and may die. Correcting the diet can be curative if the animal is not too severely affected.

**subaortic stenosis** n. a narrowing of the area just below the valve between the left ventricle of the heart and the aorta. *See* aortic stenosis.

**subchondral** adj. underneath cartilage.

**subclinical** adj. not producing observable symptoms.

**subcutaneous (SQ)** adj. underneath the skin.

**subcutis** n. the tissues that lie just under the skin.

**subinvolution of placental sites (SIPS)** n. failure of the areas in a bitch's uterus where the placentas were attached to break down normally in the weeks after birth. The disorder causes bleeding from the vulva that continues for an abnormally long period of time (e.g., over a month). Treatment can include spaying or close monitoring of the dog's condition until its next heat cycle, at which time the bleeding disappears and usually does not return.

**subluxation** n. a partial dislocation of a joint.

**submandibular** adj. underneath the lower jaw.

**submissive urination** n. a normal behavior of dogs attempting to communicate that they are not a threat and that people or other animals are dominant. Individuals will squat, dribble urine and often roll over. Most puppies outgrow submissive urination, but scolding or punishing can delay its resolution and make the behavior worse. Limiting the excitement that often accompanies bouts of urination (e.g., when family members arrive home) can be helpful. Any activity that boosts the animal's self confidence such as positive reinforcement during basic obedience training can also decrease submissive urination.

**subpalpebral lavage system** n. a device consisting of a flexible, hollow tube that can be surgically inserted through the eyelid allowing medications to be easily and frequently applied to the surface of the eye.

**subsolar** adj. underneath the sole.

**subunit vaccine** n. a type of vaccine that contains only portions of a disease-causing virus or bacteria rather the whole organism.

**suckle reflex** n. the normal, involuntary reaction of an unweaned animal to suck on a warm, soft object that is placed within its mouth.

**suction** n. the use of a device that produces negative pressure to remove fluid, gas or other substances from within the body.

**sudden acquired retinal degeneration syndrome (SARDS)** n. a disease of dogs causing blindness that develops very quickly, sometimes within a single day. Some cases have been associated with other disorders (e.g., Cushing's disease), but the cause of SARDS is not known and there is no effective treatment.

**sulcus** n. a groove.

**sulfonamide** n. a type of medicine that is most commonly used to treat some types of bacterial or protozoal infections. Sulfadimethoxine is a commonly used sulfonamide. *Also called* sulfa drug.

**summer itch** n. See *Culicoides* hypersensitivity. *Also called* summer eczema and summer dermatitis.

**summer pasture associated pulmonary disease** n. a disease of horses caused by an allergic reaction to substances (e.g., pollen and mold) associated with pastures. *See also* recurrent airway obstruction.

**summer slump** n. a disease of cattle that is seen during warm weather and is caused by ingestion of fescue grass or hay infected with a fungus. Affected animals can seek cool areas, retain their winter coats and develop poor appetites, reproductive problems and decreased weight gain and milk pro-

duction. Preventing access to infected grass or hay can reverse the disease. *See also* fescue toxicosis.

**summer sores** n. See habronemiasis.

**superficial** adj. located towards the surface of the body or other structure. *Compare* deep.

**superficial necrolytic dermatitis** n. See hepatocutaneous syndrome.

**superior** adj. above. *Compare* inferior.

**supernumerary** adj. more than the normal number, extra.

**supportive care** n. any type of attention that is needed to keep an animal's condition stable and comfortable until it has recovered from illness or injury. Supportive care can include provision of food and water, keeping an animal warm, clean and dry, providing opportunities to urinate and defecate and turning or moving animals that cannot do so themselves.

**suppurative** adj. producing pus.

**suprascapular paralysis** n. See sweeny.

**surfactant** n. a substance that helps prevent the air-filled sacs (i.e., alveoli) within the lungs from collapsing. A premature birth can occur before the fetal lungs have produced adequate amounts of surfactant to allow normal breathing.

**surgery** n. operations and manipulations used to diagnose, treat and prevent disease - **surgical** adj.

**surgical scrub** n. a thorough cleansing of the skin that will surround a surgical incision or of the hands of people involved in surgery.

**susceptible** adj. capable of becoming infected or otherwise lacking resistance to a particular condition.

**suspension** n. a combination of a liquid and an undissolved solid, which usually requires shaking to be uniformly mixed.

**suspensory apparatus** n. ligaments and small bones in a horse's lower legs that help support the back of the fetlock joint.

**suture** n. 1. thread-like material that can be used to bring tissues in close contact with one another to encourage rapid healing. 2. the area where sections of a structure (e.g., the bones of the skull) join each other.

**swamp fever** n. *See* equine infectious anemia.

**swayback** n. 1. a concave curve to the back, most frequently seen in older horses. *Compare* roach back. 2. a disorder of young animals caused by a lack of adequate amounts of copper in the diet of their mothers during pregnancy. Affected individuals can exhibit depression, diarrhea, blindness, deafness, tremors, trouble walking and paralysis. Copper supplementation can help improve the condition of animals that are not too severely affected. *See also* enzootic ataxia.

**sweeny** n. a condition characterized by a loss of muscle mass in the shoulder and a swinging of the leg to the side while in motion. The shoulder joint may appear to slip outward during weight-bearing. Causes include injury to the suprascapular nerve or any prolonged disorder that prevents

normal use of the leg. Treatment can involve rest to allow damaged nerves to heal, addressing any underlying problems and physical therapy. *Also called* suprascapular paralysis and slipped shoulder.

**sweet clover poisoning** n. *See* dicumarol poisoning.

**sweet itch** n. *See Culicoides* hypersensitivity.

**swelling** n. an enlargement of a body part that is caused by an abnormal accumulation of fluid within the tissues.

**swimmer puppy** n. a developmental abnormality of young puppies that may be caused by genetics or rapid weight gain. Affected individuals have a flattened chest and are splay-legged. Physical therapy can help many individuals regain normal orientation and use of their legs. *Also called* flat puppy syndrome.

**symblepharon** n. the condition of having one or more eyelids that are stuck to the surface of the eye.

**symmetric** adj. describes the situation in which opposite sides of a structure appear similar to each other. *Also called* symmetrical.

**sympathetic nervous system** n. part of the autonomic nervous system that acts to increase the heart rate and dilate the pupils. *Compare* parasympathetic nervous system.

**sympatholytic** adj. decreasing the activity of the sympathetic nervous system (e.g., slowing the heart rate and lowering blood pressure).

**sympathomimetic** adj. increasing the activity of the sympathetic nervous system (e.g., increasing the heart rate and raising blood pressure).

**symphysis** n. a connection that joins the right and left halves of certain structures (e.g., the mandible and pelvis).

**symptom** n. *See* clinical sign.

**symptomatic** adj. indicative of or displaying clinical signs associated with a particular disease.

**symptomatic care** n. treatment aimed not at the underlying disease but at specific clinical signs that result.

**synapse** n. the gap that lies between two nerves or between a nerve and muscle or other target tissue. Neurotransmitters carry signals across the synapse.

**synchronous diaphragmatic flutter** n. an abnormal movement of the diaphragm occurring with each heart beat that can be associated with electrolyte disturbances.

**syncope** n. a loss of consciousness that lasts for only a short period of time (i.e., fainting) and usually occurs because of a lack of adequate oxygen delivery to the brain.

**syndactyly** n. an abnormal fusion between digits.

**syndrome** n. a set of clinical signs that occur together and are recognizably associated with a particular condition.

**synechia** n. an adhesion between two normally separate structures.

**synergism** n. the combined actions of two substances (e.g., medicines) that is greater than the sum of their effects - **synergistic** adj.

**synovial cell sarcoma** n. a type of aggressive cancer affecting the bones and other tissues around a joint. Individuals develop lameness and a firm, painful swelling in the affected area. Limb amputation can extend and improve quality of life.

**synovial fluid** n. *See* joint fluid.

**synovial membrane** n. a thin layer of tissue that covers the inner surfaces of freely moveable joints and secretes joint fluid.

**synovitis** n. inflammation of a synovial membrane, which may be caused by trauma, infection or autoimmune disease.

**syphilis** n. *See* treponematosis.

**syringe** n. a device usually consisting of a barrel and plunger that can be used to inject or withdraw liquids.

**syringomyelia** n. an abnormal accumulation of cerebrospinal fluid within cavities in the spinal cord that can be caused by trauma, tumors, inflammation or birth defects. Affected individuals may have difficulty walking, weakness and pain. Treatment can include corticosteroids, surgery and addressing any underlying causes.

**systemic** adj. pertaining to the entire body, not just an isolated location. For example, systemic medications are usually given orally or by injection so that they can be absorbed into the bloodstream and carried throughout the body.

**systemic lupus erythematosus (SLE)** n. an autoimmune disease that is caused by an abnormal tendency to manufacture antibodies against cell nuclei and to produce immune complexes. Affected individuals can develop lameness, skin and oral lesions, kidney disease, bizarre behavior and other disorders. Treatment includes medications that suppress the immune system. *Compare* discoid lupus erythematosus.

**systole** n. the period of time during which the heart is contracted and pushing blood throughout the body - **systolic** adj. *Compare* diastole.

# T

**T cell** n. a type of lymphocyte (i.e., white blood cell) that is important to the normal functioning of the immune system. *Compare* B cell.

**t wave** n. a peak or trough recorded on an electrocardiogram that can change shape and size with different disorders affecting the heart.

**T₃** n. *See* triiodothyronine.

**T₃ and T₄ autoantibody test** n. a blood test that can provide useful information when a diagnosis of hypothyroidism is proving difficult.

**T₃ suppression test** n. a laboratory test measuring thyroxine levels ($T_4$) after administration of triiodothyronine ($T_3$), which can be used to help diagnose hyperthyroidism when other, more commonly used tests are inconclusive.

**T₄** n. *See* thyroxine.

**tachyarrhythmia** n. an irregular and rapid heart rhythm. *Compare* bradyarrhythmia.

**tachycardia** n. an abnormally rapid heart rate. *Compare* bradycardia.

**tachypnea** n. abnormally rapid breathing. *Compare* bradypnea.

**tack** n. saddles, bridles, halters and other equipment used in the riding, driving or handling of horses.

**tail jack** n. a technique used to prevent cattle from kicking in which the top part of the tail is grabbed and pushed firmly upwards.

**tail slip** n. a condition that can occur when a gerbil is picked up or restrained by its tail causing the skin to be pulled away from deeper structures. Tail amputation is usually necessary after tail slip has occurred.

**tamponade** n. *See* cardiac tamponade.

**tap** n. *See* centesis.

**tapetum** n. a layer of tissue that covers a structure, often referring to the membrane at the back of the eye that can reflect light - **tapetal** adj.

**tapeworm** n. a type of gastrointestinal parasite, the segments of which can sometimes be seen around the anus of infested animals. Mild tapeworm infections generally do not have a significant adverse effect on health. Animals are infected through the ingestion of insects (e.g., fleas) or tissues containing immature tapeworms. Specific types of dewormers can kill the parasites.

**tarsorrhaphy** n. a surgical procedure in which the upper and lower eyelids are sutured together. A tarsorrhaphy is often performed to protect a damaged cornea as it heals.

**tarsus** n. 1. the angular joint in the hind leg located below the tibia. *Also called* hock. 2. a piece of cartilage that supports the eyelids - **tarsal** adj.

**tartar** n. a mineralized substance that can form on teeth and promote the development of periodontal disease and other dental disorders. Physical removal of the tartar from all surfaces of the tooth is an essential part of a dental cleaning. *Also called* dental calculus.

**taurine** n. a type of amino acid. Inadequate levels of taurine in the diet can cause dilated cardiomyopathy, retinal damage and loss of vision, particularly in cats.

**tease** v. to determine if an animal is ready to breed by watching its reaction to an individual of the opposite sex.

**teat** n. a nipple.

**teat dipping** n. a liquid that can be applied to the teats of a cow or other animal producing milk to help prevent mastitis.

**Teflon® toxicosis** n. *See* polytetrafluoroethylene poisoning.

**temperature** n. a measurement of heat, such as that produced by an animal's metabolism. Normal body temperatures for a variety of species are listed in the appendices. *See also* fever.

**tendinitis** n. inflammation of a ten-

don, which is often a result of a traumatic injury. Treatment may include rest, anti-inflammatories and a gradual return to exercise.

**tendon** n. a band or sheet of fibrous connective tissue that connects muscles to bones or other structures.

**tenectomy** n. the surgical removal of a section of a tendon.

**tenesmus** n. straining to urinate or defecate.

**tenosynovitis** n. inflammation of a tendon and its surrounding sheath, which can be caused by trauma, overuse or infection. Treatment may include rest, anti-inflammatories and if infection is involved, antibiotics and surgical procedures to flush the sheath.

**tenotomy** n. a surgical incision through a tendon.

**Tensilon® test** n. a procedure used to help diagnose myasthenia gravis, which involves monitoring for improvement in muscle function after a patient is injected with the drug Tensilon®. *Also called* edrophonium test.

**tension** n. the condition of being tight or stretched. Tension on a wound can hinder healing but is sometimes unavoidable depending on the type of surgery performed or the location of an injury or incision.

**tension pneumothorax** n. a disorder that can be caused by a penetrating wound to parts of the respiratory tract allowing air to leak into the space around the lungs but not to escape back out. Affected individuals develop difficulty breathing and can die rapidly. Treatment includes procedures to remove the air from around the lungs and addressing any underlying conditions.

**teratogenic** adj. capable of causing birth defects.

**teratoma** n. a tumor that arises from abnormal development of epithelial tissues. The mass often contains hair, sweat glands and other structures normally located in the skin. Teratomas can be found in the ovaries, testicles, skin or eyes. Surgical removal is usually curative. *Also called* dermoid cyst.

**territorial aggression** n. inappropriate attacks or related behaviors (e.g., growling, hissing or snapping) that are initiated by an animal attempting to prevent people or other animals from entering a particular area. Treatment can include avoidance of situations that incite aggression and behavior modifying protocols and drugs.

**testicle** n. one of the paired male organs that produce sperm and testosterone - **testicular** adj. *Also called* testis.

**testosterone** n. a hormone produced by the testicles and to a lesser extent the adrenal glands. Testosterone stimulates the development of male characteristics, behaviors and reproductive organs.

**tetanus** n. a disease caused by toxins produced by *Clostridium tetani* bacteria, which often infect animals through wounds. Affected individuals can develop progressive stiffness, abnormal behavior, muscle spasms, sweating, rapid breathing and may die. Treatment can include administration of tetanus toxoid or antitoxin,

antibiotics, cleansing and debridement of infected tissues, sedatives and supportive care. Preventative vaccines are available.

**tetany** n. an abnormal, prolonged period of continuous muscular contraction and rigidity.

**tetralogy of Fallot** n. a birth defect in which parts of the heart and associated large blood vessels developed abnormally. Affected individuals can grow slowly, be unable to exercise normally, develop a blue color to their skin and mucous membranes, collapse and have seizures. Treatment is difficult but can include medications that improve heart function, repeated blood withdrawals and surgery.

**tetraparesis** n. *See* quadriparesis.

**tetraplegia** n. *See* quadriplegia.

**thecal cell tumor** n. *See* granulosa-theca cell tumor.

**Theiler's disease** n. a disease seen in some horses after receiving tetanus antitoxin or other injections. Some affected individuals have no history of such an injection. In either case, the animals stop eating, become jaundiced and develop bizarre behavior because of liver damage. Supportive treatment allowing time for the liver to recover can be successful. *Also called* acute hepatic atrophy, idiopathic acute hepatic disease, serum hepatitis and postvaccinal hepatitis.

**thelaziasis** n. *See* eyeworm.

**therapy** n. the treatment of disease - **therapeutic** adj.

**theriogenology** n. the science and study of animal reproduction.

**thermography** n. a diagnostic procedure that creates an image based on the amount of heat lost from body surfaces. Thermography can be used to help identify areas of inflammation.

**thermometer** n. a device that measures the temperature of its surroundings.

**thermoregulation** n. the ability of an animal to control its body temperature within a normal range.

**thiamine** n. a type of vitamin B. A lack of adequate amounts of thiamine in the diet can lead to difficulty walking, bizarre behavior, seizures and other neurological abnormalities. *See also* bracken fern poisoning and cerebrocortical necrosis.

**third degree burn** n. a severe burn that damages the skin and underlying tissues. *Compare* first and second degree burns.

**third eyelid** n. a structure that is located at the inside corner of the eye and can be raised to cover and protect the cornea. *Also called* nictitating membrane.

**third eyelid flap** n. a surgical procedure in which the third eyelid is sutured in a position covering the surface of the eye. A third eyelid flap is usually performed to protect a damaged cornea as it heals.

**third eyelid gland prolapse** n. *See* cherry eye.

**thoracic limb** n. a front leg or arm.

**thoracocentesis** n. insertion of a hollow needle through the body wall and into the chest cavity. Thoracocentesis is usually performed to remove an abnormal accumulation of air or fluid,

a sample of which may be submitted for analysis. *Also called* chest tap.

**thoracolumbar** adj. pertaining to the part of the spine and surrounding tissues that lie over the rib cage and abdomen.

**thoracostomy tube** n. *See* chest tube.

**thoracotomy** n. a surgical incision through the chest wall.

**thorax** n. the chest - **thoracic** adj.

**thoroughpin** n. a swelling located on the inside and outside of a rear leg just above the back of a horse's hock. Thoroughpin is caused by fluid accumulating within a tendon sheath but usually does not cause any lameness. If treatment is desired, withdrawal of the fluid, injection of anti-inflammatories into the tendon sheath and radiation therapy can be helpful.

**thrill** n. a palpable vibration caused by the movement of a fluid. For example, a thrill can sometimes be felt by touching the chest of an animal with a severe heart murmur.

**thrombin time (TT)** n. a test that measures the clotting ability of blood. A prolonged thrombin time indicates abnormalities affecting particular coagulation factors.

**thrombocyte** n. a cell that helps the blood to clot. *Also called* platelet.

**thrombocytopathy** n. any disorder that decreases platelet function but not platelet numbers. *Also called* thrombopathia.

**thrombocytopenia** n. a lower than normal number of platelets in circulation, which can lead to abnormal bleeding and bruising.

**thrombocytosis** n. a higher than normal number of platelets in circulation. Many cases of mild thrombocytosis have an unknown cause and are not clinically significant.

**thromboembolism** n. a blood clot that develops at one location and then breaks loose to travel to another part of the circulatory system where it becomes lodged and can disrupt blood flow.

**thrombopathia** n. *See* thrombocytopathy.

**thrombophlebitis** n. inflammation of a vein that is associated with a blood clot. Thrombophlebitis can develop with the prolonged use of intravenous catheters.

**thrombosis** n. the development of an abnormal blood clot (i.e., thrombus) within the circulatory system.

**thrombus** n. a blood clot that develops at a particular location within the circulatory system and disrupts blood flow. *Compare* embolus.

**thrush** n. 1. a fungal infection affecting parts of the digestive tract (e.g., the mouth and crop). *See also* candidiasis. 2. a disease of a horse's foot often caused by standing in wet, unsanitary conditions and the development of secondary infections. Individuals have frogs that are moist and have a dark and foul smelling discharge. Portions of the infected tissue may die and fall off. Treatment includes improved environmental conditions, removal of diseased tissues, repeated cleaning of the hooves and application of antiseptic solutions.

**thumb forceps** n. a surgical instrument that looks like a pair of tweezers and is used to grasp tissues or other objects.

**thymus** n. an organ located in the neck or chest that plays an important role in the developing immune system of young animals. The thymus shrinks once the individual reaches maturity.

**thyroglobulin autoantibody test** n. a blood test that can be used to help diagnose dogs with thyroiditis.

**thyroid gland** n. a gland located in the neck that produces hormones essential for normal growth and metabolism.

**thyroid hormone** n. the hormones thyroxine and triiodothyronine that are produced by the thryoid gland. Synthetic thyroid hormone (e.g., levothyroxine) is used in the treatment of hypothyroidism.

**thyroid-stimulating hormone (TSH)** n. *See* thyrotropin.

**thyroidectomy** n. the surgical removal of the thyroid gland.

**thyroiditis** n. a disease in which the immune system inappropriately attacks the thryoid gland causing scarring and reducing its ability to secrete thyroid hormone. Many individuals with thyroiditis will eventually develop hypothyroidism.

**thyrotoxicosis** n. *See* hyperthyroidism.

**thyrotropin** n. a hormone produced by the pituitary gland that stimulates the thyroid gland to produce thyroxine. *Also called* thyroid-stimulating hormone.

**thyroxine (T$_4$)** n. the form of thyroid hormone that is released from the thyroid gland and converted into the more active triiodothyronine in the body's tissues.

**tibia** n. the larger bone located in the lower leg between the stifle and hock.

**tibial nerve paralysis** n. a loss of function of the tibial nerve that is in the hind leg and can be damaged by a traumatic injury. Individuals have an overly flexed hock and are unable to completely extend the foot of the affected leg. Treatment includes rest and anti-inflammatories.

**tibial plateau leveling osteotomy (TPLO)** n. a surgery used to treat lameness caused by a cranial cruciate ligament rupture. The procedure involves cutting and rotating the top portion of the tibia to realign forces within the stifle, which lessens the need for a functional cranial cruciate ligament.

**tick** n. a blood-sucking insect that can attach to the skin. Tick bites often cause itching and may transmit disease.

**tick paralysis** n. a condition resulting from exposure to a toxin present in the saliva of some ticks. After being bitten, affected animals can become weak, unable to move and may die if the muscles responsible for breathing are involved. Treatment includes supportive care and tick removal.

**tick titer** n. the concentrations of antibodies against Rocky Mountain spotted fever, ehrlichiosis and Lyme disease within a blood sample. High titers can indicate current or past infection or vaccination (Lyme).

**tie** n. the period of time in a mating between a dog and bitch during which the penis is tightly held within the vagina, and the animals often stand rump to rump. The forced separation of individuals that have tied can lead to injury.

**tissue** n. an organized group of cells that together perform specialized functions.

**titer** n. the concentration of a substance within the blood. For example, a titer can be determined for antibodies against a particular disease, which can provide evidence of current or past infection or protection provided by a vaccine.

**toad poisoning** n. a disease caused by ingestion of substances secreted by the skin of toads. Affected individuals can develop profuse salivation, oral irritation, vomiting and sometimes abnormal heart rhythms and seizures, which can lead to death. Treatment may include flushing out the mouth, oxygen therapy and medications to limit drooling, normalize heart rhythms and stop seizures.

**tocopherol** n. substances that have properties similar to vitamin E.

**toe crack** n. a vertical fissure affecting the front of a horse's hoof. *See also* sand crack and grass crack.

**toe ulcer** n. a condition of cattle that is frequently associated with laminitis. A hole develops at the white line of a toe and may bleed. *See also* laminitis.

**toed-in** adj. a conformational flaw in which the feet are rotated inward.

**toed-out** adj. a conformational flaw in which the feet are rotated outward.

**tolerance** n. the ability to withstand exposure to a substance without it having a significant effect. For example, repeated administration of some types of drugs to an animal leads to tolerance and a decrease in the medicine's effectiveness.

**tone** n. the tension or firmness within the tissues of a muscle or organ.

**tonic-clonic seizure** n. *See* clonic-tonic seizure.

**tonometer** n. an instrument that measures pressure within the eye and is often used to test for glaucoma.

**tonsil** n. a small mass of tissue that is a part of the immune system, usually referring to structures located at the back of the throat.

**tonsillectomy** n. the surgical removal of a tonsil.

**tonsillitis** n. inflammation of a tonsil, which can be associated with infection.

**topical** adj. pertaining to the surface of the body or another structure.

**torpor** n. lethargy and decreased responsiveness - **torpid** adj.

**torsion** n. an abnormal twisting of a structure. Torsion of an organ (e.g., intestine, spleen or testicle) can hinder its blood supply and quickly lead to extreme pain and tissue death. Surgery is often necessary to untwist the structure and remove any irreversibly damaged tissues.

**torso** n. the body excluding the head, limbs, and tail.

**torticollis** n. an abnormal twisting of the head and neck, which can be caused by birth defects, trauma and neurologic and muscular disorders. *Also called* wryneck.

**total ear canal ablation** n. a surgery that removes the entire ear canal. A total ear canal ablation is often used to treat chronic disorders (e.g., infections) that have not responded adequately to medical treatment. The tympanic bulla should also be opened to allow removal of diseased or damaged tissues, cleansing and drainage. *Compare* lateral ear canal resection.

**total hip replacement** n. a surgical procedure most frequently used to treat dogs with osteoarthritis of one or both hips that does not respond adequately to medical therapies. The ball and socket of the hip joint are removed and replaced with devices made out of plastic and metal.

**total protein (TP)** n. *See* plasma protein.

**total solids (TS)** n. a laboratory measurement that correlates with the concentration of protein in a sample of plasma.

**touch prep** n. *See* impression smear.

**tourniquet** n. a device that can be temporarily tightened around a part of the body to limit bleeding or improve access to a vein.

**towel clamp** n. an instrument used to attach sterile draping to an animal around the site where surgery is to be performed.

**toxemia** n. a disease caused by toxins that are produced by abnormal metabolism or bacteria and released into the bloodstream. *See also* pregnancy toxemia and endotoxemia.

**toxic epidermal necrolysis** n. a disease often associated with an adverse drug reaction that can lead to skin lesions (e.g., red, raised areas and ulcers), fever and depression. Treatment includes stopping the administration of any potentially responsible drugs, supportive care and sometimes corticosteroids.

**toxicoinfectious botulism** n. a disease caused by absorption of a toxin produced by *Clostridium botulinum* bacteria infecting the tissues of an animal. Affected individuals exhibit progressive weakness and paralysis. Treatment can include antitoxin and antibiotic administration and supportive care. *Also called* shaker foal syndrome.

**toxicology** n. the science and study of poisons and the diseases that they cause.

**toxicosis** n. a disease that is caused by a poisonous substance.

**toxin** n. a poisonous substance - **toxic** adj. *Also called* toxicant.

**toxoid** n. a weakened form of a toxin injected into an animal to induce the formation of antibodies that can protect against the development of a specific disease (e.g., tetanus).

**toxoplasmosis** n. a disease caused by infection with the protozoal parasite *Toxoplasma gondii*, which is contracted through ingestion of tissues or cat feces containing the organism. Fetuses can be infected while still in the uterus. Many affected animals do not demonstrate clinical signs, but some individuals (e.g., the young or immunosuppressed) may become ill and die. Symptoms depend on where the infection localizes, but can include eye abnormalities, diarrhea, fever, difficulty breathing, jaundice, neurologic abnormalities and abortions. Treatment includes medications that kill the parasite and supportive care. Humans can contract toxoplasmosis.

**trabecular bone** n. *See* cancellous bone.

**trachea** n. the tube connecting and carrying air between the mouth or nose and the lungs.

**tracheal collapse** n. a condition primarily affecting small breed dogs in which the muscular portion of the trachea weakens, sags and narrows the passageway through which air can flow. Affected individuals develop a repetitive, dry cough with a characteristic, honking sound and may have difficulty breathing. Treatment can include bronchodilators, anti-inflammatories, antibiotics for secondary infections, cough suppressants and weight loss.

**tracheal edema syndrome** n. a condition affecting cattle that may be associated with hot weather, infections, trauma to the trachea or allergies. Affected animals develop difficulty breathing that worsens with exercise and may die quickly. Treatment can include antibiotics, anti-inflammatories and a tracheostomy.

**tracheal lavage** n. *See* transtracheal wash.

**tracheal stenosis** n. an abnormal narrowing of the trachea, which can be a congenital abnormality (e.g., brachycephalic syndrome) or a result of injury.

**tracheal wash** n. *See* transtracheal wash.

**tracheitis** n. inflammation of the trachea, which often leads to coughing and in severe cases, difficulty breathing.

**tracheobronchitis** n. inflammation of the trachea and the passageways for air within the lungs. *See also* kennel cough.

**tracheobronchoscopy** n. the use of a tubular instrument including a light source and a viewing device that is placed into the trachea and bronchi allowing the veterinarian to see abnormalities, remove foreign objects and take samples of tissue or fluid for analysis.

**tracheostomy** n. the surgical creation of a hole into the trachea through which a tube can be placed and secured to assist breathing.

**tracheotomy** n. a surgical incision into the trachea.

**trade name** n. the name given to a drug or product by a particular manufacturer. For example, Enacard® is a trade name for the generic drug enalapril.

**tranquilizer** n. a type of medication usually given to calm an anxious animal.

**transdermal** adj. through the skin.

**transect** v. to sever a structure across its width.

**transfaunation** n. the transfer of ingesta containing beneficial microorganisms from the gastrointestinal tract of one ruminant to another.

**transfusion** n. the infusion of blood or blood components (e.g., plasma) into the circulatory system. Transfusions are usually performed to replace cells or proteins that have been lost in a critically ill patient. *See also* transfusion reaction.

**transfusion reaction** n. an adverse response by the recipient of a transfusion to the donor blood. Giving blood of a different type to an animal, particularly if prior transfusions have occurred, can result in the individual's immune system attacking the foreign cells and proteins. Transfusion reactions may range from mild and reversible (e.g., fever and hives) to potentially fatal. Treatment includes stopping or slowing the transfusion, medications that decrease the immune response and supportive care.

**transient** adj. present for only a short period of time.

**transillumination** n. shining a very bright light through a part of the body to allow visualization of internal structures.

**transit time** n. the length of time required for ingested material to pass through the gastrointestinal tract. Increases and decreases in transit time can be seen with a variety of digestive disorders.

**transitional cell carcinoma** n. an aggressive cancer that most commonly affects the bladder of dogs. Individuals usually have difficulty urinating and blood in the urine. Treatment can include surgery, chemotherapy and radiation therapy to improve quality of life and survival times.

**transitional vertebra** n. an atypical vertebra with physical characteristics of nearby parts of the spine that is caused by abnormal fetal development. For example, the last lumbar vertebrae may resemble the sacrum. Most individuals have no problems associated with transitional vertebrae, though some may develop arthritis or compression of the spinal cord and require anti-inflammatories, pain relievers or surgery.

**transmissible** adj. *See* contagious.

**transmissible serositis** n. a disease of sheep, goats, calves and pigs caused by infection of their joints with *Chlamydophila psittaci*. The bacteria can also infect the gastrointestinal tract where it may or may not cause diarrhea, but it is thought that this is the source for infections within the herd. Affected animals often have a fever, swollen and painful joints, are reluctant to move and eat and may have eye infections or other disorders. Early treatment with antibiotics can be successful. *Also called* polyarthritis-serositis.

**transmissible spongiform encephalopathy** n. a type of disease thought to be caused by a prion, abnormally folded, infectious proteins. *See also* bovine spongiform encephalopathy, chronic wasting disease and scrapie.

**transmissible venereal tumor (TVT)** n. a cancer of dogs that can be spread from one individual to another through mating or other types of contact with the tumors. Affected individuals develop masses that often ulcerate and bleed around their penis or vulva and sometime around the nose, mouth and eyes. Some tumors may disappear without treatment, but most individuals require surgery, chemotherapy and/or radiation therapy to be cured.

**transplacental** adj. across the placenta.

**transplant** n. the transfer of tissues from one part of the body to another or from one animal to another. Transplants are often performed to replace an organ or tissue that is diseased or injured to the point where it no longer functions adequately for the survival or well-being of the animal. If the transplanted material comes from a different individual, rejection is possible and must be prevented with immunosuppressive drugs. *Also called* graft.

**transport tetany** n. a disorder seen after large animals have been transported for a prolonged period of time. Pregnancy, hot temperatures, stress and lack of access to food and water seem to play a role. Affected individuals can develop bizarre behavior and become stiff, unable to stand and comatose. Treatment may include supportive care and infusions of fluid, calcium, magnesium and glucose, but many animals die even with appropriate therapy.

**transtracheal wash (TTW)** n. a procedure used to take samples of mucus and cells from within the trachea. A catheter is inserted through the skin and into the trachea and a small amount of fluid is injected and subsequently withdrawn. The material is then analyzed to help determine the cause of a respiratory disorder. *Also called* transtracheal aspirate and tracheal lavage.

**transudate** n. a liquid that has leaked from blood vessels and does not contain many white blood cells or a lot of protein. Transudates can be associated with low blood albumin levels and heart or liver disease. *Compare* exudate.

**transverse** adj. at a right angle to the long axis of a structure. *Compare* longitudinal.

**trauma** n. damage to body tissues that is caused by forces originating from outside of the body - **traumatic** adj.

**traumatic gastritis** n. *See* hardware disease.

**traumatic reticuloperitonitis** n. *See* hardware disease.

**tremor** n. repeated, involuntary and rapid alternation between contraction and relaxation of a muscle. Tremors are seen with some types of neurologic diseases, poisonings and other disorders.

**tremorgenic mycotoxin** n. a type of chemical that is produced by fungal organisms usually found in spoiled food. Tremorgenic mycotoxins can cause excitement, muscle tremors, difficulty walking and seizures when ingested. Treatment includes medications and procedures that limit absorption of the toxin from the digestive tract and symptomatic and supportive care.

**trench mouth** n. *See* necrotizing ulcerative gingivostomatitis.

**trephination** n. a surgical procedure in which a circular section of tissue is removed with a round cutting instrument. Trephination of the skull can be performed to gain access to underlying structures.

**treponematosis** n. a disease of rabbits that is caused by *Treponema cuniculi* bacteria, which are transmitted through sexual contact. Affected animals develop lesions around the genitalia and sometimes the mouth, nose and eyes. Treatment with antibiotics is very successful. *Also called* syphilis, spirochetosis and vent disease.

**triage** n. a system of classifying individuals within a group of sick or injured animals so those that can most benefit from immediate treatment are given attention first.

**triceps** n. a muscle having three heads, usually referring to a muscle in the front limb that helps extend the elbow joint.

**trichobezoar** n. a mass of hair within the gastrointestinal tract that may cause vomiting and loss of appetite and weight. Treatment can include medications that lubricate and encourage the evacuation of hair, fluid therapy and surgery. *Also called* hairball.

**trichoepithelioma** n. a benign tumor arising from hair follicles. Individuals develop masses in or under their skin that can rupture and release a thick material. Surgical removal is usually curative, but new trichoepitheliomas will often arise at additional sites.

**trichomoniasis** n. a disease caused by trichomonad protozoal parasites. *Tritrichomonas foetus* in cattle causes females to be unable to maintain pregnancies. The disease is transmitted from an infected bull to cows through breeding. Treatment is difficult, but the disease can be eradicated from a herd by eliminating the infected bulls. *See also* frounce (birds).

**tricuspid valve** n. the heart valve separating the right atrium and right ventricle.

**tricuspid valve dysplasia** n. a birth defect in which the heart's tricuspid valve did not form normally. Affected individuals can have a murmur, arrhythmias, difficulty breathing, abnormal fluid accumulations and may die. No specific treatment for the underlying condition exists, but medications and other treatments that improve heart function and control fluid accumulation can be helpful.

**trigeminal nerve** n. a cranial nerve that carries sensory impulses from around the face and innervates muscles that are used during chewing.

**trigeminal neuritis** n. a disease with an unknown cause in which the trigeminal nerve stops functioning. Affected individuals cannot close their mouths, have trouble eating and drinking and may develop Horner's syndrome. Most animals recover in 3-4 weeks with supportive care.

**triglyceride** n. a compound containing fat the levels of which are often measured in the blood. *See also* lipidemia.

**trigone** n. a triangular area, often referring to the part of the bladder that surrounds the openings for the ureters and urethra.

**triiodothyronine (T$_3$)** n. the more active form of thyroid hormone that is located in tissues and created by the conversion of thyroxine released from the thyroid gland.

**triple pelvic osteotomy (TPO)** n. a surgical procedure used to treat young dogs with hip dysplasia and help prevent the development of osteoarthritis. The pelvis is cut in three places and realigned in such a way as to improve the function of the hip joint.

**triple phosphate urolith** n. *See* struvite urolith.

**trismus** n. a prolonged spasm of jaw muscles, which may prevent an animal from opening its mouth.

**trocar** n. an instrument that can be used to pierce a body part (e.g., rumen) and release gas or fluid.

**trochanteric bursitis** n. a condition of horses in which a fluid-filled sac near the hip becomes inflamed. Affected animals are lame and with time develop muscle atrophy in their hindquarters. Treatment includes rest and anti-inflammatories. *Also called* whirlbone lameness.

**trombiculosis** n. a disease caused by the bites of chiggers. Affected individuals develop skin lesions and intense itching. Medications to relieve itching can provide relief.

**trot** n. a specific way of moving in which diagonally opposed legs move forward at the same time and two distinct beats or footfalls are evident.

**trypsin-like immunoreactivity (TLI)** n. a laboratory test that can be used to help diagnose exocrine pancreatic insufficiency.

**tuberculosis (TB)** n. a contagious disease caused by certain types of *Mycobacteria* bacteria, which are most frequently transmitted through inhalation of organisms expelled from the lungs of an infected individual. Clinical signs can include weight loss, lethargy, fever, coughing, difficulty breathing, enlarged lymph nodes and other symptoms depending on where the infection localizes. Treatment is difficult, and in most cases should not be attempted because of regulatory controls and the potential for human infection.

**tucked up** adj. describes an animal with a very thin abdomen.

**tularemia** n. a disease caused by infection with *Francisella tularensis* bacteria, which can be transmitted through the bites of ticks, inhalation of the organism and contact with or ingestion of contaminated tissue. Affected individuals may develop a fever, lethargy, stiffness, coughing, diarrhea and/or urinary dysfunction, depending on where the infection localizes. Treatment with antibiotics can be successful if started early enough in the course of the disease. Humans can become infected with tularemia.

**tumor** n. an abnormal lump of tissue, most commonly referring to either a benign or malignant cancerous growth.

**turbid** adj. cloudy - **turbidity** n.

**turbinates** n. *See* nasal turbinates.

**turgid** adj. full or swollen with fluid - **turgor** n.

**twin lamb disease** n. *See* pregnancy toxemia.

**twitch** n. 1. a device used to restrain horses that applies pressure as it is tightened on the upper lip. Use of a twitch releases endorphins, natural chemicals that relieve pain and provide a sense of well-being. 2. a sudden and brief involuntary muscular contraction.

**twitchy cat disease** n. a behavioral or neurologic disease that causes cats to bite at their skin, sometimes to the point of self-mutilation and develop muscle twitches, rippling skin and abnormal behaviors. Itchy or painful diseases must be ruled out before the diagnosis of a behavioral or seizure-like disorder can be made. Treatment may include addressing any underlying diseases, corticosteroids and anti-seizure and anti-anxiety medications. *Also called* feline hyperesthesia syndrome and rolling skin disease.

**tying up** n. *See* exertional rhabdomyolysis.

**tympanic bulla** n. a hollow, bony cavity one of which is connected to each ear.

**tympanic membrane** n. the membrane that separates the outer ear from deeper structures and transmits sound waves to the bones of the middle ear. *Also called* eardrum.

**tympany** n. distension with gas. *See also* guttural pouch and ruminal tympany.

**Tyzzer's disease** n. a disease caused by infection with *Clostridium piliforme* bacteria, which may lead to fever, diarrhea, jaundice or sudden death in young and/or stressed individuals. Treatment is difficult but can include fluid therapy, glucose infusions and antibiotics.


# U

**Uberreiter's syndrome** n. *See* pannus.

**udder** n. the mammary gland of large animals.

**udder edema** n. a disorder seen most frequently in dairy cows that develops around the time of birth and causes fluid retention and swelling of the udder. Severe cases may lead to difficulties with milking and a breakdown of the ligaments that support the udder. Treatment can include massage, hot compresses, corticosteroids and medications to help decrease fluid accumulations.

**ulcer** n. a lesion in which the surface of a tissue is damaged and lost. Ulcers can affect the gastrointestinal tract, eye, skin and other tissues. *See also* corneal ulcer.

**ulcerative dermatitis** n. *See* scale rot.

**ulcerative dermatosis** n. a contagious, viral disease of sheep that causes ulcers to develop around the muzzle and lower legs or around the penile sheath and vulva. Affected animals should be isolated for several weeks until the lesions heal. Treatment can include application of topical antiseptics and supportive care. *Also called* venereal balanoposthitis and vulvitis.

**ulcerative lymphangitis** n. a disease of horses and cattle caused by infection with the bacteria *Corynebacterium pseudotuberculosis*.

Affected individuals develop abscesses and draining skin lesions on their lower legs. The infection may spread to other parts of the body. Treatment can include lancing, draining, flushing or the surgical removal of abscesses, cleaning infected skin, antibiotics and supportive care.

**ulcerative posthitis and vulvitis** n. *See* pizzle rot.

**ulcerative stomatitis** n. any of several disorders that cause oral inflammation, superficial tissue loss and discomfort. In dogs, an abnormal immune reaction to dental plaque can cause lesions to develop on the parts of the gums and lips that contact teeth. Treatment can include routine dental cleanings, improved oral hygiene, anti-inflammatories and tooth extractions. *See also* necrotizing ulcerative gingivostomatitis (dogs) and infectious stomatitis (reptiles).

**ulna** n. one of the two long bones that lie between the elbow and carpus.

**ultrasonography** n. a method of imaging the body in which high frequency sound waves are passed through a part of the body and reflected back to an instrument to be converted into detailed pictures. *Also called* sonography.

**umbilical cord** n. the tissues that carry blood and connect the fetus to the placenta.

**umbilical hernia** n. protrusion of abdominal contents through a hole in the body wall where the umbilical cord was previously attached. Genetics or trauma to this area at birth can prevent the normal closure of this structure. Affected animals have a swelling under the skin at the navel, which can sometimes be pushed back into the abdomen. Surgical repair is usually necessary.

**umbilicus** n. the scar on the abdomen that corresponds to the area where the umbilical cord was attached. *Also called* navel.

**underbite** n. the condition of having upper, front teeth that do not protrude past the lower teeth. *Compare* overbite.

**undercoat** n. the fine, insulating hairs within the coats of some animals.

**undershot jaw** n. the abnormal condition of having an upper jaw that is shorter than the lower jaw. *Also called* sow mouth and prognathism. *Compare* brachygnathism.

**undescended testicles** n. *See* cryptorchid.

**ungulate** adj. having hooves.

**unilateral** adj. involving one side. *Compare* bilateral.

**United Kennel Club (UKC)** n. an organization devoted to the registration and promotion of dogs, including spayed and neutered mixed-breed individuals, with an emphasis on performance as well as looks.

**univalent vaccine** n. a vaccine that provides protection against only one disease. *Compare* multivalent vaccine.

**unthrifty** adj. failing to grow and thrive under appropriate conditions.

**ununited anconeal process** n. a developmental disorder of dogs in which a part of the ulna involved in the elbow joint fails to attach to the rest of the bone. Affected individuals can be lame and develop osteoarthritis of the elbow at an early age. Treatment may include surgery and medications that decrease pain and inflammation.

**upper airway** n. the nasal passages, larynx, pharynx and trachea. *Compare* lower airway. *Also called* upper respiratory tract.

**upper respiratory infection (URI)** n. infection, usually with viruses or bacteria, of the nasal passages, larynx, pharynx and/or trachea but not the lungs. Affected animals cough or sneeze. Treatment can include supportive care, cough suppressants and antibiotics.

**upward fixation of the patella** n. a temporary locking of a ligament attached to the patella over a bony prominence at the bottom of the femur. Upward fixation of the patella can be caused by a lack of muscle development in the hindquarters or a genetic predisposition. Affected individuals intermittently cannot flex a hind leg and then will jerk it into a more normal position. Treatment can include exercise to improve muscle tone and surgery. *Also called* patellar luxation.

**urachus** n. the channel through which urine drains from the bladder of a fetus, through the navel and into the surrounding fluid within the uterus. The urachus should close at birth. *See also* patent urachus.

**urate** n. a breakdown product of protein metabolism. Urates form the white, more liquid portion of bird and reptile droppings. *See also* urate urolith.

**urate urolith** n. a type of stone that can form within and disrupt the function of the urinary tract. Urate uroliths may develop because of an inability of the liver to convert urate into other substances. Treatment can include diet changes, encouraging water intake, surgery or urohydropulsion to remove the stones and medications to alkalinize the urine and decrease the formation of urate.

**urea** n. a breakdown product of protein metabolism that is normally excreted in urine and can be fed to ruminants as a source of dietary nitrogen. *See also* blood urea nitrogen.

**urea poisoning** n. *See* non-protein nitrogen poisoning.

**uremia** n. *See* azotemia.

**ureter** n. the tube that carries urine from a kidney to the bladder.

**ureterolith** n. a stone that develops within a ureter and can block the flow of urine from a kidney causing abdominal pain and vomiting. Treatment includes surgery to remove the stone and sometimes the affected kidney if it is damaged and nonfunctional.

**urethra** n. the tube that carries urine from the urinary bladder to the exterior of the body.

**urethral plug** n. a mixture of mucus, protein, cells and/or crystals that can completely block the urethra thereby eliminating the ability to urinate. The condition is most often seen in male cats. *See also* blocked cat.

**urethritis** n. inflammation of the urethra, which can cause difficulty urinating.

**urethrogram** n. a radiograph that is taken after an animal has been given a contrast agent to highlight the urethra.

**urethrostomy** n. the surgical creation of an opening into the urethra through which urine can drain. *See also* perineal urethrostomy

**urethrotomy** n. a surgical incision into the urethra.

**uric acid** n. a breakdown product of protein metabolism that is normally excreted in urine. *See also* gout and urate.

**urinalysis (UA)** n. the examination of a sample of urine in the laboratory using a number of different tests and procedures (e.g., a urine dipstick and the microscopic examination of urinary sediment). A urinalysis can help diagnose urinary tract infections, kidney disease, diabetes mellitus and other disorders.

**urinary incontinence** n. the inability to control urination, which causes urine to leak at inappropriate times. Causes can include urinary tract infections, anatomic or neurologic abnormalities and hormonal diseases. Medications to tighten the sphincters that hold urine in the bladder can be helpful if the underlying disorder cannot be addressed. *See also* hormone responsive incontinence.

**urinary tract** n. the kidneys, ureters, urinary bladder and urethra, which are all associated with the production and elimination of urine.

**urinary tract infection (UTI)** n. infection, usually with bacteria, of the bladder, kidneys, ureters and/or urethra. Affected individuals can have discolored urine and urinate small amounts frequently. In most cases, an appropriate antibiotic will eliminate the infection unless treatment is stopped too soon or underlying conditions predispose the individual to relapses. *See also* pyelonephritis.

**urinate** v. pass urine from the body - **urination** n.

**urine** n. the liquid containing water and waste products that is manufactured by the kidneys and drained out of the body through the ureters, bladder and urethra.

**urine concentration** n. *See* urine specific gravity.

**urine dipstick** n. a strip of paper containing chemically treated pads that react to indicate the presence of glucose, protein, ketones and other substances when urine is applied.

**urine-marking** n. a behavior in which cats or other animals urinate or spray as a form of territorial marking or because of anxiety. Treatment includes providing multiple, well-cleaned litter boxes, preventing stressful situations (e.g., separating antagonistic cats) and behavior modifying drugs. *See also* spraying.

**urine scald** n. irritation that is caused by urine that leaks onto the skin or from prolonged contact with a contaminated environment. Treatment can include addressing any underlying conditions, topical ointments to protect the skin and antibiotics for secondary infections.

**urine specific gravity (USG)** n. a measure of the ability of the kidneys to produce concentrated urine. A high urine specific gravity can indicate dehydration and adequate kidney function while a low reading may be seen with overhydration, kidney and hormonal diseases or other disorders.

**uroabdomen** n. an accumulation of urine within the abdominal cavity, which can be caused by damage to and leakage from the bladder, urethra or ureters. *Also called* uroperitoneum.

**urobilinogen** n. a breakdown product of bilirubin the levels of which are measured in a urine sample and can rise with increased red blood cell destruction or liver disease.

**urogenital** adj. pertaining to the reproductive and urinary tracts.

**urogram** n. a radiograph of the urinary tract that is taken after an animal has been given a contrast agent by either intravenous injection or infusion into the bladder. *See also* excretory urogram.

**urohydropulsion** n. a procedure used to remove small stones from the bladder or urethra. In voiding urohydropulsion, the bladder is filled with fluid and pressure applied to the abdomen to push the liquid and stones out through the urethra. Retrograde urohydropulsion is used to flush a stone lodged in the urethra back into the bladder where it can be surgically removed.

**urolith** n. an accumulation of minerals and other substances that clump together to form a hard object within the urinary tract. Uroliths often are associated with bloody urine, straining or the inability to urinate and infections. Some types can be dissolved with special diets or medications while others must be removed surgically. *See also* struvite, calcium oxalate, urate and cystine uroliths.

**uroperitoneum** n. *See* uroabdomen.

**urospermia** n. the abnormal presence of urine within the ejaculate, which can decrease fertility.

**urovagina** n. an accumulation of urine within the vagina, which is often caused by anatomical changes in older females and can limit their ability to maintain a pregnancy.

**urticaria** n. a condition characterized by raised, red and frequently itchy areas that form on the skin often in response to an allergic reaction. Treatment can include avoidance of potential allergens, antihistamines and corticosteroids.

**uterine inertia** n. the condition in which uterine contractions are too weak to lead to a successful birth. Uterine inertia may be caused by prolonged labor or conditions (e.g., low blood calcium levels) that hinder the process. Treatment includes medications that stimulate contractions and addressing any underlying conditions.

**uterine tube** n. the passageway through which an egg released by the ovary travels to the uterus. *Also called* oviduct and fallopian tube.

**uterus** n. the abdominal organ of female mammals that contains, protects and nourishes a developing embryo and fetus - **uterine** adj.

**uvea** n. a layer of tissues within the eye. The iris is the most recognizable part of the uvea.

**uveitis** n. inflammation of the uvea, which may be associated with infection, trauma or the presence of substances (e.g., lens protein leaking from a cataract) that stimulate the immune system. Affected animals often have red, cloudy and painful eyes, small pupils and ocular drainage. Treatment depends on the underlying cause but can include antibiotics, anti-inflammatories and drugs to dilate the pupil. *See also* recurrent and anterior uveitis.

**uveodermatologic syndrome** n. a disease of dogs in which the immune system inappropriately attacks parts of the eye and skin. Affected individuals can develop uveitis, blindness and whitening of the skin and hair. Treatment with immunosuppressive drugs can control the disease. *Also called* Vogt-Koyanagi-Harada-like syndrome.

# V

**vaccination** n. introduction of a vaccine into an animal's body with the goal of preventing disease. *Also called* immunization.

**vaccination schedule** n. the optimal timetable for giving vaccines to an animal in order to provide maximum protection. *Also called* immunization schedule.

**vaccine** n. a substance (e.g., inactivated microorganisms) that is given to an animal to stimulate the immune system to develop protective mechanisms against a particular disease.

**vaccine reaction** n. any unwanted response of an animal to vaccination. Vaccine reactions can range from mild and self-limiting (e.g., fever and discomfort at injection sites) to rare but potentially fatal allergic reactions that can cause difficulty breathing, low blood pressure and collapse.

**vagal indigestion** n. a disorder most commonly seen in cattle that causes animals to gradually develop distention of the rumen or other parts of the digestive tract and have a poor appetite and scant fecal production. Lesions affecting the vagus nerve (e.g., inflammation and scarring after a case of hardware disease) are often to blame. Treatment can include surgery, transfaunation, antibiotics and supportive and symptomatic care. *See also* hardware disease.

**vagal maneuver** n. the application of pressure to the eye or part of the carotid artery in the upper neck to stimulate the vagus nerve and slow the heart rate.

**vagina** n. the passageway within the female reproductive tract that lies between the cervix and the outside of the body - **vaginal** adj.

**vaginal cytology** n. the microscopic examination of a sample of cells taken from within the vagina, applied to a glass slide and stained. Vaginal cytology can be used to help diagnose infections and determine the stage of a bitch's reproductive cycle. *Also called* vaginal smear.

**vaginal hyperplasia** n. a disorder of bitches that is most frequently seen as they are coming into heat and causes a mass to develop within the vagina and sometimes protrude from the vulva. The condition usually resolves as the animal progresses through its reproductive cycle. Treatment can include keeping the mass clean and moist, surgery to remove severely damaged tissues and ovariohysterectomy. *Also called* vaginal edema and vaginal fold prolapse.

**vaginitis** n. inflammation of the vagina, which is usually associated with infection. *See also* puppy vaginitis.

**vaginoscopy** n. the use of an instrument (e.g., an endoscope) to allow visualization of the inside of the vagina and sometimes to perform minor procedures.

**vagolytic** adj. *See* anticholinergic.

**vagus nerve** n. a long cranial nerve that is involved with the function of the larynx, pharynx and organs in the chest and abdomen. Lesions affecting the vagus nerve can cause difficulty swallowing and respiratory, cardiac and digestive disorders - **vagal** adj.

**valgus** adj. describes an abnormal bending of a leg away from an animal's midline. Disorders of the bones or soft tissues of joints are the most common causes for a valgus deformity. Young animals may be born with this disorder, or it may develop with growth. Treatment can include splints, casts, exercise restriction and surgery. *Compare* varus.

**valley fever** n. *See* coccidioidomycosis.

**valve** n. a structure in the body that promotes flow of a fluid in one direction.

**varus** adj. describes an abnormal bending of a leg towards an animal's midline. Disorders of the bones or soft tissues of joints are the most common causes for a varus deformity. Young animals may be born with this disorder, or it may develop with growth. Treatment can include splints, casts, exercise restriction and surgery. *Compare* valgus.

**vas deferens** n. *See* ductus deferens.

**vascular** adj. pertaining to a blood vessel or the supply of blood.

**vascular ring anomaly** n. *See* persistent right aortic arch.

**vascularization** n. the development of new blood vessels.

**vasculitis** n. inflammation of a blood vessel or vessels.

**vasculopathy** n. any disorder affecting blood vessels.

**vasoactive** adj. dilating or constricting a blood vessel.

**vasoconstriction** n. a narrowing of the diameter of blood vessels, which can decrease blood flow to a part of the body or raise blood pressure. *Compare* vasodilation.

**vasodilation** n. a widening of the diameter of blood vessels, which can increase blood flow to a part of the body or lower blood pressure. *Compare* vasoconstriction.

**vasopressin** n. *See* antidiuretic hormone.

**vasospasm** n. a sudden narrowing of a blood vessel that can decrease blood flow to a part of the body.

**vector** n. an object or organism (e.g.,

insect) that can passively carry and transmit disease-causing microorganisms.

**vein** n. a vessel carrying blood towards the heart - **venous** adj. *Compare* artery.

**Velpeau sling** n. a type of bandage that is applied to keep the elbow and carpus flexed and prevent weight-bearing and unwanted movement of a front limb.

**vena cava** n. one of the large blood vessels draining blood from the front and back of the body to the heart.

**vena cava syndrome** n. *See* caval syndrome.

**venereal** adj. transmitted through sexual contact.

**venereal balanitis** n. *See* coital exanthema.

**venereal balanoposthitis and vulvitis** n. *See* ulcerative dermatosis.

**Venezuelan equine encephalomyelitis (VEE)** n. a viral disease of horses that is transmitted by the bite of infected mosquitos. Affected individuals can develop fever, depression, difficulty walking and swallowing, head pressing, circling, wandering, weakness, seizures and may die. There is no specific treatment for the virus, but supportive care is essential. Vaccination and mosquito control can help prevent the disease.

**venipuncture** n. *See* phlebotomy.

**venom** n. a poisonous substance produced and secreted by some types of animals (e.g., certain snakes). Bites or stings that inject venom can cause local tissue damage and/or potentially fatal reactions throughout the body.

**venous** adj. pertaining to a vein or veins.

**vent** n. an opening through which material can be expelled. *See also* cloaca.

**vent disease** n. *See* treponematosis.

**ventilate** v. 1. to exchange gasses between the lungs and the outside environment. 2. to provide fresh air to the interior of a building - **ventilation** n.

**ventilation-perfusion mismatch** n. a condition in which lesions affecting the airways and/or circulatory system within the lungs prevent efficient transfer of gasses and cause low blood oxygen levels.

**ventral** adj. situated towards the bottom side of the body - **ventrum** n. *Compare* dorsal.

**ventricle** n. 1. one of the muscular chambers of the heart that pushes blood to the lungs (i.e., right ventricle) or body (i.e., left ventricle). 2. a chamber in the brain filled with cerebrospinal fluid - **ventricular** adj.

**ventricular fibrillation** n. uncoordinated, ineffective and rapid contractions of the heart's ventricles that can quickly lead to death. Treatment includes defibrillation and medications to initiate a more normal heart rhythm.

**ventricular flutter** n. abnormally rapid contractions of the heart's ventricles that usually occur just before

the heart stops beating. Emergency treatment with antiarrhythmic drugs and defibrillation is necessary.

**ventricular premature contraction (VPC)** n. *See* premature ventricular contraction.

**ventricular septal defect (VSD)** n. an abnormal hole in the portion of the heart that separates the right and left ventricles. Affected individuals develop heart enlargement, a murmur and heart failure if the hole is large enough. Treatment can include vasodilators and surgery to close the defect or otherwise improve heart function.

**ventriculus** n. the muscular portion of a bird's stomach that helps grind food. *Also called* gizzard.

**verminous** adj. caused by or pertaining to animals, especially worms, that can be detrimental to health - **vermin** n.

**verminous bronchitis and pneumonia** n. *See* lungworm.

**vertebra** n. one of the bones that surrounds, supports and protects the spinal cord - **vertebrae** pl., **vertebral** adj.

**vertebral canal** n. *See* spinal canal.

**vertebral column** n. *See* spinal column.

**vertebral heart score (VHS)** n. a method of assessing the size of a heart by comparing it to a particular vertebra on a chest radiograph.

**vertical transmission** n. the passage of disease-causing microorganisms or other pathogens from a dam to her offspring during pregnancy, birth or lactation. *Compare* horizontal transmission.

**vesicle** n. 1. a pocket of serum that forms under the surface of a tissue (i.e., a blister). 2. a structure that can hold fluid - **vesicular** adj.

**vesicular stomatitis (VS)** n. a contagious, viral disease affecting horses, cattle, pigs and sometimes other species that causes blisters, ulcers and other lesions most commonly located around the feet, nose, mouth and teats. Most cases resolve uneventfully within a week or two. Because of the similarity of vesicular stomatitis to other, more serious diseases (e.g., foot and mouth disease), suspected cases must be reported to the appropriate regulatory agencies. People can become infected with the virus.

**vestibular system** n. the parts of the brain and inner ear that are responsible for the sense of balance.

**vestibular disease** n. a disorder affecting the vestibular system, which can cause a head tilt, circling, difficulty walking, rolling, vomiting and abnormal eye movements. Some individuals may have inner ear infections, lesions (e.g., tumors) within the brain or other identifiable disorders, but many cases have no known cause. Treatment for idiopathic vestibular disease is usually not necessary as most animals return to normal within a few weeks. Severely affected animals can benefit from anti-nausea medications and supportive care and may retain a mild head tilt and slight loss of balance.

**vestigial** adj. present in a small, underdeveloped and usually nonfunctional state.

**veterinarian** n. a person who has been trained and has received an advanced degree in the medical and surgical treatment of animals.

**veterinary medical doctor (VMD)** n. *See* doctor of veterinary medicine.

**veterinary-client-patient relationship** n. the legal requirement for a veterinarian to have sufficient knowledge of an animal's condition and an association with the owner to diagnose and treat an individual or herd.

**viable** adj. capable of surviving.

**vibriosis** n. a disease caused by infection with *Campylobacter* or *Vibrio* bacteria. Infection of the gastrointestinal tract causes diarrhea in many species. Some animals may carry and shed the bacteria in their feces without becoming ill themselves and are a source of infection for other animals or people. Treatment with antibiotics can be successful. Infection of the genital tract can cause sheep to abort and cows to lose their pregnancies early in gestation. Vaccinations and antibiotics can help eliminate the disease from cattle and sheep herds. *Also called* campylobacteriosis.

**vibrissa** n. a whisker - **vibrissae** pl.

**vice** n. an unwanted and potentially dangerous or destructive habit.

**villonodular synovitis** n. a disease of horses with an unknown cause. Affected individuals develop inflammation and masses within one or both front fetlock joints, which produces lameness. Treatment can include surgery and radiation therapy.

**viral hemorrhagic disease** n. *See* rabbit calicivirus.

**viremia** n. the presence of viruses within the bloodstream.

**viricidal** adj. having the ability to kill viruses.

**virilization** n. the development of typically male characteristics. Some types of hormonal or other disorders can induce virilization of female animals. *Also called* masculinization.

**virology** n. the science and study of viruses and the diseases that they cause.

**virulence** n. the ability of a microorganism to infect an animal causing disease and/or death - **virulent** adj.

**virus** n. an infectious particle that contains DNA or RNA but not the systems necessary for replication. Viruses must invade an organism and use its cells to reproduce - **viral** adj.

**visceral** adj. pertaining to a large organ of the abdominal or chest cavity.

**viscerotropic velogenic Newcastle disease (VVND)** n. an especially severe strain of Newcastle disease, which is caused by a contagious virus infecting birds. Affected individuals can develop sneezing, nasal discharge, difficulty breathing, neurologic abnormalities, diarrhea, tissue swelling and often die. Treatment should not be attempted, and appropriate regulatory agencies must be contacted. *Also called* exotic Newcastle disease.

**viscus** n. one of the large organs of the abdominal or chest cavities - **viscera** pl.

**visual evoked potential** n. a method of testing for blindness that measures the brain's responsiveness to a flashing light or other visual stimulus.

**vital signs** n. the temperature, pulse rate and respiration rate of a patient. *Also called* cardinal signs.

**vitamin** n. a substance that contains carbon and is required in the diet in small amounts for normal body function.

**vitamin A** n. a fat-soluble vitamin that is essential to the normal growth and maintenance of epithelial tissues (e.g., skin and hooves), eyes and bones. *See also* hypervitaminosis A.

**vitamin B** n. a group of water-soluble vitamins that have many important functions within the body. *See also* biotin, folate, niacin, riboflavin and vitamin $B_{12}$.

**vitamin $B_{12}$** n. a vitamin that is especially important to the development of red blood cells. Inadequate vitamin $B_{12}$ levels in the diet can cause anemia. *Also called* cyanocobalamine.

**vitamin C** n. a water-soluble vitamin that is an essential part of the diet in some species (e.g., guinea pigs) because these animals are unable to make it within their bodies. *Also called* ascorbic acid. *See also* scurvy.

**vitamin D** n. a fat-soluble vitamin that is essential to normal growth and maintenance of bones. *See also* hypervitaminosis D.

**vitamin E** n. a fat-soluble vitamin that is an important antioxidant.

Dietary insufficiencies of vitamin E can lead to disorders affecting muscles (e.g., white muscle disease) and the neurologic system.

**vitamin K** n. a group of fat-soluble vitamins that are essential to the ability of blood to clot normally.

**vitiligo** n. the progressive and patchy loss of pigment in the skin and hair. There is no effective treatment, but the disorder does not adversely affect most animals. *See also* Arabian fading syndrome.

**vitrectomy** n. the surgical removal of the vitreous body.

**vitreocentesis** n. the insertion of a hollow needle into the eye to remove a sample of the vitreous body.

**vitreous body** n. the thick, clear material that fills the eye's vitreous chamber. *Also called* vitreous humor.

**vitreous chamber** n. the portion of the eye that lies behind the lens and in front of the retina.

**vocal cords** n. the bands of tissue within the larynx that can vibrate and produce sounds. *Also called* vocal folds.

**vocalization** n. sounds intentionally produced by an animal as a form of communication.

**Vogt-Koyanagi-Harada-like (VKH) syndrome** n. *See* uveodermatologic syndrome.

**voice box** n. *See* larynx.

**voice change** n. an alteration in the tone or other quality of an animal's vocalizations, which can be a sign of disorders affecting the larynx.

**void** v. to eliminate waste material from the body (e.g., to urinate) - **voided** adj.

**volume expansion** n. intravenous fluids or transfusions that are given to increase the volume of circulating blood. Volume expansion is often used to treat shock or dehydration.

**voluntary muscle** n. *See* striated muscle.

**volvulus** n. an abnormal twisting of a part of the gastrointestinal tract. Volvulus of an organ can hinder its blood supply and quickly lead to extreme pain and tissue death. Surgery is often necessary to untwist the structure and remove any irreversibly damaged tissues. *See also* gastric dilatation and volvulus.

**vomeronasal organ** n. an area in the nasal cavity that identifies chemical signals (e.g., pheromones) produced by another individual of the same species.

**vomit** v. to expel ingesta out of the stomach and through the mouth or nose.

**vomitoxin** n. a substance produced by a fungus that can grow on grain and cause an unwillingness to eat, weight loss and vomiting in animals exposed to infected feed.

**vomitus** n. the material expelled out of the stomach by vomiting.

**von Willebrand's disease** n. a genetic disease causing a failure to produce a blood coagulation factor, which leads to an increased tendency to bleed. A transfusion with fresh blood or plasma can effectively treat an episode of bleeding.

**vulva** n. the external tissues located at the end of the female reproductive tract - **vulvar** adj.

**vulvitis** n. inflammation of the vulva. *See also* ulcerative dermatosis.

**vulvovaginitis** n. inflammation of the vagina and vulva.

# W

**walk** n. a specific, slow way of moving in which four distinct beats or footfalls are evident.

**walking dandruff** n. *See* cheyletiellosis.

**walleye** n. 1. an opaque, white discoloration of the cornea. 2. an iris that is partially or completely white or light colored because it is lacking in normal pigments. 3. a condition in which one eye is rotated so that it appears to be looking in an abnormal direction.

**wanderer** n. a newborn foal that did not have adequate oxygen delivered to its brain during the birthing process. *See also* neonatal maladjustment syndrome.

**warble** n. 1. the larva of a *Cuterebra* fly that usually causes a lump with a central hole in the skin of an infested animal. Manual removal of the larva and cleansing of the area is curative. The larva can sometimes migrate to other organs, causing a wide range of problems. *Also called* bot and cuterebriasis. 2. the larva of a *Hypoderma* or *Dermatobia* fly that can infest cattle. Adult flies lay their eggs on a cow's hair, usually around the legs. The larvae hatch and migrate throughout the body eventually ending up under the skin where they form a lump with a central hole. Many medications and insecticides will kill the larvae as they migrate within the body. *Also called* cattle grub and hypodermosis.

**warfarin poisoning** n. *See* anticoagulant rodenticide toxicity.

**wart** n. a small, raised skin mass often with a cauliflower-like surface. *See also* papilloma, sebaceous adenoma and sebaceous epithelioma.

**wasting** n. the loss of large amounts of fat and/or muscle mass from the body.

**water deprivation test** n. a procedure that can help diagnose cases of diabetes insipidus or psychogenic polydipsia when other, more common causes of increased thirst and urination are ruled out. Water is withheld until the individual is mildly dehydrated or begins to produce concentrated urine. Close monitoring is essential to prevent severe dehydration.

**waterbelly** n. a condition in which fluid accumulates in the abdominal cavity. Waterbelly usually refers to a disorder most commonly affecting male goats in which a stone blocks the urethra, prevents urination and causes the bladder to rupture and leak urine. Treatment is difficult but includes surgically repairing the bladder, relieving or bypassing the urinary obstruction, flushing out the abdomen and medications or diet changes that can prevent recurrence of the stones.

**water-soluble vitamins** n. vitamins (e.g., C and B) that can be dissolved in water and easily eliminated from the body in the urine. Animals cannot store large amounts of these vitamins and require a fairly regular supply in their diet. *Compare* fat-soluble vitamins.

**wattle** n. a fleshy fold of tissue that hangs under the lower jaw of some species (e.g., turkeys and goats).

**wave mouth** n. an abnormal condition in which a horse's teeth are unevenly worn creating an undulating chewing surface and difficulty eating. Treatment can include routine dental floating and diet changes.

**waxing up** n. a symptom occurring in a mare within a few hours to days of her giving birth. A thick, waxy substance is secreted from and sticks to the ends of her teats.

**wean** v. 1. to stop a young animal from nursing and usually separate it from the dam. 2. to gradually taper the administration of or access to a particular substance.

**weanling** n. a young horse that has been weaned but is not yet one year old.

**weaving** n. an undesirable habit of horses during which they stand in place and rhythmically sway their heads from side to side. Boredom or anxiety is thought to initiate many cases of weaving. Treatment can include relieving stress (e.g., providing companionship or more time at pasture), dietary and bedding changes and adding an unbreakable mirror to the inside of stalls.

**weightbearing** n. the degree to which an animal is willing or able to support itself on a particular leg.

**West Nile encephalomyelitis** n. a viral disease that is most commonly seen in horses and transmitted by the bite of infected mosquitos. Affected individuals can develop fever, loss of appetite, depression, difficulty walking, muscle tremors, abnormal behavior, other neurologic signs and may die. There is no specific treatment for the virus, but supportive care is essential. Vaccines available for horses and mosquito control can help prevent the disease.

**Western equine encephalomyelitis (WEE)** n. a viral disease of horses that is transmitted by the bite of infected mosquitos. Affected individuals can develop fever, depression, difficulty walking and swallowing, head pressing, circling, wandering, weakness, seizures and may die. There is no specific treatment for the virus, but supportive care is essential. Vaccination and mosquito control can help prevent the disease. Birds are also susceptible to the virus and may develop neurologic abnormalities.

**wet dewlap** n. a condition of female rabbits in which chronic dampness of the dewlap from water bowls or dental disorders leads to inflammation and infection of the skin. Treatment can include antiseptics, antibiotics and addressing the underlying condition. *Also called* moist dermatitis.

**wet tail** n. *See* proliferative enteritis (hamsters) and Tyzzer's disease (gerbils).

**wether** n. a male sheep that was castrated at a young age.

**wet-to-dry bandage** n. a type of bandage that is used to reduce the amount of wound contamination. A damp piece of gauze is placed over the lesion, covered with absorbent material and allowed to dry. When the bandage is removed, debris is captured in the gauze.

**wheal** n. *See* hive.

**wheelbarrowing** n. a procedure used to test neurologic function. The animal is held up by the hind end and forced to walk forward on its front legs.

**wheeze** n. an abnormal, high-pitched sound that is usually heard when an animal exhales and is caused by partial obstruction of an airway (e.g., asthma).

**whelp** v. to give birth to puppies.

**whipworm** n. a type of parasite that attaches to the wall of the large intestine and is transmitted through the ingestion of eggs within the environment. Whipworms can cause diarrhea that may contain blood. Some types of dewormers can kill the parasites.

**whirlbone lameness** n. *See* trochanteric bursitis.

**white blood cell (WBC)** n. a type of cell that helps identify and remove potentially harmful microorganisms or other materials (e.g., cancerous or damaged cells) from the body. *Also called* leukocyte.

**white line** n. the connection between the wall and the sole of the hoof.

**white line disease** n. a disease in which the connection between the wall and sole of the hoof weakens allowing separation of these structures. Debris collects in the resulting cavity, which may cause lameness and infections that can travel up the foot. Damp conditions, overgrown hooves and laminitis encourage the development of white line disease. Treatment can include draining abscesses, removing foreign material from within the hoof, soaking the foot in antiseptic solutions, therapeutic hoof trimming and shoeing and addressing any underlying conditions.

**white matter** n. the portion of the brain and spinal cord composed primarily of the long, thin axons of nerves that transmit signals throughout the body. *Compare* gray matter.

**white muscle disease** n. a disorder of muscles that is caused by a deficiency of vitamin E and selenium in the diet. Affected animals, including young born to females fed a deficient diet, can develop difficulty walking, breathing and eating. Sudden death is possible when the muscles of the heart are involved. Treatment includes vitamin E and selenium supplements. *Also called* nutritional myopathy and stiff lamb disease.

**whole blood** n. blood that can be used for a transfusion from which no elements (e.g., plasma) have been removed.

**windgalls** n. fluid-filled swellings around a horse's fetlock that are associated with the joint (i.e., articular windgalls) or tendon sheaths (i.e., tendinous windgalls). Causes can include injury or overwork. Most cases are not associated with lameness, do not require any treatment and may resolve with time. *Also called* windpuffs.

**windsucking** n. *See* cribbing and pneumovagina.

**windswept** adj. describes a conformational abnormality in which one leg is bent to the inside and the limb on the opposite side of the body is bent to the outside. Most windswept animals developed the condition while in the uterus and their legs will straighten with time and restricted exercise. *See also* angular limb deformity.

**winging** n. an undesirable pattern of movement in which a leg is swung too far to the inside or outside of the body when it is moved forward.

**winking** n. the opening and closing of a mare's vulva that can be seen when she is in heat and approached by a male.

**withdrawal reflex** n. the normal, involuntary response of pulling a leg away when a painful stimulus (e.g., a pinch) is applied to the foot.

**withdrawal time** n. the length of time that must pass after an animal has been treated with a particular medicine before it can be used for meat or to produce milk for human consumption. Withdrawal times reduce consumers' exposure to drugs and drug residues.

**withers** n. the raised area over top of an animal's shoulders where the neck joins the chest.

**wobbler syndrome** n. a disorder seen most often in young dogs and horses in which the spinal cord in the neck is compressed causing pain and difficulty walking. *See also* cervical spondylomyelopathy (dog) and cervical stenotic myelopathy (horse).

**wolf tooth** n. a small tooth located in front of the upper chewing teeth in some horses. Wolf teeth usually fall out as the animal matures but can be removed if they remain and are problematical (e.g., interfere with the bit).

**wooden tongue** n. *See* actinobacillosis.

**Wood's lamp** n. a light source of a certain wavelength that causes some substances (e.g., fluorescein dye and ringworm) to glow.

**wool block** n. *See* gastric stasis.

**wool sucking** n. an undesirable behavior affecting some cats in which they chew or suck on cloth or other objects. Many cases seem to originate from early weaning. Severely affected animals may eat the foreign material and develop gastrointestinal disorders. Treatment can include stress relief (e.g. separating antagonistic cats), keeping food available at all times and behavior modifying drugs.

**worming** n. *See* deworming.

**wound** n. an injury to a body surface that is caused by an external force.

**wrist** n. *See* carpus.

**wry mouth** n. a condition, usually genetic, in which the left and right sides of the jaw grow unevenly. Wry mouth prevents the animal's teeth from aligning properly, which can hinder the ability to chew. Some cases may resolve as an individual matures while other animals require tooth extractions or orthodontic techniques. *Also called* wry bite.

**wryneck** n. *See* torticollis.

## X -Y - Z

**xanthoma** n. a benign, fatty mass that is usually yellow and located in or under the skin. Xanthomas may be caused by poor nutrition or abnormal fat metabolism. Treatment can include improving the animal's diet, vitamin A supplements and surgical removal.

**xanthomatosis** n. a disorder in which fatty substances are deposited throughout the body because of a disease that adversely affects the metabolism of fat (e.g., diabetes mellitus). *See also* xanthoma.

**xerograph** n. a type of radiograph that gives a very detailed image but requires special equipment.

**xerophthalmia** n. a lack of normal tear production producing a dry and inflamed eye. Potential causes are a dietary deficiency of vitamin A and keratoconjunctivitis sicca. Treatment can include lubricating eye drops and addressing any underlying conditions. *Also called* dry eye.

**xerostomia** n. a lack of normal saliva production, which produces a dry mouth and difficulty eating. Radiation therapy, the use of some drugs and immune mediated or other diseases can cause xerostomia. Treatment includes oral rinses and addressing any underlying disorders.

**x-ray** n. *See* radiograph.

**yearling** n. an animal that is between one and two years of age.

**yeast** n. a one-celled fungal organism, some species of which can cause disease in animals.

**yellow fat disease** n. inflammation of fat that is seen most frequently in animals fed a diet high in unsaturated fatty acids (e.g., fish) and low in vitamin E. Affected individuals develop a fever and are in pain, especially when touched. Treatment includes dietary changes and vitamin E supplements.

**yellow-star thistle poisoning** n. a fatal disease of horses that eat yellow-star thistle plants for an extended period of time. The plant's toxin damages a portion of the brain and causes abnormal chewing motions, other movements of lips and tongue and an inability to eat, drink and fully close the mouth. There is no treatment.

**yolk sac** n. a structure attached to a developing fetus that provides nourishment and circulatory support.

**zearalenone** n. *See* estrogenism.

**zinc** n. an element that is an important part of the diet and essential to the health of the skin. *See also* parakeratosis and zinc-responsive dermatosis.

**zinc phosphide toxicosis** n. ingestion of zinc-phosphide containing rodent poisons that can cause vomiting, abdominal pain, bizarre behavior, difficulty breathing, seizures and death in exposed animals. Treatment includes medications that raise the pH of the stomach and body and supportive and symptomatic care.

**zinc responsive dermatosis** n. a disorder in which affected animals develop crusting and flaking of the skin, particularly around the face, feet and legs. Some cases are related to a genetic need for increased amounts of zinc while others are caused by over-supplementation with calicum or a dietary zinc deficiency. Treatment with zinc supplements can be very successful.

**zinc sulfate fecal exam** n. the placement of a sample of feces in a liquid containing zinc sulfate, which encourages parasite eggs to rise to the surface. A glass cover slip collects the eggs and is placed on a slide to be examined under the microscope.

**zinc toxicosis** n. ingestion of sufficient quantities of zinc to cause disease. Animals are exposed by ingesting pennies, batteries, metallic wire and hardware, ointments or other substances containing zinc. Affected individuals may develop vomiting, diarrhea, loss of appetite, lethargy, jaundice and seizures. Treatment can include fluid therapy, transfusions, oxygen therapy, surgery or endoscopy to remove the source of zinc and the use of medications that bind to and enhance the elimination of zinc from the body.

**Zollinger-Ellison syndrome** n. a condition most commonly affecting dogs in which a tumor in the pancreas secretes gastrin leading to an overproduction of stomach acid and severe ulceration of the upper gastrointestinal tract. *See also* gastrinoma.

**zoonotic** adj. describes the ability of a disease to pass from an animal to a human - **zoonosis** n.

**zygomycosis** n. a disease caused by infection with a *Zygomycetes* fungus, most often causing lesions around the nose, mouth or skin of horses. Treatment includes surgical removal of the affected areas and drugs to kill the fungus.

# APPENDICES

## COMMONLY PRESCRIBED DRUGS

It is important to remember that any individual animal can have an unusual reaction to any drug, including a potentially serious allergic reaction. This table does not describe all possible uses, side effects or names of the listed drugs. Many other drugs are used to treat veterinary patients. Inclusion of a medicine does not constitute endorsement of the product.

| Drug | Other Common Names | Major Uses | Possible Side Effects |
|---|---|---|---|
| Acarexx® | ivermectin | kills ear mites | rare |
| acepromazine | PromAce® | sedation, prevents motion sickness | low blood pressure, low heart rate, extension of the penis (horse), third eyelid elevation |
| acetaminophen | Tylenol® | pain relief | extremely toxic to cats; kidney, liver, gastrointestinal, and blood disorders rare but possible in other species |
| Actigall® | See ursodiol | | |
| activated charcoal | Toxiban® | prevents absorption of toxins from the gastrointestinal tract | vomiting, diarrhea, stains feces black |
| Adequan® | See polysulfated glycosaminoglycan | | |
| Advantage® | See imidacloprid | | |
| Albon® | See sulfadimethoxine | | |
| albuterol | Proventil®, Ventolin® | dilates airways | increased heart rate, tremors, excitement |
| altrenogest | Regu-Mate® | prevents heat cycles, maintains pregnancy | rare when used at recommended doses. Latex gloves should always be worn when handling this drug, and pregnant women and people affected by a variety of other health problems should not handle altrenogest at all. |
| aluminum hydroxide | many antacids | reduces phosphorous levels, decreases rumen and stomach acidity | constipation |
| amikacin | | kills some types of bacteria | potentially irreversible damage to kidneys, hearing and sense of balance |
| aminophylline | | dilates airways | excitement, vomiting, diarrhea, high heart rate, increased appetite, thirst and urination |
| amitraz | Mitaban®, Taktic®, Preventic® | kills Demodex mange mites, ticks and some other insects | sedation, can be poisonous to cats and rabbits |

| Drug | Other Common Names | Major Uses | Possible Side Effects |
|---|---|---|---|
| amitriptyline | Elavil® | treats a variety of behavior problems and may help relieve some types of chronic pain, itching or feline urinary disease | sedation |
| ammonium chloride | Uroeze® | acidifies urine, dissolves struvite crystals | vomiting, diarrhea, loss of appetite, lowering of the body's pH |
| amoxicillin | Amoxi-Tab®, Amoxi-Drop® | kills some types of bacteria | vomiting, diarrhea, loss of appetite |
| amoxicillin with clavulanic acid | Clavamox®, Augmentin® | kills some types of bacteria | vomiting, diarrhea, loss of appetite |
| Amoxi-Drop® | See amoxicillin | | |
| Amoxi-Tab® | See amoxicillin | | |
| ampicillin | Polyflex® | kills some types of bacteria | vomiting, diarrhea, loss of appetite |
| Anipryl® | See selegiline | | |
| Antirobe® | See clindamycin | | |
| Antisedan® | See atipamezole | | |
| Antizol-Vet® | See fomepizole | | |
| apomorphine | | induces vomiting | excessive vomiting |
| aspirin | | pain relief, reduces inflammation, reduces tendency of blood to clot | gastrointestinal ulcers, blood loss, vomiting, loss of appetite, cats are especially sensitive |
| Atarax® | See hydroxyzine | | |
| atipamezole | Antisedan® | reverses effects of medetomidine, detomidine and xylazine | rare but occasional vomiting, excitement, drooling, tremors |
| Atopica® | See cyclosporine | | |
| atropine | | increases heart rate, lessens drooling and respiratory secretions, antidote to some poisons, dilates airways | rare except with high doses |
| atropine for eyes | | dilates pupil, relieves pain associated with some types of eye disease | topical irritation, salivation, glaucoma, low tear production, colic (horse) |
| Augmentin® | See amoxicillin with clavulanic acid | | |
| azathioprine | Imuran® | suppresses the immune system | low blood cell counts, infections, vomiting, diarrhea, liver disease |
| azithromycin | Zithromax® | kills some types of bacteria | vomiting, liver disease |
| Azium® | See dexamethasone | | |

# Appendix I- Commonly Perscribed Drugs

| Drug | Other Common Names | Major Uses | Possible Side Effects |
|---|---|---|---|
| Bactrim® | *See* trimethoprim with sulfamethoxazole | | |
| Banamine® | *See* flunixin meglumine | | |
| Baytril® | *See* enrofloxacin | | |
| Baytril Otic® | enrofloxacin with silver sulfadiazine | kills some types of bacteria and yeast in the ear | may damage inner ear if ear drum is ruptured |
| Benadryl® | *See* diphenhydramine | | |
| Betadine® | *See* povidone-iodine | | |
| betamethasone | | reduces inflammation, itching and allergies | low adrenal gland function, increased thirst, urination and hunger, many others |
| bethanechol | | increases contractility of the urinary bladder | vomiting, diarrhea, salivation, loss of appetite |
| bisacodyl | Dulcolax® | laxative | diarrhea, gastrointestinal cramps |
| bismuth subsalicylate | Pepto-Bismol® | reduces diarrhea, helps eliminate *Helicobacter* infections of the stomach wall | darkens stools, may cause side effects similar to those of aspirin if high doses are used |
| Bloat Release® | *See* docusate | | |
| Brethine® | *See* terbutaline | | |
| bromide | *See* potassium bromide | | |
| Buprenex® | *See* buprenorphine | | |
| buprenorphine | Buprenex® | pain relief | low respiratory rate, sedation |
| Buscopan® | *See* N-butylscopol-ammonium bromide | | |
| BuSpar® | *See* buspirone | | |
| buspirone | BuSpar® | treats a variety of behavior problems | rare but abnormal behavior, low heart rate, vomiting and diarrhea are possible |
| bute | *See* phenylbutazone | | |
| butorphanol | Torbutrol®, Torbugesic® | sedation, pain relief, suppresses coughs | over-sedation, loss of appetite |
| Capstar® | *See* nitenpyram | | |
| Carafate® | *See* sucralfate | | |
| Cardizem® | *See* diltiazem | | |
| Cardoxin® | *See* digoxin | | |

| Drug | Other Common Names | Major Uses | Possible Side Effects |
|---|---|---|---|
| carprofen | Rimadyl® | pain relief, reduces inflammation | vomiting, diarrhea, loss of appetite, liver disease, kidney disease |
| Cefa-Drops® | See cefadroxil | | |
| cefadroxil | Cefa-Tabs®, Cefa-Drops® | kills some types of bacteria | vomiting, diarrhea, loss of appetite |
| Cefa-Tabs® | See cefadroxil | | |
| cefazolin | Kefzol® | kills some types of bacteria | rare |
| cefpodoxime | Simplicef® | kills some types of bacteria | vomiting, diarrhea, loss of appetite |
| ceftiofur | Naxcel® | kills some types of bacteria | rare |
| cephalexin | Keflex® | kills some types of bacteria | vomiting, diarrhea, loss of appetite |
| Cestex® | See epsiprantel | | |
| chloramphenicol | | kills some types of bacteria | vomiting, diarrhea, loss of appetite, low blood cell counts. It is often recommended that latex gloves be worn when handling chloramphenicol to prevent potential side effects in people. |
| chlorhexidine | Nolvasan® | reduces numbers of microorganisms on body surfaces | can cause deafness if applied to an ear with a ruptured ear drum |
| chlorpheniramine | Chlor-Trimetron® | relieves symptoms of allergies | sedation, vomiting, diarrhea, loss of appetite |
| chlorpromazine | See chlorpheniramine | reduces vomiting | low blood pressure, low heart rate |
| Chlor-Trimetron® | See chlorpheniramine | | |
| chondroitin sulphate | Cosequin®, GlycoFlex® | promotes healthy cartilage and joint fluid, relieves osteoarthritis and pain | rare diarrhea |
| cimetidine | Tagamet® | reduces stomach acid, heals gastrointestinal ulcers | rare |
| Cipro® | See ciprofloxacin | | |
| ciprofloxacin | Cipro® | kills some types of bacteria | damage to cartilage in growing animals, vomiting, diarrhea, loss of appetite |
| cisapride | | promotes movement of food and feces through the gastrointestinal tract | diarrhea |
| Clavamox® | See amoxicillin with clavulanic acid | | |
| clemastine fumarate | Tavist® | relieves symptoms of allergies | sedation |
| clenbuterol | | dilates airways | increased heart rate, tremors, excitement, sweating |

# Appendix I- Commonly Perscribed Drugs

| Drug | Other Common Names | Major Uses | Possible Side Effects |
|---|---|---|---|
| clindamycin | Antirobe® | kills some types of bacteria | vomiting, diarrhea, loss of appetite |
| Clomicalm® | See clomipramine | | |
| clomipramine | Clomicalm® | treats a variety of behavior problems | sedation, vomiting, diarrhea, loss of appetite, liver disease |
| cloprostenol | Estrumate® | induces heat, abortion or birth and treats uterine infections | Pregnant women and people affected by respiratory disorders should use caution when handling cloprostenol to prevent potential side effects. |
| codeine | | pain relief, cough suppressant, reduces diarrhea | sedation, excitement (cats), vomiting, constipation, loss of appetite |
| Colace® | See docusate | | |
| Conofite® | See miconazole | | |
| Cosequin® | glucosamine with chondroitin sulfate | promotes healthy cartilage and joint fluid, relieves osteoarthritis and pain | rare diarrhea |
| Cosopt® | timolol maleate with dorzolamide | reduces eye pressure | topical irritation |
| cyclosporine | Atopica®, Sandimmune® | suppresses the immune system | vomiting, diarrhea, loss of appetite |
| cyclosporine for eyes | Optimmune® | increases tear production, suppresses the immune system | rare |
| Cydectin® | See moxidectin | | |
| Cytotec® | See misoprostol | | |
| Deccox® | See decoquinate | | |
| decoquinate | Deccox® | helps eliminate coccidia | rare |
| Dectomax® | See doramectin | | |
| Demerol® | See meperidine | | |
| Denosyl® | See s-adenosyl-methionine | | |
| Depo-Medrol® | See methyl-prednisolone | | |
| deracoxib | Deramaxx® | pain relief, reduces inflammation | vomiting, diarrhea, loss of appetite, liver disease, kidney disease |
| Deramaxx® | See deracoxib | | |
| Dermagen® | nystatin with neomycin, thiostrepton and triamcinolone | kills some types of bacteria and yeast and relieves itching | rare |

290

| Drug | Other Common Names | Major Uses | Possible Side Effects |
|---|---|---|---|
| DES | See diethylstilbestrol | | |
| deslorelin | Ovuplant® | induces ovulation | inflammation over site of implant |
| desoxycortico-sterone pivalate | DOCP, Percorten-V® | treats Addison's disease by increasing sodium and lowering potassium levels | rare unless overdosed |
| detomidine | Dormosedan® | sedation, pain relief | low heart rate, sweating |
| dexamethasone | Azium® | reduces inflammation, reduces immune response, relieves itching and allergies, treats some types of cancer, many other uses | low adrenal gland function, increased thirst, urination and hunger, many others |
| diazepam | Valium® | relieves anxiety, relaxes muscles, stimulates the appetite, controls seizures | sedation, liver disease (cats), tremors (horses), behavior changes, excitement (dogs) |
| diclofenac | Surpass® | relieves local areas of pain and inflammation | rare |
| diclofenac for eyes | Voltaren® | reduces inflammation | can hinder healing from infection |
| Dicural® | See difloxacin | | |
| diethylstilbestrol | DES | improves urinary incontinence and benign prostatic hypertrophy, induces heat and abortion | low blood cell counts (possibly fatal), uterine infections, many others |
| difloxacin | Dicural® | kills some types of bacteria | damage to cartilage in growing animals, vomiting, diarrhea, loss of appetite |
| Diflucan® | See fluconazole | | |
| digoxin | Lanoxin®, Cardoxin® | slows heart rate and increases the strength of heart muscle contractions | arrhythmias, vomiting, diarrhea, loss of appetite |
| diltiazem | Cardizem® | treats some types of abnormal heart rhythms, high blood pressure and hypertrophic cardiomyopathy | slow heart rate, vomiting |
| dimethyl sulfoxide | DMSO, Domoso® | reduces swelling, relieves pain and inflammation, promotes absorption of other drugs | strong odor to breath, topical irritation, easily absorbed through skin (always wear rubber gloves) and can carry unwanted substances into circulation. When given IV, it can damage red blood cells (horses). |
| dinoprost | Lutalyse® | synchronizes heat cycles within a herd, treats uterine infections, promotes abortion | abdominal pain, vomiting, defecation, increased heart and respiratory rates, salivation, incoordination and many others |

| Drug | Other Common Names | Major Uses | Possible Side Effects |
|---|---|---|---|
| diphenhydramine | Benadryl® | relieves symptoms of allergies, motion sickness and some types of nausea, treats anaphylaxis | sedation |
| DMSO | See dimethyl sulfoxide | | |
| dobutamine | | increases heart muscle contractions and blood pressure | abnormal heart rhythms, high blood pressure |
| DOCP | See desoxycortico-sterone pivalate | | |
| docusate | DSS, Bloat Release®, Ex-Lax® | laxative | diarrhea, gastrointestinal cramps |
| Domitor® | See medetomidine | | |
| Domoso® | See dimethyl sulfoxide | | |
| domperidone | | promotes lactation and normal gestation length in pregnant mares exposed to fescue | leakage of milk |
| Dopram® | See doxapram | | |
| doramectin | Dectomax® | kills many internal and external parasites | rare unless overdosed |
| Dormosedan® | See detomidine | | |
| dorzolamide | Trusopt®, Cosopt® | reduces eye pressure | topical irritation |
| doxapram | Dopram® | stimulates breathing | high blood pressure, abnormal heart rhythms, seizures, high respiratory rates |
| Doxirobe® | See doxycycline | | |
| doxycycline | Doxirobe® | kills some types of bacteria | vomiting, damage to the esophagus, discoloration of growing teeth |
| Droncit® | See praziquantel | | |
| Drontal® | praziquantel and pyrantel | kills many internal parasites, including tapeworms | salivation (cat) |
| Drontal Plus® | praziquantel with pyrantel and febantel | kills many internal parasites, including tapeworms | rare but loss of appetite and energy, vomiting and diarrhea are possible |
| DSS | See docusate | | |
| Dulcolax® | See bisacodyl | | |
| Duragesic® | See fentanyl | | |
| ECP® | See estradiol | | |
| Elavil® | See amitriptyline | | |

# Appendix I- Commonly Perscribed Drugs

| Drug | Other Common Names | Major Uses | Possible Side Effects |
|---|---|---|---|
| Enacard® | See enalapril | | |
| enalapril | Enacard®, Vasotec® | dilates blood vessels and lowers blood pressure | vomiting, diarrhea, loss of appetite |
| enrofloxacin | Baytril® | kills some types of bacteria | damage to cartilage in growing animals, vomiting, diarrhea, loss of appetite |
| epinephrine | | treats anaphylaxis and stimulates the heart to beat | abnormal heart rhythms, anxiety, vomiting |
| eprinomectin | Ivomec® Eprinex® | kills many internal and external parasites | rare |
| epsiprantel | Cestex® | kills tapeworms | rare |
| Equimax® | ivermectin with praziquantel | kills many internal parasites including tapeworms | rare unless overdosed |
| Equimectrin® | ivermectin | kills many internal parasites | rare unless overdosed |
| Eqvalan® | ivermectin | kills many internal parasites | rare unless overdosed |
| erythromycin | | kills some types of bacteria, promotes movement of food through the gastrointestinal tract | vomiting, diarrhea, loss of appetite |
| estradiol | ECP® | induces heat or abortion and treats uterine infections (cattle) | low blood cell counts, uterine infections (especially dogs and cats) |
| Estrumate® | See cloprostenol | | |
| etodolac | EtoGesic® | pain relief, reduces inflammation | vomiting, diarrhea, loss of energy, low blood protein levels |
| EtoGesic® | See etodolac | | |
| Ex-Lax® | See docusate | | |
| famotidine | Pepcid® | reduces stomach acid, heals gastrointestinal ulcers | rare |
| Feldene® | See piroxicam | | |
| fenbendazole | Panacur®, Safe-Guard® | kills many internal parasites | rare |
| fentanyl | Duragesic® | pain relief | low heart and respiratory rates, abnormal behavior |
| fipronil | Frontline® | kills fleas and ticks | rare |
| firocoxib | Previcox® | pain relief, reduces inflammation | vomiting, diarrhea, loss of appetite, blood in stool |
| Flagyl® | See metronidazole | | |
| florfenicol | Nu-Flor® | kills some types of bacteria | loss of appetite, diarrhea |
| Florinef® | See fludrocortisone | | |

293

| Drug | Other Common Names | Major Uses | Possible Side Effects |
|---|---|---|---|
| Flovent® | See fluticasone | | |
| fluconazole | Diflucan® | treats a variety of fungal infections | loss of appetite |
| fludrocortisone | Florinef® | treats Addison's disease by increasing sodium and lowering potassium levels | rare unless overdosed |
| flunixin meglumine | Banamine® | pain relief, reduces inflammation | gastrointestinal ulcers, kidney failure |
| fluoxetine | Prozac® | treats a variety of behavioral problems | loss of appetite, abnormal behavior |
| fluticasone | Flovent® | relieves airway inflammation | rare |
| fomepizole | Antizol-Vet® | treats antifreeze toxicosis | rare |
| Frontline® | See fipronil | | |
| Frontline Plus® | fipronil with methoprene | kills fleas and ticks | rare |
| Fulvicin® | See griseofulvin | | |
| furosemide | Salix®, Lasix® | removes fluid from the body, reduces bleeding from the nose of racehorses | dehydration, electrolyte imbalances |
| GastroGard® | See omeprazole | | |
| Genesis® | triamcinolone | relieves local areas of itching and inflammation | rare |
| gentamicin | Gentocin® | kills some types of bacteria | potentially irreversible damage to kidneys, hearing and sense of balance (does not apply to topical products) |
| Gentocin® | See gentamicin | | |
| Gentocin Durafilm® | gentamicin with betamethasone | kills some types of bacteria and relieves inflammation of the eye | corneal ulcers, topical irritation |
| GlaucTabs® | See methazolamide | | |
| glipizide | Glucotrol® | lowers blood sugar | vomiting, low blood sugar, liver damage |
| Glucophage® | See metformin | | |
| glucosamine | Cosequin®, GlycoFlex® | promotes healthy cartilage and joint fluid, relieves osteoarthritis and pain | rare diarrhea |
| Glucotrol® | See glipizide | | |
| GlycoFlex® | glucosamine with chondroitin sulfate | promotes healthy cartilage and joint fluid, relieves osteoarthritis and pain | rare diarrhea |
| glycopyrrolate | | increases heart rate, lessens drooling and respiratory secretions | salivation, glaucoma, low tear production, colic (horse) |

# Appendix I- Commonly Perscribed Drugs

| Drug | Other Common Names | Major Uses | Possible Side Effects |
|---|---|---|---|
| griseofulvin | Fulvicin® | treats ringworm | vomiting, diarrhea, loss of appetite, low blood cell counts |
| guaifenesin | | relaxes muscles | rare unless overdosed |
| halothane | | general anesthetic | low blood pressure, low respiratory and heart rates, abnormal body temperature |
| Heartgard® | ivermectin | prevents heartworm disease and kills some internal parasites | rare unless overdosed |
| heparin | | decreases blood clotting | bleeding |
| hetastarch | | promotes the ability of fluids to remain in circulation | decreased blood clotting, vomiting |
| hyaluronic acid | Legend® | decreases joint inflammation | temporary increase in joint inflammation, joint infections if improperly injected |
| hydrocortisone | | reduces inflammation, reduces immune response, relieves itching, many other uses | low adrenal gland function, increased thirst, urination and hunger, infections, many others |
| hydroxyzine | Atarax® | relieves symptoms of allergies | sedation |
| imidacloprid | Advantage® | kills fleas | rare |
| Immiticide® | See melarsomine | | |
| Imodium® | See loperamide | | |
| Imuran® | See azathioprine | | |
| insulin | Vetsulin®, many other types | lowers blood sugar | dangerously low blood sugar |
| Interceptor® | See milbemycin | | |
| ipecac syrup | | induces vomiting | excessive vomiting |
| isoflurane | | general anesthetic | low blood pressure, low respiratory and heart rates, abnormal body temperature |
| isoxsuprine | | vasodilator used to treat navicular disease | rare when given orally |
| itraconazole | Sporanox® | treats a variety of fungal infections | loss of appetite, liver damage, skin lesions |
| ivermectin | Ivomec®, Eqvalan®, Heartgard®, Equimectrin®, Rotectin®, Acarexx®, Zimecterin®, Equimax® | kills many internal and external parasites (see specific trade name for details) | dependent on animal species and parasite being treated (see specific trade name for details) |

| Drug | Other Common Names | Major Uses | Possible Side Effects |
|---|---|---|---|
| Ivomec® | ivermectin | kills many internal and external parasites | rare unless overdosed and dependent on animal species and parasite being treated |
| Ivomec® Eprinex® | See eprinomectin | | |
| K9 Advantix® | imidacloprid and permethrin | kills fleas and ticks, repels mosquitoes | drooling, vomiting, diarrhea, tremors, changes in behavior, extremely toxic to cats |
| Keflex® | See cephalexin | | |
| Kefzol® | See cefazolin | | |
| ketamine | | short acting general anesthetic, pain relief | high blood pressure, drooling, low respiratory rate, vomiting, stiffness, jerking, seizures |
| ketoconazole | Nizoral® | treats a variety of fungal infections | vomiting, diarrhea, loss of appetite, liver damage |
| Ketofen® | See ketoprofen | | |
| ketoprofen | Ketofen® | pain relief, reduces inflammation | gastrointestinal ulcers, kidney and liver damage |
| LA200® | See oxytetracycline | | |
| Lactated Ringers Solution | LRS | replaces fluid and electrolytes | overhydration |
| lactulose | | reduces blood ammonia levels, laxative | diarrhea, gastrointestinal cramps |
| Lanoxin® | See digoxin | | |
| Lasix® | See furosemide | | |
| latanaprost | Xalantan® | reduces eye pressure | constricted pupil, topical irritation |
| Laxatone® | petrolatum | laxative | rare |
| L-deprenyl | See selegiline | | |
| Legend® | See hyaluronic acid | | |
| levamisole | Levasole® | kills many internal parasites, stimulates the immune system | excitability, drooling, vomiting, diarrhea |
| Levasole® | See levamisole | | |
| Levotabs® | See levothyroxine | | |
| levothyroxine | Thyrotabs®, Levotabs®, Soloxine®, Thyrozine® | replaces thyroid hormone | rare unless overdosed |
| lidocaine | | local anesthetic, treats some abnormal heart rhythms, promotes postoperative gastrointestinal function (horse) | rare unless overdosed |
| lime sulfur | | treats topical fungal infections, parasites and itching | smells like rotten eggs and can stain fur |
| Liquamycin® | See oxytetracycline | | |

| Drug | Other Common Names | Major Uses | Possible Side Effects |
|------|-------------------|------------|----------------------|
| loperamide | Imodium® | reduces diarrhea | constipation, sedation, bloat |
| LRS | See Lactated Ringers Solution | | |
| lufenuron | Program® | flea control | rare |
| Lutalyse® | See dinoprost | | |
| lysine | | treat herpesvirus in cats | rare |
| Lysodren® | See mitotane | | |
| mannitol | | promotes production of urine, reduces pressure within the eye and brain | fluid and electrolyte imbalances |
| marbofloxacin | Zeniquin® | kills some types of bacteria | damage to cartilage in growing animals, vomiting, diarrhea, loss of appetite |
| Marquis® | See ponazuril | | |
| medetomidine | Domitor® | sedation, pain relief | low heart and respiratory rates, low body temperature |
| Medrol® | See methyl-prednisolone | | |
| megestrol acetate | Ovaban® | delays heat cycles, treats benign prostatic hypertrophy, false pregnancy and behavioral and skin disorders | adrenal disease, diabetes mellitus, uterine disorders, many others |
| melarsomine | Immiticide® | kills adult heartworms | pain and swelling at the injection site, coughing, loss of energy and appetite |
| meloxicam | Metacam® | pain relief, reduces inflammation | gastrointestinal ulcers, vomiting, loss of appetite, kidney damage |
| meperidine | Demerol® | pain relief, sedation | over-sedation, low respiratory rates, vomiting |
| Metacam® | See meloxicam | | |
| Metamucil® | See psyllium | | |
| metformin | Glucophage® | lowers blood sugar | loss of energy and appetite, vomiting, weight loss |
| methazolamide | GlaucTabs®, Neptazane® | lowers eye pressure | vomiting, diarrhea, loss of appetite, sedation, low blood cell counts |
| methimazole | Tapazole® | reduces thyroid hormone levels | loss of appetite, vomiting, loss of energy, low blood cell counts |
| methocarbamol | Robaxin® | relaxes muscles | sedation, weakness, drooling, vomiting |
| methyl-prednisolone | Medrol®, Depo-Medrol® | reduces inflammation, reduces immune response, relieves itching and allergies, many other uses | low adrenal gland function, increased thirst, urination and hunger, infections, many others |

| Drug | Other Common Names | Major Uses | Possible Side Effects |
|---|---|---|---|
| metoclopramide | Reglan® | reduces vomiting, promotes movement of food through the gastrointestinal tract | abnormal behavior, constipation |
| metronidazole | Flagyl® | kills some types of bacteria and protozoal parasites | neurologic problems |
| miconazole | Conofite® | treats some types of topical fungal infections | rare |
| Milbemite® | milbemycin | kills ear mites | rare |
| milbemycin | Interceptor®, Milbemite®, Sentinel® | prevents heartworm disease and kills some internal and external parasites | rare unless overdosed |
| misoprostol | Cytotec® | reduces stomach acid, heals gastrointestinal ulcers, pregnancy termination | diarrhea, gastrointestinal cramps, vomiting |
| Mitaban® | See amitraz | | |
| mitotane | Lysodren® | reduces adrenal gland function | loss of energy and appetite, weakness, vomiting, diarrhea |
| morphine | | pain relief, sedation | behavioral changes, low respiratory and heart rates, panting, vomiting, diarrhea, constipation, abnormal body temperature |
| moxidectin | ProHeart®, Cydectin®, Quest® | kills a variety of internal and external parasites, prevents heartworm disease | rare unless overdosed. See also ProHeart®. |
| Mycitracin® | bacitracin with neomycin and polymyxin B | kills some types of bacteria on the eye | topical irritation |
| Mydriacyl® | See tropicamide | | |
| N-butylscopol-ammonium bromide | Buscopan® | relieves spasmodic colic in horses | high heart rate |
| Navigator® | See nitazoxanide | | |
| Naxcel® | See ceftiofur | | |
| Nemex® | See pyrantel | | |
| Neobacimyx® | bacitracin with neomycin and polymyxin B | kills some types of bacteria on the eye | topical irritation |

| Drug | Other Common Names | Major Uses | Possible Side Effects |
|---|---|---|---|
| Neobacimyx-H® | bacitracin with neomycin, polymyxin B and hydrocortisone | kills some types of bacteria and relieves inflammation of the eye | topical irritation, corneal ulcers |
| Neo-Predef® | neomycin with isoflupredone | kills some types of bacteria and relieves inflammation of the eye | topical irritation, corneal ulcers |
| Neptazane® | See methazolamide | | |
| Nilstat® | See nystatin | | |
| nitazoxanide | Navigator® | treats EPM and potentially other infectious diseases | fever, loss of appetite, loss of energy, diarrhea, colic, laminitis |
| nitenpyram | Capstar® | kills fleas | rare |
| Nitro-bid® | See nitroglycerin | | |
| nitroglycerin | Nitro-bid® | dilates blood vessels, improves heart function | rash, low blood pressure |
| Nizoral® | See ketoconazole | | |
| Nolvasan® | See chlorhexidine | | |
| Nu-Flor® | See florfenicol | | |
| Numorphan® | See oxymorphone | | |
| nystatin | Nilstat® | kills the fungus *Candida* | loss of appetite, vomiting, diarrhea |
| omeprazole | GastroGard® | reduces stomach acid, heals gastrointestinal ulcers | rare |
| Ophthaine® | See proparacaine | | |
| Optimmune® | See cyclosporine for eyes | | |
| Orbax® | See orbifloxacin | | |
| orbifloxacin | Orbax® | kills some types of bacteria | rare, possible vomiting, diarrhea, loss of appetite |
| Otomax® | gentamicin with betamethasone and clotrimazole | kills some types of bacteria and yeast and relieves itching and inflammation | may damage inner ear if ear drum is ruptured |
| Ovaban® | See megestrol acetate | | |
| Ovuplant® | See deslorelin | | |
| Oxyglobin® | | carries oxygen in the bloodstream | discolored tissues and urine, vomiting, diarrhea, loss of appetite |
| oxymorphone | Numorphan® | pain relief, sedation | behavioral changes, low respiratory and heart rates, constipation |

| Drug | Other Common Names | Major Uses | Possible Side Effects |
|---|---|---|---|
| oxytetracycline | LA200®, Terramycin®, Liquamycin® | kills some types of bacteria | discoloration of growing teeth, bone damage in growing animals, kidney and liver damage, vomiting, diarrhea, loss of appetite |
| oxytocin | Pitocin® | causes uterine contractions and involution, promotes lactation | rare unless overdosed |
| Panacur® | See fenbendazole | | |
| pancrelipase | Viokase®, Pancrezyme® | replaces pancreatic digestive enzymes | rare but diarrhea and gastrointestinal cramps are possible |
| Pancrezyme® | See pancrelipase | | |
| Panmycin® | See tetracycline | | |
| Panolog® | nystatin with neomycin, thiostrepton and triamcinolone | kills some types of bacteria and yeast and relieves itching | rare when applied to skin, may cause damage if ear drum ruptured and ointment reaches inner ear |
| paroxetine | Paxil® | treats a variety of behavioral problems | loss of appetite, abnormal behavior |
| Paxil® | See paroxetine | | |
| penicillin | | kills some types of bacteria | vomiting, diarrhea, loss of appetite |
| pentobarbital | | euthanasia, anesthesia, controls seizures | low respiratory rate and body temperature |
| Pentothal® | See thiopental | | |
| pentoxifylline | Trental® | promotes blood flow through small vessels | vomiting, loss of appetite, excitement |
| Pepcid® | See famotidine | | |
| Pepto-Bismol® | See bismuth subsalicylate | | |
| Percorten-V® | See desoxycortico- sterone pivalate | | |
| pergolide | Permax® | controls symptoms of equine metabolic syndrome and equine Cushing's disease | rare |
| Permax® | See pergolide | | |
| permethrin | common in many insecticides | kills many external parasites | drooling, vomiting, diarrhea, tremors, changes in behavior, extremely toxic to cats |
| phenobarbital | | controls seizures | sedation, increased thirst, urination, appetite and liver enzyme levels |

| Drug | Other Common Names | Major Uses | Possible Side Effects |
|---|---|---|---|
| phenylbutazone | bute | pain relief, reduces inflammation | gastrointestinal ulcers, kidney damage, diarrhea, loss of appetite, low protein levels |
| phenylpropanolamine | PPA, Proin® | reduces urine leakage from bladder | changes in behavior, high blood pressure, loss of appetite, rarely stroke |
| phytonadione | See vitamin K | | |
| piroxicam | Feldene® | treats some types of cancer, pain relief, reduces inflammation | gastrointestinal ulcers, kidney damage, vomiting, diarrhea, loss of appetite |
| Pitocin® | See oxytocin | | |
| Polyflex® | See ampicillin | | |
| polysulfated glycosaminoglycan | PSGAG, Adequan® | decreases joint inflammation | if injected into a joint, temporary increase in inflammation and infections if improperly injected |
| ponazuril | Marquis® | treats EPM | rashes. Other side effects may become evident as more horses are treated with this drug. |
| Posilac® | See recombinant bovine somatotropin | | |
| potassium bromide | bromide | controls seizures | sedation, vomiting, loss of appetite, respiratory disease (cats) |
| povidone-iodine | Betadine® | reduces numbers of microorganisms on body surfaces | rare |
| PPA | See phenylpropanolamine | | |
| praziquantel | Droncit®, Drontal®, Drontal Plus® Quest Plus®, Equimax®, Zimecterin Gold® | kills tapeworms | rare but loss of appetite and energy, vomiting, diarrhea and salivation are possible |
| prednisolone | | reduces inflammation, reduces immune response, treats some types of cancer, relieves itching and allergies, many other uses | low adrenal gland function, increased thirst, urination and hunger, infections, many others |
| prednisone | | reduces inflammation, reduces immune response, treats some types of cancer, relieves itching and allergies, many other uses | low adrenal gland function, increased thirst, urination and hunger, infections, many others |
| Preventic® | See amitraz | | |
| Previcox® | See firocoxib | | |

# Appendix I- Commonly Perscribed Drugs

| Drug | Other Common Names | Major Uses | Possible Side Effects |
|---|---|---|---|
| Primor® | See sulfadimethoxine with ormetoprim | treats some abnormal heart rhythms | vomiting, diarrhea, loss of appetite, low blood pressure, abnormal heart rhythms |
| procainamide | | | |
| Program® | See lufenuron | | |
| ProHeart® | moxidectin | prevents heartworm disease and kills some internal parasites | As of 2005, questions have arisen over the safety of ProHeart®, which is currently not available for use. |
| Proin® | See phenylpropanolamine | | |
| PromAce® | See acepromazine | | |
| proparacaine | Ophthaine® | topical anesthetic for eye | rare with short term use |
| propofol | | short acting general anesthesia | low respiratory rate, seizures |
| propranolol | | treats some abnormal heart rhythms | low heart rate, loss of energy, low blood pressure, worsening heart failure |
| Proventil® | See albuterol | | |
| Prozac® | See fluoxetine | | |
| PSGAG | See polysulfated glycosaminoglycan | | |
| psyllium | Vetasyl®, Metamucil® | laxative, removes sand from the gastrointestinal tract (horse), lessens diarrhea | flatulence, constipation |
| pyrantel | Nemex®, Strongid® | kills some intestinal parasites | rare |
| pyrethrin | common in many insecticides | kills many external parasites | drooling, vomiting, diarrhea, tremors, changes in behavior, extremely toxic to cats |
| Quest® | See moxidectin | | |
| Quest Plus® | moxidectin with praziquantel | kills many internal parasites, including tapeworms | rare |
| ranitidine | Zantac® | reduces stomach acid, heals gastrointestinal ulcers, promotes flow of food and feces through the gastrointestinal tract | rare |
| recombinant bovine somatotropin | Posilac® | increases milk production in dairy cows | infections of the mammary glands, lameness and infertility |
| Reglan® | See metoclopramide | | |

# Appendix I- Commonly Perscribed Drugs

| Drug | Other Common Names | Major Uses | Possible Side Effects |
|---|---|---|---|
| Regu-Mate® | See altrenogest | | |
| Revolution® | See selamectin | | |
| rifampin | | used in conjunction with other drugs to treat infections (e.g. *Rhodococcus equi*) | red staining to tears, urine, sweat and saliva |
| Rimadyl® | See carprofen | | |
| Robaxin® | See methocarbamol | | |
| romifidine hydrochloride | Sedivet® | sedation, pain relief | low heart rate, sweating, low blood pressure |
| Rompun® | See xylazine | | |
| Rotectin® | ivermectin | kills many internal parasites | rare unless overdosed |
| s-adenosyl-methionine | SAMe, Denosyl® | helps protect the liver from damage, treats a variety of liver diseases and osteoarthritis | rare |
| Safe-Guard® | See fenbendazole | | |
| Salix® | See furosemide | | |
| SAMe | See s-adenosyl-methionine | | |
| Sandimmune® | See cyclosporine | | |
| Sedivet® | See romifidine hydrochloride | | |
| selamectin | Revolution® | kills a variety of internal and external parasites, prevents heartworm disease | rare |
| selegiline | L-deprenyl, Anipryl® | improves canine cognitive dysfunction, may alleviate symptoms of Cushing's disease | vomiting, diarrhea, loss of appetite, abnormal behavior |
| Sentinel® | milbemycin with lufenuron | prevents heartworm disease, kills some internal parasites, controls fleas | rare |
| sertraline | Zoloft® | treats a variety of behavioral problems | loss of appetite, abnormal behavior |
| sevoflurane | | general anesthetic | low blood pressure, low respiratory and heart rates, abnormal body temperature |
| Simplicef® | See cefpodoxime | | |
| sodium bicarbonate | | increases body and urine pH | abnormal body pH, electrolyte imbalances, congestive heart failure |
| Soloxine® | See levothyroxine | | |
| Sporanox® | See itraconazole | | |

# Appendix I- Commonly Perscribed Drugs

| Drug | Other Common Names | Major Uses | Possible Side Effects |
|---|---|---|---|
| stanozolol | Winstrol® | improves appetite, weight gain and strength, increases red blood cell production | liver damage (especially cats) |
| Strongid® | See pyrantel | | |
| sucralfate | Carafate® | heals ulcers in the gastrointestinal tract | constipation |
| sulfadimethoxine | Albon® | treats some bacterial and protozoal (e.g. *Coccidia*) infections | low tear production (dog), liver damage (dog), vomiting, diarrhea, loss of appetite, low blood cell counts, urine crystals |
| sulfadimethoxine with ormetoprim | Primor® | treats some bacterial and protozoal diseases | low tear production (dog), liver damage (dog), vomiting, diarrhea, loss of appetite, low blood cell counts, urine crystals |
| sulfasalazine | | improves inflammatory bowel disease | low tear production |
| Sumycin® | See tetracycline | | |
| Surpass® | See diclofenac | | |
| Synotic® | fluocinolone with DMSO | relieves ear itching and inflammation due to allergies | rare |
| tacrolimus | | increases tear production | topical irritation |
| Tagamet® | See cimetidine | | |
| Taktic® | See amitraz | | |
| Tapazole® | See methimazole | | |
| Tavist® | See clemastine fumarate | | |
| Telazol® | See tiletamine with zolazepam | | |
| Temaril-P® | trimeprazine with prednisolone | relieves symptoms of allergies | sedation, low blood pressure, abnormal heart rhythm, abnormal body temperature, low adrenal gland function, increased thirst, urination and hunger, infections |
| tepoxalin | Zubrin® | pain relief, reduces inflammation | vomiting, diarrhea, loss of appetite |
| terbutaline | Brethine® | dilates airways | increased heart rate, tremors, abnormal behavior |
| Terramycin® | See oxytetracycline | | |
| Terramycin® for eyes | oxytetracycline with polymyxin B | kills some types of bacteria on the eye | topical irritation (especially cats) |

| Drug | Other Common Names | Major Uses | Possible Side Effects |
|---|---|---|---|
| tetracycline | Panmycin®, Sumycin® | kills some types of bacteria | discoloration of growing teeth, bone damage in growing animals, kidney and liver damage, vomiting, diarrhea, loss of appetite |
| theophylline | | dilates airways | excitement, vomiting, diarrhea, increased appetite, thirst and urination, increased heart rate |
| thiopental | Pentothal® | short-acting general anesthetic | abnormal heart rhythms (dog); low respiratory rate (cat); excitement, difficulty walking (horse) |
| Thyrotabs® | See levothyroxine | | |
| Thyrozine® | See levothyroxine | | |
| tiletamine with zolazepam | Telazol® | sedation, anesthesia | low respiratory rate, high heart rate, abnormal behavior, drooling, kidney damage (rabbit) |
| timolol maleate | Timoptic®, Cosopt® | reduces eye pressure | rare |
| Timoptic® | See timolol maleate | | |
| Torbugesic® | See butorphanol | | |
| Torbutrol® | See butorphanol | | |
| Toxiban® | See activated charcoal | | |
| tramadol | Ultram® | pain relief | abnormal behavior, vomiting, loss of appetite, diarrhea, constipation |
| Trental® | See pentoxifylline | | |
| Tresaderm® | thiabendazole with dexamethasone and neomycin | kills ear mites, some types of bacteria and yeast and relieves itching in the ear | topical irritation |
| triamcinolone | Vetalog®, Genesis® | reduces inflammation, reduces immune response, relieves itching and allergies, many other uses | low adrenal gland function, increased thirst, urination and hunger, infections, many others |
| Tribrissen® | See trimethoprim with sulfadiazine | | |
| trifluridine | Viroptic® | treats viral infections of the eye | topical irritation |
| trimethoprim with sulfadiazine | Tribrissen® | treats some bacterial and protozoal diseases | low tear production (dog), liver damage (dog), vomiting, diarrhea, loss of appetite, low blood cell counts, urine crystals |
| trimethoprim with sulfamethoxazole | Bactrim® | treats some bacterial and protozoal diseases | low tear production (dog), liver damage (dog), vomiting, diarrhea, loss of appetite, low blood cell counts, urine crystals |
| tropicamide | Mydriacyl® | dilates pupil | topical irritation, salivation, glaucoma |

| Drug | Other Common Names | Major Uses | Possible Side Effects |
|---|---|---|---|
| Trusopt® | See dorzolamide | | |
| Tumil-K® | potassium | increases potassium levels in the body | vomiting, diarrhea, loss of appetite, abnormally high potassium levels |
| Tylan® | See tylosin | | |
| Tylenol® | See acetaminophen | | |
| tylosin | Tylan® | kills some bacteria | loss of appetite, diarrhea |
| Ultram® | See tramadol | | |
| Uroeze® | See ammonium chloride | | |
| ursodiol | Actigall® | promotes flow of bile through the liver | can worsen liver disease and cause pain |
| Valium® | See diazepam | | |
| Vasotec® | See enalapril | | |
| Ventolin® | See albuterol | | |
| Vetalog® | See triamcinolone | | |
| Vetasyl® | See psyllium | | |
| Vetsulin® | See insulin | | |
| Viokase® | See pancrelipase | | |
| Viroptic® | See trifluridine | | |
| vitamin K | phytonadione | reduces bleeding caused by a lack of vitamin K | rare when given correctly |
| Voltaren® | See diclofenac for eyes | | |
| Winstrol® | See stanozolol | | |
| Xalantan® | See latanaprost | | |
| xylazine | Rompun® | sedation, pain relief | vomiting (especially cats), low heart rate, low respiratory rate, urination, sweating (horses), salivation (cattle), bloat |
| Yobine® | See yohimbine | | |
| yohimbine | Yobine® | reverses effects xylazine, treats side effects of amitraz | rare but occasional vomiting, excitement, drooling, tremors |
| Zantac® | See ranitidine | | |
| Zeniquin® | See marbofloxacin | | |
| Zimecterin® | ivermectin | kills many internal parasites | rare unless overdosed |
| Zimecterin Gold® | ivermectin with praziquantel | kills many internal parasites, including tapeworms | rare unless overdosed |

# Appendix I- Commonly Perscribed Drugs

| Drug | Other Common Names | Major Uses | Possible Side Effects |
|------|--------------------|-----------|-----------------------|
| Zithromax® | *See* azithromycin | | |
| Zoloft® | *See* sertraline | | |
| Zubrin® | *See* tepoxalin | | |

## ACRONYMS AND ABBREVIATIONS

Full definitions can be found in the body of the dictionary.

| | | | | |
|---|---|---|---|---|
| °C | degrees Celsius | | CBC | complete blood count |
| °F | degrees Fahrenheit | | cc | cubic centimeter, same as milliliter |
| AAFCO | Association of American Feed Control Officials | | CD/T | vaccine given to sheep, goats and cattle to protect against enterotoxemia and tetanus |
| ACE | angiotensin converting enzyme or acepromazine | | CERF | canine eye registry foundation |
| ACTH | adrenocorticotrophic hormone | | CHF | congestive heart failure |
| AD | right ear | | CID | combined immunodeficiency |
| ADH | antidiuretic hormone | | CL | caseous lymphadenitis |
| ADR | ain't doing right. See NDR. | | cm | centimeter |
| AI | artificial insemination | | CNS | central nervous system |
| AIHA | autoimmune hemolytic anemia | | CO₂ | carbon dioxide |
| AKC | American Kennel Club | | COPD | chronic obstructive pulmonary disease |
| ALP | alkaline phosphatase | | CP | conscious proprioception |
| ALT | alanine aminotransferase | | CPK | creatinine phosphokinase |
| ANA | antinuclear antibodies | | CPR | cardiopulmonary resuscitation |
| AP | anterior-posterior - a view of a leg from the front to the back, often used when taking x-rays | | CRF | chronic renal failure |
| | | | CRT | capillary refill time |
| APHIS | Animal and Plant Health Inspection Service | | CSF | cerebrospinal fluid |
| | | | CT | computed tomography |
| ARF | acute renal failure | | cysto | cystocentesis |
| AS | left ear | | D/C | discontinue |
| AST | aspartate aminotransferase | | DA | displaced abomasum |
| AU | both ears | | DAPP | distemper, canine adenovirus, parainfluenza and parvovirus vaccine given to dogs |
| BAR | bright, alert and responsive | | | |
| BCS | body condition score | | DEA | Drug Enforcement Agency |
| BFD | budgerigar fledgling disease | | DHLPP | distemper, hepatitis, leptospirosis, parainfluenza and parvovirus vaccine given to dogs |
| BID | twice daily, every 12 hours | | | |
| BLV | bovine leukemia virus | | | |
| BP | blood pressure | | DHLPPC | distemper, hepatitis, leptospirosis, parainfluenza, parvovirus and coronavirus vaccine given to dogs |
| BPH | benign prostatic hyperplasia | | | |
| BPM | beats or breaths per minute - unit of measurement for heart and respiratory rates | | | |
| | | | DHPP | distemper, hepatitis, parainfluenza and parvovirus vaccine given to dogs |
| BSE | bovine spongiform encephalopathy | | | |
| BST | bovine somatotropin | | DIC | disseminated intravascular coagulation |
| BUN | blood urea nitrogen | | | |
| BVD | bovine viral diarrhea | | diff | differential complete blood count |
| Bx | biopsy | | DJD | degenerative joint disease |
| C & S | culture and sensitivity | | DKA | diabetic ketoacidosis |
| CAE | caprine arthritis-encephalitis | | DLE | discoid lupus erythematosus |
| cap | capsule | | DLH | domestic long hair |

| | |
|---|---|
| DNA | deoxyribonucleic acid |
| DNR | do not resuscitate - a medical order preventing intervention in case of cardiopulmonary arrest |
| DOA | dead on arrival |
| DSH | domestic short hair |
| DTM | dermatophyte test media |
| DV | dorsal-ventral - a view of the body from the back towards the belly, often used when taking x-rays |
| DVM | doctor of veterinary medicine |
| Dx | diagnosis |
| ECG | electrocardiogram |
| Echo | echocardiography |
| EDTA | a type of anticoagulant often used to prevent blood samples from clotting |
| EEE | Eastern equine encephalitis |
| EENT | eyes, ears, nose and throat |
| EHV | equine herpes virus |
| EIA | equine infectious anemia |
| EKG | electrocardiogram |
| ELISA | enzyme-linked immunosorbent assay |
| EOD | every other day |
| EPI | exocrine pancreatic insufficiency |
| EPM | equine protozoal myeloencephalitis |
| F | female |
| F/S | spayed female |
| FDA | Food and Drug Administration |
| FeLV | feline leukemia virus |
| FHO | femoral head ostectomy |
| FIP | feline infectious peritonitis |
| FIV | feline immunodeficiency virus |
| Flu | influenza |
| FLUTD | feline lower urinary tract disease |
| FNA | fine needle aspirate |
| FORL | feline oral resorptive lesion |
| FUO | fever of unknown origin |
| FUS | feline urologic syndrome |
| FVRCP | feline viral rhinotracheitis, calicivirus and panleukopenia vaccine |
| Fx | fracture |
| g | gram |
| GDV | gastric dilatation and volvulus |
| GFR | glomerular filtration rate |
| GI | gastrointestinal |
| GME | granulomatous meningoencephalitis |

| | |
|---|---|
| gt(t) | drop(s) |
| $H_2O$ | water |
| $H_2O_2$ | hydrogen peroxide |
| HBC | hit by car |
| HCT | hematocrit |
| HDDS | high dose dexamethasone suppression test |
| Hgb | hemoglobin |
| HR | heart rate |
| HW | heartworm |
| Hx | history |
| HYPP | hyperkalemic periodic paralysis |
| I | iodine |
| $I_{131}$ | radioactive iodine |
| IBD | inflammatory bowel disease |
| IBR | infectious bovine rhinotracheitis |
| IC | intracardiac |
| ICH | infectious canine hepatitis |
| ICU | intensive care unit |
| ID | intradermal |
| IFA | immunofluorescent antibody assay |
| IgA | immunoglobulin A |
| IgE | immunoglobulin E |
| IgG | immunoglobulin G |
| IgM | immunoglobulin M |
| IM | intramuscular |
| IMHA | immune mediated hemolytic anemia |
| IMT | immune mediated thrombocytopenia |
| IN | intranasal |
| IOP | intraocular pressure |
| IP | intraperitoneal |
| IV | intravenous |
| IVDD | intervertebral disk disease |
| K | potassium |
| KC | kennel cough |
| kcal | kilocalorie |
| KCl | potassium chloride |
| KCS | keratoconjunctivitis sicca |
| kg | kilogram |
| L | liter |
| lb(s) | pound(s) |
| LDA | left displaced abomasum |
| LDSS | low dose dexamethasone suppression test |
| LH | luteinizing hormone |
| LRS | lactated ringers solution |
| LSA | lymphosarcoma |

| | |
|---|---|
| LVT | licensed veterinary technician |
| M | male |
| M/C | castrated male |
| M/N | neutered male |
| mcg | microgram |
| MDP | minimum data base |
| mg | milligram |
| MIC | minimum inhibitory concentration |
| ml | milliliter |
| MLV | modified live virus |
| mm | mucous membrane or millimeter |
| MRI | magnetic resonance imaging |
| N | nitrogen or normal |
| N/A | not applicable |
| Na | sodium |
| NaCl | sodium chloride |
| NAF | no abnormalities found |
| NDR | not doing right - a temporary diagnosis used to describe an animal that is unwell, but the specific problem has not yet been uncovered |
| NG tube | nasogastric tube |
| NPO | nothing by mouth |
| NRBC | nucleated red blood cell |
| NSAID | nonsteroidal anti-inflammatory drug |
| NSF | no significant findings |
| O$_2$ | oxygen |
| OB | obstetrics |
| OCD | osteochondritis dissecans |
| OD | right eye |
| OFA | Orthopedic Foundation for Animals |
| OHE | ovariohysterectomy |
| OPP | ovine progressive pneumonia |
| OR | operating room |
| OS | left eye |
| OTC | over-the-counter |
| OU | both eyes |
| oz | ounce |
| P | pulse rate |
| PA | posterior-anterior - a view of a leg from the back to the front often used when taking x-rays |
| PBFD | psittacine beak and feather disease |
| PCV | packed cell volume |
| PD | polydipsia |
| PDA | patent ductus arteriosus |
| PE | physical examination |

| | |
|---|---|
| PHF | Potomac horse fever |
| PLI | pancreatic lipase immunoreactivity |
| PLR | pupillary light reflexes |
| PMI | point of maximal intensity |
| PMN | polymorphonuclear neutrophil |
| PNS | peripheral nervous system |
| PO | by mouth |
| PP | plasma protein |
| PRA | progressive retinal atrophy |
| PRN | as needed |
| PT | prothrombin time |
| PTT | partial thromboplastin time |
| PU | perineal urethrostomy or polyuria |
| PU/PD | polyuria/polydipsia |
| PVC | premature ventricular complex |
| q | every (e.g. q4hrs, every 4 hours) |
| QAR | quiet, alert and responsive |
| QD | once daily, every 24 hours |
| QID | four times daily, every 6 hours |
| QOD | every other day |
| R | respiratory rate |
| RAO | recurrent airway obstruction |
| RBC | red blood cell |
| RDA | right displaced abomasum |
| REM | rapid eye movement |
| Rhino | equine rhinopneumonitis |
| RNA | ribonucleic acid |
| ROM | range of motion |
| RR | respiratory rate |
| Rv | rabies virus |
| RVT | registered veterinary technician |
| Rx | prescription |
| S/R | suture removal |
| SAP | serum alkaline phosphatase |
| SARDS | sudden acquired retinal degeneration syndrome |
| SC | under the skin |
| SCC | somatic cell count |
| SIBO | small intestinal bacterial overgrowth |
| SID | once daily, every 24 hours |
| SLE | systemic lupus erythematosus |
| SLUD | salivation, lacrimation, urination and defecation - clinical signs associated with certain types of poisonings |
| SOAP | subjective, objective, assessment, plan - a way of organizing medical records |

# Appendix II- Acronyms and Abbreviations

| | |
|------|------------------------------|
| SQ | under the skin |
| stat | immediately |
| Sx | surgery |
| T | tetanus or temperature |
| $T_3$ | triiodothyronine |
| $T_4$ | thyroxine |
| tab | tablet |
| TB | tuberculosis |
| tbsp | tablespoon |
| Tet | tetanus |
| TID | three times daily, every 8 hours |
| TLI | trypsin-like immunoreactivity |
| TMR | total mixed ration |
| TNTC | too numerous to count |
| TP | total protein |
| TPLO | tibial plateau leveling osteotomy |
| TPR | temperature, pulse and respiration rates |
| tsp | teaspoon |
| TT | thrombin time |

| | |
|------|------------------------------|
| TTW | transtracheal wash |
| TVT | transmissible venereal tumor |
| Tx | treatment |
| U/S | ultrasound |
| UA | urinalysis |
| µg | microgram |
| µl | microliter |
| URI | upper respiratory infection |
| USG | urine specific gravity |
| UTI | urinary tract infection |
| VD | ventral-dorsal - a view of the body from the belly towards the back, often used when taking x-rays |
| VEE | Venezuelan equine encephalitis |
| VMD | veterinary medical doctor |
| VPC | ventricular premature contraction |
| WBC | white blood cell |
| WEE | Western equine encephalitis |
| WNL | within normal limits |

## WEIGHTS, MEASURES AND CONVERSIONS

**Temperature**
To convert Fahrenheit (□°F) to Celsius (°C)
Subtract 32 from the temperature in °F then multiply the result by 0.555
To convert Celsius to Fahrenheit
Multiply the temperature in °C by 1.8 then add 32

**Weight**
To convert pounds to kilograms
Divide the weight in pounds by 2.2
To convert kilograms to pounds
Multiply the weight in kilograms by 2.2
To convert weight in ounces to grams
Multiply the weight in ounces by 28.4
To convert grams to weight in ounces
Divide the weight in grams by 28.4
1 pound (lb) = 16 ounces (oz)
1 kilogram (kg) = 1000 grams (g)
1 gram = 1000 milligrams (mg)
1 mg = 1000 micrograms (µg)
1 grain (gr) = 64.8 mg

**Fluids**
To convert fluid ounces to milliliters
Multiply the amount in ounces by 29.625
To convert milliliters to fluid ounces
Divide the amount in milliliters by 29.625
1 cup = 8 fluid ounces (oz)
1 liter (L) = 1000 milliliter (ml)
1 ml = 1000 microliters (µl)
1 ml = 1 cubic centimeter (cc)
1 teaspoon (tsp) = 5 ml
1 tablespoon (tbsp) = 15 ml

**Length**
To convert inches into centimeters
Multiply the length in inches by 2.54
To convert centimeters into inches
Divide the length in centimeters by 2.54
1 yard = 3 feet
1 foot = 12 inches
1 meter = 100 centimeters
1 centimeter = 10 millimeters

## NORMAL PHYSIOLOGIC PARAMETERS

| species | average life expectancy (years) | heart rate (beats per minute) | respiration rate (breaths per minute) | body temperature (°F) | body temperature (°C) |
|---|---|---|---|---|---|
| Amazon | 15 (max. 80) | 125-160 | 15-45 | | |
| budgerigar | 6 (max. 18) | 260-270 | 60-75 | | |
| canary | 5-15 (max. 25) | 265-325 | 60-80 | | |
| cat | 10-15 | 120-170 | 20-40 | 100-103.1 | 37.8-39.5 |
| chicken | 10-11 | 220-360 | 12-37 | | |
| chinchilla | 9-17 | 100-150 | 40-80 | 98.6-100.4 | 37-38 |
| cockatiel | 6 (max. 32) | 210-220 | 40-50 | | |
| cockatoo | 15 (max. 60+) | 125-170 | 15-40 | | |
| conure | 10 (max. 35) | 165-220 | 30-50 | | |
| cow | 15-25 | 40-80 | 12-36 | 100-102.5 | 37.8-39.2 |
| dog | 10-12 | 70-120 | 20-34 | 99.5-102.5 | 37.5-39.2 |
| ferret | 5-11 | 200-400 | 33-36 | 100-104 | 37.8-40 |
| finch | 5 (max. 17) | 300-350 | 90-110 | | |
| gerbil | 2-3.5 | 260-600 | 85-160 | 100.7 | 38.2 |
| goat | 8-15 | 70-110 | 15-40 | 101.5-103.5 | 38.6-39.7 |
| guinea pig | 5-6 | 240-310 | 42-105 | 99-103.1 | 37.2-39.5 |
| hamster | 1.5-3 | 310-471 | 38-110 | 99.7 | 37.6 |
| hedgehog | 4-8 | 180-280 | 25-50 | 95.7-98.6 | 35.4-37 |
| horse | 20-25 | 28-40 | 10-14 | 99-101.3 | 37.2-38.5 |
| lovebird | 4 (max. 12) | 240-250 | 50-60 | | |
| macaw | 15 (max. 50+) | 115-135 | 20-25 | | |
| mouse | 1-3 | 427-697 | 91-216 | 98.9 | 37.1 |
| pig | 10-20 | 70-120 | 32-58 | 100-102 | 37.8-38.9 |
| prairie dog | 8-10 | 83-318 | not reported | 95.7-102.3 | 35.4-39 |
| rabbit | 7-13 | 120-150 | 30-60 | 101.3-104 | 38.5-40.0 |
| rat | 2-3.5 | 313-493 | 71-146 | 99.9 | 37.7 |
| sheep | 8-15 | 60-120 | 12-72 | 102-103.5 | 38.9-39.7 |
| sugar glider | 10-12 | 200-300 | 16-40 | 89.6 cloacal 97.3 rectal | 32 cloacal 36.3 rectal |

Data compiled from *Large Animal Internal Medicine* by Bradford P. Smith (Mosby, 1996), *Plumb's Veterinary Drug Handbook* by Donald C. Plumb (Blackwell Publishing, 2005), *Duke's Physiology of Domestic Animals* by Melvin J. Swenson, William O. Reece (Cornell university, 1993), *Ferrets, Rabbits, and Rodents* by Katherine E. Quesenberry, James W. Carpenter (Saunders, 2003), *Exotic Companion Medicine Handbook* by Cathy A. Johnson-Delaney (Zoological Education Network, 2000) and personal observations.

## Appendix V-

## NORMAL REPRODUCTIVE PARAMETERS

| species | age of sexual maturity | time in heat | estrous cycle duration | pregnancy length (days) |
|---|---|---|---|---|
| cat | 4-10 months | 2-19 days | 4-30 days ovulates when bred | 58-70 |
| chinchilla | 7-10 months | not reported | 30-50 days | 105-118 |
| cow | 8-13 months | 18 hours | 21 days | 271-310 |
| dog | 6-12 months | 7- 42 days (proestrus and estrus) | 5-8 months but variable | 58-71 |
| ferret | 6-12 months | variable | ovulates when bred | 41-42 |
| gerbil | 9-18 weeks | 12-18 hours | 4-7 days | 23-26 |
| goat | 8-9 months | 40 hours | 20 days | 146-155 |
| guinea pig | 2-3 months | 6-11 hours | 15-17 days | 59-72 |
| hamster | 6-8 weeks | 8-26 hours | 4-5 days | 15-18 |
| hedgehog | 2-6 months (female) 6-8 months (male) | not reported | not reported | 34-37 |
| horse | 12-18 months | 5-6 days | 21 days | 310-374 |
| mouse | 6 weeks | 9-20 hours | 4-5 days | 19-21 |
| pig | 6-7 months | 45 hours | 21 days | 113-115 |
| prairie dog | 1-3 years | not reported | 2-3 weeks | 34-37 |
| rabbit | 22-52 weeks | variable | ovulates when bred | 30-33 |
| rat | 4-5 weeks | 9-20 hours | 4-5 days | 21-23 |
| sheep | 8-9 months | 36 hours | 17 days | 143-155 |
| sugar glider | 8-12 months (female) 12-15 months (male) | not reported | 29 days | 15-17, in pouch additional 70 |

Data compiled from *Large Animal Internal Medicine* by Bradford P. Smith (Mosby, 1996), *Plumb's Veterinary Drug Handbook* by Donald C. Plumb (Blackwell Publishing, 2005), *Duke's Physiology of Domestic Animals* by Melvin J. Swenson, William O. Reece (Cornell university, 1993), *Ferrets, Rabbits, and Rodents* by Katherine E. Quesenberry, James W. Carpenter (Saunders, 2003), *Exotic Companion Medicine Handbook* by Cathy A. Johnson-Delaney (Zoological Education Network, 2000) and personal observations.

# SOURCES FOR MORE INFORMATION

## Veterinary Dictionaries and Manuals Written for Professionals

These resources are technically written but provide definitions and explanations to most words encountered in the veterinary profession.

*Saunders Comprehensive Veterinary Dictionary.* D.C. Blood, V.P. Studdert (W.B. Saunders, 1999)

*Merck Veterinary Manual*, Cynthia M. Kahn, Scott Line (John Wiley & Sons, 2005)

## Handbooks, Manuals and Guides to Animal Care and Diseases

These books are sources for more detailed information on the veterinary care, diseases and treatment of animals.

### General Resources

*Veterinary Guide for Animal Owners: Cattle, Goats, Sheep, Horses, Pigs, Poultry, Rabbits, Dogs, Cats,* C.E. Spaulding, Jackie Clay (Rodale Press, 2001)

*Keeping Livestock Healthy: A Veterinary Guide to Horses, Cattle, Pigs, Goats & Sheep*, N. Bruce Haynes (Storey Publishing, 2001)

*The Pill Book Guide to Medication for Your Dog and Cat,* by Kate Roby, Lenny Southam (Bantam Books, 1998)

### Horses

*UC Davis School of Veterinary Medicine Book of Horses: A Complete Medical Reference Guide for Horses and Foals*, Mordecai Siegal (HarperResource, 1996)

*Horse Owner's Veterinary Handbook*, James M. Giffin, Tom Gore (Howell Book House, 2002)

**Dogs**

*Dog Owner's Home Veterinary Handbook*, James M. Giffin, Lisa D. Carlson (Howell Book House, 1999)

*Hound Health Handbook: The Definitive Guide to Keeping Your Dog Happy, Healthy & Active*, Betsy Brevitz (Workman Publishing Company, 2004)

**Cats**

*The Cornell Book of Cats: A Comprehensive and Authoritative Medical Reference for Every Cat and Kitten*, Mordecai Siegal (Villard Books, 1997)

*Cat Owner's Home Veterinary Handbook,* Delbert G. Carlson, James M. Giffin (Howell Book House, 1995)

**Other Species**

*The Complete Pet Bird Owner's Handbook,* Gary Gallerstein (Avian Publications, 2003)

*The Biology, Husbandry and Health Care of Reptiles and Amphibians* (3 volumes), Lowell J. Ackerman (TFH Publications, 1997)

*Ferrets for Dummies,* Kim Schilling (For Dummies, 2000)

TFH Publications' *Proper Care of* series includes comprehensively written books on rabbits, rats, guinea pigs, hamsters, snakes and other mammals, birds and fish.

**Internet Resources**

The web site *VeterinaryPartner.com* is an excellent and growing source for information on the care, behavior, diseases and drugs used in treatment of dogs, cats, reptiles and small mammals. http://www.veterinarypartner.com

*NetVet* and the *Electronic Zoo* offer exhaustive listings of veterinary and animal resources available online. http://netvet.wustl.edu

Cornell University's feline health center has excellent descriptions of health problems and treatment options that are written for cat owners. http://www.vet.cornell.edu/FHC/

The American Animal Hospital Association's online pet care library has dozens of articles covering the care of dogs, cats and exotic animals. http://healthypet.com

The American Veterinary Medical Association's care for pets page contains information on many aspects of animal ownership. http://www.avma.org/care4pets

The American Association of Equine Practioners' web page for horse owners has a "horse health" link providing excellent information. http://www.myhorsematters.com

The magazine *The Horse* has a web site that contains informative and accurate articles about the health care of horses. http://www.thehorse.com

The web site *PetPlace.com* has a lot of detailed information regarding a variety of issues affecting many species. http://www.petplace.com

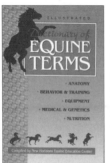
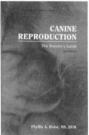
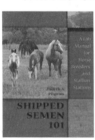
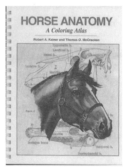
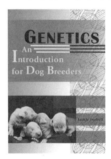